Procedures
for Primary Care
Providers

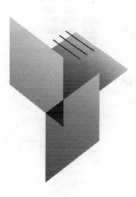

Procedures for Primary Care Providers

Denise L. **Robinson**, RN, PhD, FNP

Professor
Director, MSN Program
Northern Kentucky University
Highland Heights, Kentucky
and
Family Nurse Practitioner
Northern Kentucky Family Health Centers, Inc.
Covington, Kentucky

Cheryl L. **McKenzie**, RN, CS, FNP, MN

Associate Professor
Department of Nursing
Northern Kentucky University
Highland Heights, Kentucky
and
Family Nurse Practitioner
Northern Kentucky Family Health Centers, Inc.
Dayton, Kentucky

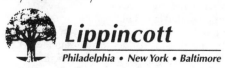

Lippincott
Philadelphia • New York • Baltimore

Acquisitions Editor: Lisa Stead
Editorial Assistant: Claudia Vaughn
Project Editor: Nicole Walz/Barbara Ryalls
Senior Production Manager: Helen Ewan
Production Coordinator: Pat McCloskey
Design Coordinators: Susan Hermansen/Carolyn O'Brien
Cover/Interior Design: BJ Crimm
Indexer: Ellen Brennan

9 8 7 6 5 4 3 2 1

Library of Congress Cataloging in Publications Data

Robinson, Denise L.
    Procedures for primary care providers / Denise L. Robinson, Cheryl
L. McKenzie.
        p.   cm.
    Includes bibliographical references and index.
    ISBN 0-7817-1968-2 (alk. paper)
    1. Primary care (Medicine)   I. McKenzie, Cheryl.   II. Title.
    [DNLM: 1. Primary Health Care—methods.   W 84.6 R659p 1999]
    R729.R63   1999
    362.1—dc21
    DNLM/DLC   99-34310
    for Library of Congress   CIP

Care has been taken to confirm the accuracy of the information presented and to describe generally accepted practices. However, the authors, editors, and publisher are not responsible for errors or omissions or for any consequences from application of the information in this book and make no warranty, express or implied, with respect to the content of the publication.

The authors, editors, and publisher have exerted every effort to ensure that drug selection and dosage set forth in this text are in accordance with current recommendations and practice at the time of publication. However, in view of ongoing research, changes in government regulations, and the constant flow of information relating to drug therapy and drug reactions, the reader is urged to check the package insert for each drug for any change in indications and dosage and for added warnings and precautions. This is particularly important when the recommended agent is a new or infrequently employed drug.

Some drugs and medical devices presented in this publication have Food and Drug Administration (FDA) clearance for limited use in restricted research settings. It is the responsibility of the health care provider to ascertain the FDA status of each drug or device planned for use in his or her clinical practice.

Karen Barnett, MSN, CFNP
Instructor, College of Nursing
Family Nurse Practitioner Program
University of New Mexico
Albuquerque, New Mexico

Kathleen U. Boggs, PhD, FNP–C
Associate Professor
University of North Carolina at Charlotte
Charlotte, North Carolina

Delores W. Clark, RN, BSN, MSN, FNP, CPNP
Director of Pediatric Nurse Practitioner Program
Director of Center for Health Services
University of Texas at Arlington School of Nursing
Arlington, Texas

Kathryn Fiandt, DNS, C–FNP
Assistant Professor
Coordinator of Family Nurse Practitioner Program
College of Nursing
University of Nebraska Medical Center
Omaha, Nebraska

Frances Francabandera, EdD, RN, FNP
Associate Professor
Department of Nursing
Kean University
Union, New Jersey

Patricia Lynn Giurgevich, EdD, MN, ARNP
Assistant Professor
School of Health Sciences
Seattle Pacific University
Seattle, Washington

Thomasine D. Guberski, PhD, CRVA
Associate Professor and Program Director
Adult Primary Care Nurse Practitioner
University of Maryland School of Nursing
Baltimore, Maryland

Mary Louise Keller, PhD, CRNP
Associate Professor/Chairperson
Department of Nursing
Edinboro University of Pennsylvania
Edinboro, Pennsylvania

Rosemary Ligouri, ARNP, PhD, CPNP
Assistant Professor
College of Nursing
University of Oklahoma
Tulsa, Oklahoma

Kathleen M. Miller, RN, MA, MS, CNAA, CS, FNP
Assistant Professor
Coordinator of Family Nurse Practitioner Program
Molloy College
Rockville Center, New York

Ingrid P. Pearson, MS, RN, CPNP
Assistant Professor of Nursing
Medical University of South Carolina
Charleston, South Carolina

Karen A. Plager, DSNc, RNC, FNP
Assistant Professor
Department of Nursing
Northern Arizona University
Flagstaff, Arizona

Avis Johnson-Smith, RN, MSN, CPNP, FNP–C, CNS
Family Nurse Practitioner Director and Assistant Professor
Albany State University College of Health Professions
Albany, Georgia
Pediatric Nurse Practitioner
Mitchell County Pediatrics
Camilla, Georgia

Melinda M. Swenson, PhD, RNCS, FNP
Associate Professor
Director, Family Nurse Practitioner Major
Indiana University School of Nursing
Indianapolis, Indiana

Benita Walton-Moss, DNS, RNCS, FNP
Assistant Professor
Johns Hopkins University School of Nursing
Baltimore, Maryland

CONTRIBUTORS

Janet L. Andrews, RNC, WHNP, PhD
Assistant Professor
School of Health Sciences
Georgia College State University
Milledgeville, Georgia
Cervical Cap Fitting, Diaphragm Fitting, Gonorrhea and Chlamydia, Pap Smear

Kim Hudson Benton, RNC, MS
Assistant Professor
Department of Family Health
School of Health Sciences, Division of Nursing
Georgia College State University
Milledgeville, Georgia
Female Condom, Wet Mount

Sandra Chaisson Brown, DNS, RN, FNP
Associate Professor and Chair
Graduate Nursing Program
Southern University and Agricultural and Mechanical College
Baton Rouge, Louisiana
Basic Electrocardiogram Interpretation

Laura L. Flesch, RN, MSN
Registered Nurse, Level III
Trauma Center
Emergency Department
Children's Hospital Medical Center
Cincinnati, Ohio
Simple Lacerations

Cindy Gastrich, MSN, BSN, RN
Director, Nursing
Department of Ambulatory Patient Care Services
The University Hospital of Cincinnati
Cincinnati, Ohio
Fungal Scraping, Herpes Scraping, Scabies Scraping

C. E. Hartman, PA–C
Physician Assistant
Internal Medicine Clinic
Fort Worth, Texas
Fishhook Removal

Marilyn Jacobs, RNC, MSN, WHNP
Associate Professor
Department of Nursing
Missouri Southern State College
Joplin, Missouri
Treatment of Condyloma Acumination

Cheryl Pope Kish, EdD, RNC, WHCNO, SANE
Professor and Coordinator
Graduate Programs in Health Science
School of Health Sciences
Georgia College and State University
Milledgeville, Georgia
Depo Provera, Sexual Abuse

Mary D. Knudston, MSN, NP
Associate Clinical Professor
Director of FNP Program
Department of Family Medicine
University of California, Irvine
Irvine, California
Norplant Insertion and Removal

Steven D. Martin, RN, MSN, FNP
Staff RN, Emergency Department
St. Elizabeth Medical Center
Edgewood, Kentucky
Nurse Practitioner
Cardiology Associates
Edgewood, Kentucky
Specimen Collection: Stool Cultures, Voided Urine, Urine Analysis; Treatment of Epistaxis, Peak Flowmeter, Nebulizer and Metered-Dose Inhaler, Spirometry

Todd Martin, RN, MSN, FNP
Assistant Director, Emergency Nursing
Children's Hospital Medical Center
Cincinnati, Ohio
Avulsed Tooth, Cerumen Removal, Corneal Abrasion, Ear Irrigation, Foreign Body: Ear, Foreign Body: Eye, Fracture Immobilization, Hair Tourniquet, Tick Removal

Cheryl L. McKenzie, RN, CS, FNP, MN
Associate Professor
Department of Nursing
Northern Kentucky University
Highland Heights, Kentucky
Child Restraints, Glucose Testing, Tympanometry
Co-Author for: *Specimen Collection: Stool Cultures,*

Voided Urine, Urine Analysis, Treatment of Epistaxis, Peak Flowmeter Measurement, Nebulizer and Metered-Dose Inhaler, Spirometry

Michael J. Morgan, PhD, MPH, RN, CS
Graduate Program Director
University of Wisconsin, Oshkosh
Oshkosh, Wisconsin
Anoscopy, Foreign Body: Mouth, Foreign Body: Nose

Roger D. Porter, DPM
Director of Northern Kentucky Family Footcare
Surgical Privileges at St. Elizabeth and St. Luke's Hospital
Crescent Springs, Kentucky
Corn and Callus Management, Toenail Removal Procedures

Mollie Poyton, BSN, RN
Graduate Assistant
Northern Kentucky University
Department of Nursing
Highland Heights, Kentucky
Abscess: Incision and Drainage, Ring Removal

Susan Rivers-Payne, RN, MSN, CNS
Clinical Nurse Specialist
Department of Nursing Administration
Good Samaritan Hospital
Cincinnati, Ohio
Unna Boot

Denise L. Robinson, RN PhD, FNP
Associate Professor

Director, MSN Program
Northern Kentucky University
Highland Heights, Kentucky
Family Nurse Practitioner
Department of Plastic and Reconstructive Surgery
The Plastic Surgery Group
Cincinnati, Ohio
Skin Lesions Removal, Simple Lacerations, Local Anesthesia for Lacerations

Charles Volpenheim, ADN, PA-C
Physician Assistant
Department of Adult Medicine
Group Health Associates
Cincinnati, Ohio
Skin Lesions, Subungal Hematoma

Karen M. Wigger, ARNP, CPSN
Nurse Practitioner
Department of Plastic and Reconstructive Surgery
The Plastic Surgery Group
Cincinnati, Ohio
Local Anesthesia for Lacerations, Skin Lesions, Lacerations

Michael Zychowicz, MSN, NP, CCRN
Nurse Practitioner
Department of Orthopedic Surgery
State University of New York, Health Science Center at Syracuse
Syracuse, New York
Arthrocentesis, Corticosteroid Joint Injection, Trigger Point Injection

DEDICATIONS

Thanks to all of my family
for their patience and understanding during
the writing and editing of this book.
Their support and love has helped me
grow throughout the year.

—DR

I would like to thank my husband Jeffrey,
and my daughters Caitlyn, Samantha, and Salena.
Their support was invaluable during
the editing of this book.

—CMcK

PREFACE

The purpose of this text is to provide a succinct and illustrated resource of procedures that primary care providers might encounter in practice. This book is designed for nurse practitioner and physician assistant students as well as the experienced provider. It is not meant to serve as the only exposure or guide in performing these procedures (see a further discussion of learning procedures in the Introduction). It is assumed that the primary care provider will use this text as a foundation for new procedures (along with a mentor or a teacher), and as a review if the procedure has not been performed in a while.

Since most people are visual learners (a picture is worth a thousand words), illustrations provide graphic detail on how to do the procedures.

Because the aim of the text is to both teach and provide guidelines for practice, users are referred to additional readings for more in depth information. National guidelines or standards are incorporated into each procedure as appropriate.

Several unique features have been incorporated into this book to make accessing information easy and fast:

Alphabetical ordering of content within each section.

Step–by–step approach to the procedure: identification of equipment needed, breaking down the procedure into steps, and identifying special considerations that may apply in each situation.

Important information is identified using ALERT boxes to direct your attention to crucial material.

Follow-up care and referral information is included for every procedure.

Appropriate patient education for each procedure is identified.

Developmental considerations related to age, gender, or pregnancy is identified as to its influence on the procedure.

Identification of CPT coding and the average reimbursement rate for each procedure.

The procedures were written by primary care providers with a wide variety of experience: plastic surgery, emergency department, orthopedic, cardiology, podiatry, and women's health, as well as family care. These varied experiences add to the value of the book since the writers are out in the field doing the procedures about which they have written.

Information that transcends the individual procedures is presented prior to the procedures, such as restraint of children, discussion of procedures needed for primary care practice, and laboratory governmental processes.

We encourage all primary care providers to seek opportunities to learn at the "hands of an experienced teacher" and get adequate opportunities to practice prior to implementing these procedures with patients. We also ask you to share your expertise with those who are seeking the assistance of experienced mentors. We think you will find this text useful in those endeavors.

ACKNOWLEDGMENTS

Thanks to the primary care providers who shared their busy lives with us by writing these procedures. We also thank Northern Kentucky Family Health Center, Inc., for providing us with the opportunity to maintain a part time practice and serve as preceptors for students in a great clinical setting. We appreciate their sharing of various resources related to procedure cost and reimbursement. We would like to acknowledge Lisa Stead for her support during this project, and Claudia Vaughn for her assistance in finding the "right" illustration, and her help with the many other steps during the book editorial process.

DR and CMcK

CONTENTS

Introduction: Procedures and Clinical Laboratory Procedures: Implications for Primary Care Providers

Traditionally, procedures have not been a major component of nurse practitioner programs, yet many nurse practitioners are finding that integrating procedures into their primary care case load is necessary and cost saving. Skills in procedures have been emphasized historically in physician assistant programs, and are considered an integral part of their role in practice.

Smithing and Wily (1996) advocate a core set of procedures that are essential for primary care providers. These basic skills serve as a foundation for many other specialized procedures that can be added as the need arises within the particular clinical setting.

WE BELIEVE THE FOLLOWING PROCEDURES SHOULD BE CONSIDERED CORE PROCEDURES:
- local anesthesia
- simple interrupted suturing
- skin staple placement
- removal of skin lesions (shave biopsy, punch biopsy, elliptical biopsy, cryodesiccation)
- collection of specimens for microscopy
- fracture immobilization
- ear, nose, and throat (ENT) procedures (ear irrigation, cerumen removal, removal of foreign body (FB) in eye, nose, ear)
- wound care (Unna boot, corn, and callus care)
- gynecology procedures (Pap smear, cultures, depo provera injection, initial assessment of alleged sexual abuse to determine if further evaluation is needed)
- specialized examination techniques (anoscopy, audiometry, tympanogram)
- respiratory procedures (peak flow monitoring, nebulizer, inhaler use)
- basic x-ray interpretation
- basic electrocardiogram (EKG) interpretation

DEVELOPMENT OF BASIC CORE SKILLS

Development of core competencies enables the performer to manipulate equipment skillfully, in a manner that produces the desired goal. Included within the skills are manual dexterity, good eye-hand coordination, and the ability to troubleshoot when equipment is not working properly.

The primary care provider should learn the basic core procedures/skills by reading step-by-step instructions and by watching an experienced, skilled provider perform the procedure. The experienced mentor/preceptor should then review the steps of the procedure, and guide the nurse practitioner (NP) or physician assistant (PA) as they perform the procedure for the first time (and additional times, if learner or teacher deem necessary). Many skills, while taught in NP or PA programs, will still require exposure and development of expertise during the clinical practicum or on the job as a primary care provider.

A SUGGESTED SYSTEM ON HOW TO APPROACH A NEW SKILL IS DELINEATED BELOW:

- If manual dexterity is required in the skill/procedure, practice the skill until you feel confident.
- Familiarize yourself with the procedure (read the step-by-step instructions) and the equipment needed to perform the procedure. If available, watch a videotape demonstrating the skill. Watching someone else perform the procedure is probably the most helpful way to learn the steps and techniques needed.
- Identify someone who is an expert in performing the procedure and willing to share his/her expertise.
- Seek assistance if you feel unsure of how to proceed, or if it has been a long time since you have performed the procedure (even though you were once proficient).

MAINTENANCE OF BASIC CORE SKILLS

Core skills that a primary care provider keeps honed are based on the premise that the skill is used frequently enough to keep mastery of the skills. There should be an adequate number of patients who require the procedure. Consider a mechanism to review or practice procedures on a regular basis to keep your skills proficient. A few more specialized procedures are included in this text since they "logically" may be the ones that an NP or PA adds to their armamentarium. These skills and procedures will require specialized training and guidance.

LIMITATIONS OF PROCEDURES THAT CAN BE PERFORMED

There is no standardized list of procedures that NPs and PAs can perform. Each state will determine the scope of practice for the various providers. Be sure to check the states' regulations as they pertain to performing procedures. These regulations are legal standards which identify the *minimum* level of practice deemed essential for the safety of patients. In most cases, the regulations do not specifically identify procedures which can or cannot be performed. Rather, a more general statement related to the scope of practice and educational preparation is found.

Physician assistants are able "to provide any legal medical service which is delegated to them by the supervising physician when the service is within their skills, forms a component of the physician's scope of practice, and is provided with the supervision of a physician" (AAPA, 1998, pg vii). The American Academy of Physician Assistants does not recommend the use of a list of specific tasks since it may be overly restrictive. Each state determines its own legislative regulations, and may vary from state to state.

Nurse practitioner scope of practice and legal authority for practice varies from state to state. There is little consistency in the form of scope of practice, or prescriptive privileges or third-party reimbursement. The American Nurses Association (ANA) recommends using a broad scope of practice, with the specific regulation of specialities left to the professional organizations. The ANA standards of care identify that nurse practitioners "prescribe pharmacologic and non-pharmacologic treatments in the direct management of acute and chronic illness and disease" (ANA, 1996, pgs 3–4). The ability of the nurse practitioner to perform procedures is based on his/her educational background, and the clinical experience needed to perform the procedure competently.

CLINICAL LABORATORY PROCEDURES

The Clinical Laboratory Improvement Amendment (CLIA) of 1988 has had a profound impact on the types of laboratory procedures that are now performed in primary care offices. This law resulted from an examination of quality of the services provided in a variety of settings. CLIA set standards designed to improve quality, and included specifications for quality control, quality assurance, personnel, proficiency testing, and inspection (Mastrangela, 1993; NANP, 1994).

Waived tests are considered those that are inherently accurate, risk free to the patient, or those available over the counter. For tests that are considered waived, a certificate of waiver must be obtained. It is assumed that the manufacturer's instructions are followed when performing these tests. Tests that are waived from CLIA requirements include:

Test	Current Procedural Terminology (CPT)
Dipstick or tablet U/A	81002
Fecal occult blood testing	82270
Ovulation test using color comparison	84830
Erythrocyte sedimentation rate	85651
Hemoglobin copper sulfate (nonautomated)	83026
Spun microhematocrit	85013
Blood glucose using glucose testing devices for home use	82962
Strep A test	86588QW
Urine pregnancy using color comparison	81025

Tests that are considered a higher level of complexity are classified into two levels: moderate and high complexity (this includes approximately 10,000 other tests and procedures). Laboratory procedures that can be performed in the office are determined by CLIA status. CLIA status is determined by the number of lab tests done, and the number of subspecialties for which the tests are done. The amount paid for certification increases with an increased volume and complexity of performed tests.

Another category of laboratory procedures includes provider performed microscopy procedures (PPMP). This classification includes procedures that are not subject to scheduled inspections, and puts the burden of proficiency testing, quality assurance, and quality control on the individual who performs the microscopy. Quality control specifies that instructions, how the tests are performed, and who is performing the tests, be clearly defined for all PPMP. A written plan for quality assurance designed to monitor and evaluate the quality of PPMP should also be in place.

Procedures that are considered PPMP include:

Procedure	Coding
We mounts (vaginal, cervical, or skin specimens)	Q0111
All potassium hydroxide (KOH) preparations	Q0112
Pinworm examination	Q0113
Fern test	Q0114
Postcoital direct qualitative examination of vaginal or cervical mucus	Q0115
Urinalysis (microscopy only)	CPT 81015
Urinalysis by dipstick	CPT 81000
Nasal smear for eosinophils	CPT 89190
Fecal leukocyte examination	G0026
Semen analysis, presence or motility of sperm, excluding Huhner test	G0027

BIBLIOGRAPHY

American Academy of Physician's Assistants. (1998). *Physician Assistants: State laws and regulations* (7th ed). Alexandria, VA: American Academy of Physician's Assistants.

American Medical Association. (1998). *Physicians' current procedural terminology: CPT.* Chicago: American Medical Association.

Lowe, S. & Saxe, J. M. (1999). *Microscopic procedures for primary care providers.* Philadelphia: Lippincott Williams & Wilkins.

Mastrangelo, R. (1993). CLIA '88. Advance for Nurse Practitioners, Vol. 2, 13–15.

National Association of Nurse Practitioners in Reproductive Health. (1994). Clinical laboratory improvement amendments of 1988. Personal communication, 10-31-94.

Pearson, L. (1998). Annual update of how each state stands on legislative issues affecting APN. Nurse Practitioner, 23(1): 14–66.

Smithing, R., & Wiley, M. (1996). Nurse practitioner-performed procedures. *Nurse Practitioner,* 21(8): 106–107.

chapter
1

Specimen Collection: Stool Cultures and Rectal Swabs (pinworm microscopy, rectal smear)

CPT Coding:

87045 Stool Culture ($38–$46)
87177 Ova and Parasites, Feces ($32–$39)

DEFINITION

Collected for identification of parasites, viruses, and organisms in the intestinal tract.

INDICATION

• For a routine stool culture, the stool is examined to detect and to rule out *Salmonella, Shigella, Campylobacter, Yersinia,* enteropathogenic *Escherichia* coli, and pure cultures of Staphylococcus (Fischbach, 1996).

PATIENT EDUCATION

• Explain the purpose and procedure for obtaining stool specimens.
• A freshly passed stool is best.

ASSESSMENT

1. Perform history and physical examination to determine need for testing.
2. Determine if patient can cooperate with testing.

 ALERT: *Observe universal precautions.*

STOOL CULTURE

Equipment
• Specimen container with label
• Tongue depressor or spatula
• Gloves

PROCEDURE	SPECIAL CONSIDERATIONS
Instruct the patient to defecate into a clean, dry container. The entire stool volume should be collected.	Do not obtain stool from toilet bowl or mix urine with stool. This may cause inaccurate results if protozoa are present. Do not put toilet paper into collection container; the paper may contain bismuth, which will interfere with results (Fischbach, 1996).
Transfer a portion (1 to 2 teaspoons) of the stool into the specimen container by using a clean tongue depressor or spatula.	The entire stool volume should be collected and measured. Send only specified amount needed for each test.
Properly label the sealed specimen container. The type of test should be written on the requisition.	
Send or take the labeled specimen to the laboratory immediately.	If there is a delay, try to place the specimen for parasite examination in a warm place.
If more than one specimen is to be sent, number appropriately.	Refrigerate specimens for other examinations until delivered to the laboratory.

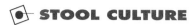 RECTAL SWAB SMEAR

Equipment
• Rectal swab with transport medium
• Gloves

PROCEDURE	SPECIAL CONSIDERATIONS
Insert swab into rectum (3 cm or more); rotate swab to obtain fecal material.	This is an alternative to the above mentioned procedure. Rectal swabs are inferior to defecated specimens because they reach only the anal canal.

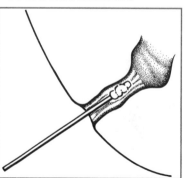

(procedure continued)

| PROCEDURE | SPECIAL CONSIDERATIONS |

Place the swab into appropriate medium to prevent drying.

Label the specimen; send to laboratory.

If a delay longer than 2 hours is expected, the specimen should be placed into a transport medium such as Cary-Blair (Fischbach, 1996).

Illustration from: Fischbach, F. [1996] A manual of laboratory and diagnostic tests, (5th ed.). Philadelphia: Lippincott-Raven.)

CELLOPHANE TAPE TEST

Equipment
• Gloves
• Cellophane tape
• Microscope
• Xylene
• Forceps

| PROCEDURE | SPECIAL CONSIDERATIONS |

Apply a strip of tape to the end of a tongue depressor.

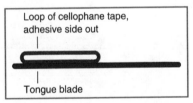

Loop of cellophane tape, adhesive side out

Tongue blade

Spread the buttocks and apply the adhesive side of the tape to the perianal area.

Rotate the tape in a circular manner to include the entire anal area.

Apply a microscope slide to the adhesive side of the tape.

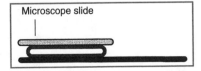

Microscope slide

The tape test is indicated in cases of suspected enterobiasis (pinworms). Best to perform test in morning before patient has bathed or had bowel movement.

Do not use micropore or adhesive tape (Fischbach, 1996).

(procedure continued) ──

| **PROCEDURE** | **SPECIAL CONSIDERATIONS** |

Cut tongue blade from remaining tape.

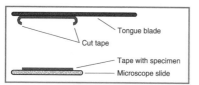

Pull up one edge of tape attached to slide using forceps.

Apply a small drop of xylene under tape edge.

Examine specimen under low power, then confirm with high power.

The xylene will clear the adhesive, increasing the chance of ova identification. **Fumes from xylene may be toxic, need ventilation and decreased exposure** (Lowe & Saxe, 1999).

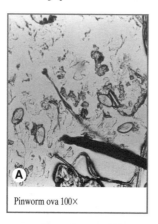

Pinworm ova 100×

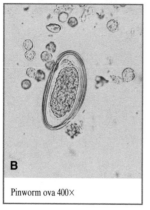

Pinworm ova 400×

(procedure continued)

PROCEDURE	SPECIAL CONSIDERATIONS
May need to repeat the above-mentioned procedure on consecutive days.	Need to obtain a series of negative tests to rule out pinworms.

Illustration from: Lowe, S. & Saxe, J [1999]. Microscopic procedures for primary care providers. Philadelphia: Lippincott Williams & Wilkins.

ALTERNATIVE PROCEDURE

• There are kits available for pinworm examination; follow manufacturer's instructions.

FOLLOW-UP

• Interpret test outcomes.
• Monitor for intestinal infection.
• Counsel appropriately: medication, diet, and hygiene regimen.

BIBLIOGRAPHY

American Medical Association. (1998). *Physicians' current procedural terminology: CPT.* Chicago: American Medical Association.

Fischbach, F. (1996). *A manual of laboratory diagnostic tests.* (5th ed). Philadelphia: Lippincott-Raven.

Healthcare Consultants of America. (1998). *1998 Physicians' fee and coding guide.* Augusta, GA.

Lowe, S. & Saxe, J. M. (1999). *Microscopic procedures for primary care providers.* Philadelphia: Lippincott Williams & Wilkins.

chapter 2

Specimen Collection: Voided Urine and Catheterization

CPT Coding:

53670 Urine Catheterization ($37–$44)

 ## DEFINITION

Several methods are available for obtaining a urine specimen. Some techniques are more accurate as well as more expensive. Some methods cause significant discomfort for the patient.

 ## INDICATIONS

• Can be used as a screening test or to monitor physiologic functioning. (See Chapter 3: Urine Analysis.)

 ## PATIENT EDUCATION

• Explain the purpose and procedure of the test to the patient.
• Give specific directions related to the method used to obtain specimen.

ASSESSMENT

1. Perform history and physical examination as appropriate to hypothesized diagnoses.
2. Determine if patient can cooperate with testing.

 ## DEVELOPMENTAL CONSIDERATIONS

• Urine collection in children poses a different challenge. Restraint may be necessary to perform the procedure to obtain accurate results.

 ## EQUIPMENT

• Specimen container (clean or sterile)
• Disposable wipes

- Urine bottle with preservative (for 24-hour urine only)
- Specimen container
- Gloves
- Catheter with lubricant (for catheterized specimen)
- Urine bag for pediatric patients

    See table below for specifics about when to use the equipment or check specimen.

PROCEDURE	SPECIAL CONSIDERATIONS
Random specimen Collect urine at any time of the day or night.	
Fasting specimen Instruct patient to void 4 hours or more after eating; discard urine. Collect next voided urine.	
Postprandial specimen Instruct patient to void after eating; collect specimen.	
Clean-catch midstream specimen Patient should wash hands. Open package of disposable wipes, placing them on a clean, dry surface.	In adults, this method may be as reliable as a catheterized specimen. This method may be useful with a cooperative child who is toilet trained.
Remove lid from specimen container, and place it flat side down.	Do not touch the inside of the container or lid.
Insruct female patient to sit as far back on the toilet as possible.	
Instruct her to spread her labia apart with one hand; continue doing this for the entire procedure.	
Use disposable wipe to clean the area between the labia around the urethra from top to bottom, using a new wipe for each stroke.	
Instruct male patient to cleanse the head of the penis from the urethral opening toward the shaft with the disposable wipe. Discard wipe.	If uncircumcised male, pull foreskin back first. To prevent contamination of secretions from prostate, do not collect last few drops of urine. Avoid touching skin with the container.

(procedure continued) ————————————————————————————

PROCEDURE	SPECIAL CONSIDERATIONS
Instruct patient to void a small amount into toilet first.	
Then hoid specimen container below the urine stream and catch 1 to 2 ounces (30–60 ml) of urine in the container.	
Place the lid on the container and return specimen to appropriate area.	

24-Hour specimen

Instruct patient to discard first morning specimen.	Urine collection bottle must be refrigerated at all times.
Collect all urine for exactly 24 hours.	Need to repeat procedure if all urine is not collected.
Instruct female to void in specified container first.	
Transfer urine to collection bottle; avoid spillage.	
Males may urinate directly into collection bottle (Fischbach, 1996).	

Catheterized specimen

Restrain patient as necessary.	Most accurate method for obtaining urinalysis or urine culture in neonates or infants
Use sterile technique.	
Cleanse area.	
Use appropriate catheter.	
Obtain sterile urine specimen.	
Send to laboratory or perform office analysis.	

Urine bag specimen

Cleanse area.	May be useful in children for chemical analysis of urine.
Apply bag.	
Remove bag once urine is obtained.	
Place bag in specimen container.	
Perform analysis.	
	Do not use this method if child has a fever or if a UTI is suspected. It is not as reliable as a catheterized specimen.

(procedure continued)

PROCEDURE	**SPECIAL CONSIDERATIONS**

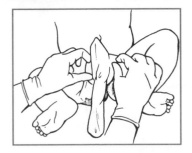

FOLLOW-UP

- Interpret test outcomes, and treat patient appropriately.
- If analysis will not be performed in office laboratory within an hour, then will need to refrigerate specimen.

BIBLIOGRAPHY

American Medical Association. (1998). *Physicians' current procedural terminology: CPT.* Chicago: American Medical Association.

Fischbach, F. (1996). *A manual of laboratory diagnostic tests* (5th ed). Philadelphia: Lippincott-Raven.

Healthcare Consultants of America. (1998). *1998 Physicians' fee and coding guide.* Augusta, GA.

Lowe, S. & Saxe, J.M. (1999). *Microscopic procedures for primary care providers.* Philadelphia: Lippincott Williams & Wilkins.

chapter 3

Urine Analysis With Microscopy and Urine Culture

CPT Coding:

81015 Urinalysis (UA), microscopic only ($11–$15)
87086 Culture, bacterial, urine; quantitative colony count ($30–$38)

 DEFINITIONS

Microscopy identifies the type and approximate number of formed elements present in a urine specimen, thus providing information useful for both prognosis and diagnosis. Microscopic UA is done by a variety of methods. Traditionally, the most common laboratory technique of microscopic UA for clinical purposes has been the examination of unstained, centrifuged urine.

Urinalysis detects abnormalities in kidney function and conditions that may affect the urinary tract.

 INDICATIONS

- Evaluate for renal function and for disease pathology.
- Check for presence of red blood cells (RBCs), white blood cells (WBCs), epithelial cells, casts, crystals, and bacteria.

 PATIENT EDUCATION

- Explain the purpose and procedure of the test to the patient.
- Explain about the cleansing procedure and its importance (see Chapter 2 for complete explanation).
- Collect specimen in a clean, disposable impervious plastic container only.
- Urine specimens should be collected in the morning whenever possible.

 DIPSTICK ANALYSIS

- Dipstick tests are available for urinalysis; these devices are useful because they don't require a laboratory and can be read immediately.

EQUIPMENT

- Clean, dry urine container (use sterile if doing a culture)
- Reagent strips
- Gloves

PROCEDURE	SPECIAL CONSIDERATIONS
Put on gloves, then completely dip the reagent areas of the dipstick into the urine. While removing, run the edge of the strip against the rim of the container to remove excess urine.	If a female patient is menstruating, a tampon should be inserted into the vagina.
Hold the strip in the horizontal position to prevent possible mixing of chemicals from adjacent reagent areas and/or contaminating the hands with urine.	The tests normally included in a dipstick urine are odor, appearance, color, nitrites, leukocytes. pH, specific gravity, protein, glucose, urobilinogen, and blood.
The tip is impregnated with chemicals that react with specific substances in the urine to produce colored end products.	A dipstick urine test can be done on a minute amount of urine if the patient is unable to urinate enough for a specimen.
The depth of color produced is related to the concentration of the substance in the urine. The reaction rates are standard for each dipstick, and color changes **must be matched at the correct time** after each stick is dipped into the urine specimen. Hold strip close to the color blocks and match carefully.	**Avoid laying the strip directly on the color chart, because this will result in the urine soiling the chart.**
Maintain sterile conditions if a urine culure will be sent after the dipstick testing. If testing cannot be done within an hour after voiding, refrigerate the specimen immediately and let it return to room temperature before testing.	The urine container (not the lid) must have a label affixed containing (at the minimum) the patients name, time, and date of collection.

ALERT: Nitrate test results are optimized by using a first morning specimen or one that has incubated in the bladder for 4 hours or more. It is especially important to use fresh urine to obtain optimal results with the tests for bilirubin and urobilinogen because these compounds are very unstable when exposed to room temperature and light.

Prolonged exposure of urine to room temperature may result in microbial proliferation, with resultant changes in pH. A shift to alkaline pH may cause false-positive results with the protein test area. Urine containing glucose *may decrease in pH because organisms metabolize the glucose. Bacterial growth from contaminating organisms may cause false-positive blood reactions from peroxidases produced.*

Glucose and ketone test areas are so sensitive that overtiming by only 1 to 3 seconds will demonstrate falsely high amounts of the substance.

URINE MICROSCOPY

Equipment
• Gloves
• Microscope
• 10-mL urine specimen
• Slide and coverslip

PROCEDURE	SPECIAL CONSIDERATIONS

Preparation of spun urine:
Put on a pair of gloves. To obtain the sediment, place 10 to 15 mL of thoroughly mixed urine in a centrifuge tube and centrifuge for 5 minutes at the standard speed of 1500 revolutions per minute (rpm).

Pour off the supernate fluid. The supernate is the clear fluid in the tube after it has been centrifuged.
Leave the several drops of urine that remain along the side of the tube to flow back down into the sediment, then tap the tube with your fingers to mix the contents.
Place a drop of this sediment on a slide and cover with a coverslip. The slide is now ready to be examined.

Position the slide on the microscope stage. Remove gloves and wash your hands.
Adjust the lower power lens of the microscope and examine the slide for casts in at least 10 different fields; then examine for other elements that are present in just a few fields.

Reduce the light to a minimum by almost completely closing the diaphragm beneath the stage on the microscope, and scan the entire slide to obtain an overall picture of the sedi-

Using spun urine is recommended because the urine is concentrated. It may distort the formed elements depending on the volume of the specimen, the time and speed of centrifugation, the fragility of the formed elements, and the size of the field.

Examination of unspun, unstained urine placed on a regular microscope slide is a qualitative method sometimes used in the diagnosis of UTI. Using one organism / hpf as a positive result, the sensitivity and specificity in detecting >10⁵ CFU/ml are between 60% and 90%.
Others have used >1 WBC/low-powered field as a criterion for infection.

The low-power lens (10×) is used to find and count casts. The high-power lens (40×) is used to identify WBCs, RBCs, and bacteria.

(procedure continued)

PROCEDURE	SPECIAL CONSIDERATIONS

ment. You must vary the intensity of the light source so that correct identification of various components may be obtained.

Next, adjust the microscope to identify the specific types of cells such as RBCs, crystals, and other elements present in the sediment. Further identification of the various types of casts should also be done at this time.

Estimate the approximate number of the various structures identified. Casts are counted per low-power field; epithelial cells, WBCs, and RBCs are reported in terms of cells in hpf (for example, 10 to 15 WBCs/hpf).

To determine the number of elements present, count the number of each type seen in at least 10 fields. The average of this number is then used for the reported value.

The other elements (crystals, bacteria, parasites, and spermatozoa) are reported as none, rare, occasional, frequent, many, or numerous.

CFU, Colony-forming units; hpf, high-powered field; RBCs, red blood cells; UTI, urinary tract infection; WBCs, white blood cells.

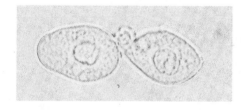

Figure 3-1 Transitional epithelial cell. (Lowe, S. & Saxe, J. [1999]. *Microscopic procedures for primary care providers.* Philadelphia: Lippincott Williams & Wilkins.)

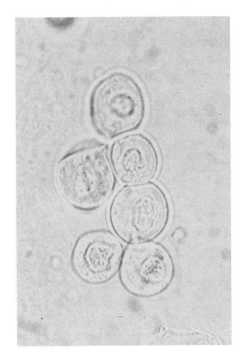

Figure 3-2 Renal tubular epithelial cell. (Lowe, S. & Saxe, J. [1999]. *Microscopic procedures for primary care providers.* Philadelphia: Lippincott Williams & Wilkins.)

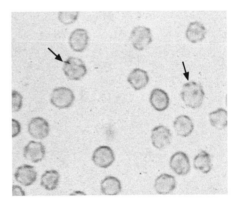

Figure 3-3 Red blood cells. Arrows indicate crenated cells. (Lowe, S. & Saxe, J. [1999]. *Microscopic procedures for primary care providers.* Philadelphia: Lippincott Williams & Wilkins.)

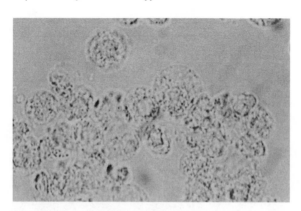

Figure 3-4 White blood cells enlarged to show detail. (Lowe, S. & Saxe, J. [1999]. *Microscopic procedures for primary care providers.* Philadelphia: Lippincott Williams & Wilkins.)

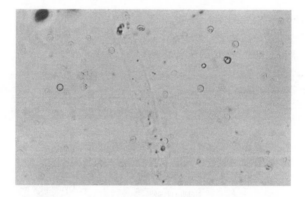

Figure 3-5 Hyaline cast and red blood cell. (Lowe, S. & Saxe, J. [1999]. *Microscopic procedures for primary care providers.* Philadelphia: Lippincott Williams & Wilkins.)

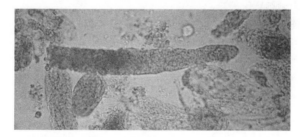

Figure 3-6 Granular casts. (Lowe, S. & Saxe, J. [1999]. *Microscopic procedures for primary care providers.* Philadelphia: Lippincott Williams & Wilkins.)

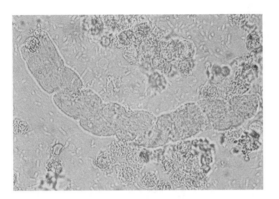

Figure 3-7 Broad waxy cast. (Lowe, S. & Saxe, J. [1999]. *Microscopic procedures for primary care providers.* Philadelphia: Lippincott Williams & Wilkins.)

◨— NORMAL VALUES OF URINALYSIS AND MICROSCOPY

General Characteristics and Measurements	Chemical Determinations	Microscopic Examination of Sediment
Color: yellow-amber indicates a high specific gravity and small output of urine.	Glucose: negative	Casts negative: occasional hyaline casts
	Ketones: negative	
	Blood: negative	Red blood cells negative or rare
	Protein: negative	Crystals negative
Turbidity: clear to slightly hazy	Bilirubin: negative	
	Urobilinogen: 0.1–1	White blood cells negative or rare
Specific gravity: 1.015–1.025 with normal fluid intake	Nitrate for bacteria: negative	
pH: 4.6–4.8 - average person has a pH of about 6 (acid)	Leukocyte estrase: negative	

SIGNIFICANCE OF ELEMENTS FOUND IN URINARY SEDIMENT OF MICROSCOPIC EXAMINATION

Element	Significance
RBC	Bleeding in urinary tract
Red cell cast	Acute glomerulonephritis, lupus, Goodpasture's syndrome, renal infarction, subacute bacterial endocarditis
Hemoglobin cast	Glomerulitis or hemoglobinuria due to intravascular hemolysis
WBC cast (nucleated cells present)	Acute pyelonephritis, interstitial pyelonephritis, lupus nephritis.
Oval fat body	Heavy proteinuria, indicating nephrotic syndrome
Waxy casts (broad, structureless, refractile, sharply outlined)	Severe tubular atrophy, renal failure, renal parenchymal disease
Many WBCs	UTI
Many granular casts	Nephrotic syndrome, pyelonephritis, glomerulonephritis, transplant rejection, lead toxicity
Bacteria	UTI
Epithelial cell (may be hard to distinguish from WBC cast)	Tubular necrosis, cytomegalovirus infection, toxicity from heavy metals, salicylates, transplant rejection
Hyaline	Normal in people after strenuous exercise, congestive heart failure, diabetic nephropathy, chronic renal failure
Cystine crystals	Diagnostic for cystinuria found in patients with disorder of amino acid metabolism
Calcium phosphate	Alkaline urine
Calcium oxalate and uric acid	May appear in normal urine as it cools
$MgNH_4PO_4$ (struvite or triple phosphate)	UTI

RBC, red blood cell; UTI, urinary tract infection; WBC, white blood cell.
Adapted from Fischbach, F. (1996). A Manual of laboratory and diagnostic tests, (5th ed.), pp 191–201. Philadephia: Lippincott-Raven.

 ALERT: The microscopic findings of the urine sediment should always be correlated with the dipstick findings.

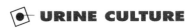 URINE CULTURE

Equipment
- Gloves
- Midstream urine specimen (3–5 mL)
- Sterile container

PROCEDURE	SPECIAL CONSIDERATIONS
Follow directions for how your lab wants urine cultures sent: ie, in cup versus test tube.	If the specimen is collected for diagnosis of cytomegalovirus, it should be kept at room tempature. If refrigerated, the cytomegalovirus will be destroyed. Whenever possible, specimens should be obtained before antibiotic or antimicrobial therapy begins.

 ALERT: *The urine culture sample should not be taken from a urinal, indwelling catheter collection bag, or bedpan and should not be brought from home. The urine needs to be collected directly into the sterile container that will be used for culture.*

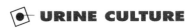 ALTERNATIVE PROCEDURES

- Catheterization, suprapubic, or indwelling catheter aspiration are alternative methods for producing urine specimens (see Chapter 2).

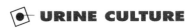 SIGNIFICANCE OF URINE CULTURE

A count of 100,000 (10^5) or more bacteria per milliliter indicates infection. A bacterial count of fewer than 10,000 bacteria per milliliter does not necessarily indicate infection but possible contamination.

Using a colony count of 10^5 may miss a urinary tract infection (UTI) in about 50% of women. A colony count of 10^2 in a symptomatic female is considered to be sufficient to be diagnosed as a UTI (Hancock & Selig, 1994)

The following organisms, when present in the urine in sufficient titers, may be considered pathogenic:

- *Escherichia coli*
- Enterococci
- *Neisseria gonorrhoeae*

- *Klebsiella-Enterobacter-Serratia* species
- *Mycobacterium tuberculosis*
- *Proteus* species
- *Pseudomonas aeruginosa*
- Staphylococci: coagulase positive and coagulase negative
- Streptococci: beta-hemolytic, usually group B
- *Trichomonas vaginalis*
- *Candida albicans* and other yeasts

FOLLOW-UP

- Interpret test outcomes, treat, and counsel appropriately.

BIBLIOGRAPHY

American Medical Association. (1998). *Physicians' current procedural terminology: CPT.* Chicago: American Medical Association.

Barkin, Roger M. (1997). *Concepts and clinical practice: Pediatric emergency medicine* (2nd ed.). St. Louis: Mosby.

Fischbach, F. (1996). *A manual of laboratory diagnostic tests,* (5th ed.). Philadelphia: Lippincott-Raven.

Hancock, L. & Selig, P. (1994). Medical problems in primary care. In E. Youngkin & M. Davis (Eds.), *Women's health.* Norwalk, CT: Appleton & Lange.

Healthcare Consultants of America. (1998). *1998 Physicians' fee and coding guide.* Augusta, GA: Author.

Lowe, S. & Saxe, J. M. (1999). *Microscopic procedures for primary care providers.* Philadelphia: Lippincott Williams & Wilkins.

chapter
4

Abscess: Incision and Drainage

CPT Coding:

10060 Incision and drainage of abscess, simple or single ($91–$108)
10061 Incision and drainage of abscess, complicated or multiple ($261–$316)
10080-10081 Incision and drainage of pilonidal cyst, simple;
complicated ($106–$129; $226–$269)

 ## DEFINITION

Localized induration and fluctuance due to inflammation of the soft tissue.

 ## INDICATIONS

- To relieve pain and allow healing of a cutaneous abscess.
- To promote healing by secondary intention.

 ## PATIENT EDUCATION

- Explain procedure to patient and provide comfort measures.
- Instruct patient to keep dressing clean and dry until seen by a health care professional in 1 to 2 days. Client may shower but should not immerse wound by taking a bath or soaking the wound.
- Client may change outer dressing only if it becomes wet or dirty. Client should not change or reinsert packing.
- After packing is removed, warm water soaks several times a day will promote healing.
- After packing is removed, the wound should be cleansed with mild soap and water three times a day and a clean dressing should then be applied. If recommended to client, instruct in use of topical antibiotic ointment.
- Instruct client to call if he or she experiences fever, chills, uncontrolled bleeding, increased redness, increased swelling, or increased pain.
- The wound should heal in 7 to 10 days in most cases.

 ## ASSESSMENT

1. Obtain history from client. Specifically determine if the client is immuno-compromised, diabetic, or if he or she has any allergies to latex or medica-

tion. Also determine whether or not the client is a candidate for endocarditis prophylaxis.

2. Assess site for redness, swelling, red streaking, pain, and fluctuance.
3. Obtain a temperature and heart rate.
4. Determine necessity of incision and drainage. Small boils that have not caused a tightening of the skin or surrounding cellulitis, however uncomfortable, may be treated with warm compresses and topical ointment.

Figure on page 27 shows most likely places where abscesses occur.

ALERT: Pilonidal abscesses develop in the sacral area when a pilonidal cyst becomes infected. They may be incised and drained for comfort. If the abscess recurs and is considered to be chronic, the cyst should be resected by a surgeon.

5. Determine whether referral is necessary. Consider referral if the abscess is in close proximity to a major vessel, a nerve, or a tendon, particularly if it is an abscess on the hand. Also consider referral for a recurrent pilonidal abscess, because it may be treated definitively with resection of the cyst and closure. A rectal abscess should be drained in the operating room. Refer a patient with a facial abscess to a plastic surgeon.

ALERT: A felon is a trabeculated abscess in the pulp of the distal finger. It is evidenced by severe pain, heat, and redness. Immediate incision and drainage is indicated for prevention of osteitis. The incision should be made vertically over the center of the abscess, and sufficiently deep as to divide all the fibrous septa. This wound is not packed. This wound may warrant referral to a plastic or hand surgeon. Upper figure on page 28 illustrates technique for incision of felon.

☉ DEVELOPMENTAL CONSIDERATIONS

Child: Client must not move during incision and drainage. Consider restraint as appropriate. Instruct client regarding procedure using age-appropriate language and description. Instruct parent or guardian regarding procedure, aftercare, and follow-up.

☉ EQUIPMENT

- Disposable waterproof pads, pillows, light source
- Scissors, 2 × 2 or 4 × 4 gauze, topical antiseptic solution such as povidone-iodine (Betadine)
- Gloves, local anesthetic, needles, syringe
- #11 scalpel; consider protective equipment such as eyewear

- Hemostats or cotton swabs
- Syringe, large-bore peripheral intravenous (PIV) cannula (optional), normal saline solution
- Iodoform gauze packing strips such as Nu-Gauze, forceps, gauze dressing of adequate size to cover wound, tape
- Sharps container

PROCEDURE	SPECIAL CONSIDERATIONS
Position patient for procedure. Provide comfort measures as appropriate, and position light scource.	
Place disposable waterproof pads around treatment area to protect client during irrigation.	This is a clean, not sterile, procedure.
Prepare the skin. Cut closely any hairs in the area of the incision. Saturate several pieces of gauze with antiseptic solution and scrub in circular motion from center of site outward.	Razors can impair skin integrity by creating miniscule cuts and abrasions. Scissors are preferable.
Instill local anesthetic.	Avoid injecting into the abscess cavity. Inject into the tissue immediately surrounding the abscess, as well as the tissue over the abscess.

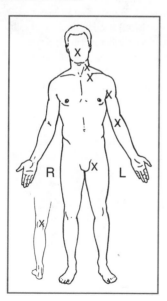

(procedure continued)

PROCEDURE ──── (**SPECIAL CONSIDERATIONS**)

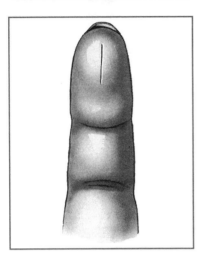

Incise the abscess. Hold the scalpel at a 90-degree angle and incise parallel to the skin lines. Do not hold the skin taut. Expel purulent material by applying manual pressure with a gauze.

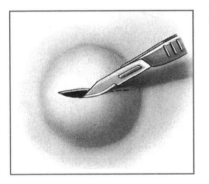

Purulent material will likely exude from the site of the incision as soon as it is incised. If a culture is indicated (as for an immunosuppressed client), it should be obtained at this time. If unable to manually expel purulence, consider choice of incision site and depth of incision. Repeat if necessary. Client should experience some pain relief at this time.

(procedure continued)

PROCEDURE	**SPECIAL CONSIDERATIONS**

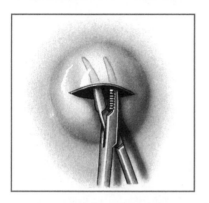

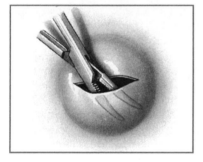

Consider sending a culture of wound purulence.

Break up pockets and adhesions by exploring abscess with hemostats or cotton swabs.	Septi and loculations (pockets) are common in cutaneous abscesses.
Expel remaining purulence.	
Irrigate wound. Remove the needle from a intravenous cannula and attach to syringe for use in irrigating.	This step is considered optional.
Prepare packing material. Pack wound loosely. Leave a short wick to facilitate removal.	**TIP:** Loosen and unfold packing material to increase surface area. The gauze serves to help prevent the incision from sealing over and helps facilitate drainage.
Apply external dressing.	

(procedure continued)

PROCEDURE	SPECIAL CONSIDERATIONS

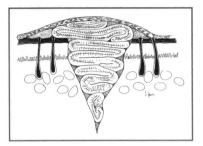

Evaluate client tolerance of procedure.	Consider antibiotic therapy if there is a large area of cellulitis, if the client is immunosuppressed, diabetic, or if the patient has a cardiac condition indicating endocarditis prophylaxis.
Reposition for comfort if necessary, and dispose of sharp items in the appropriate receptacles. Instruct client in care of abscess and necessary follow-up. Evaluate effectiveness of client teaching.	

Illustrations 1 to 5 from Lohr, J. A. (1991). Pediatric outpatient procedures. Philadelphia: J.B. Lippincott Company. Illustration 6 from Simon, R. & Brenner, B. (1994). Emergency procedures and techniques, (3rd Ed.). Baltimore: Williams & Wilkins.

FOLLOW-UP

- Client should be evaluated in 1 to 2 days, at which time the packing should be removed. As long as purulent material remains evident, the wound should be repacked and re-evaluated every 1 to 2 days. When purulence is no longer evident, the packing should be discontinued.
- Provide close follow-up care for clients at high risk for complications, such as diabetics and immunocompromised clients.

COMPLICATIONS

- Poor healing: Healing generally occurs in approximately 1 to 3 weeks. Consider consultation with a wound care nurse if healing is slow or poor. Assess client's aftercare regimen and reinforce teaching as necessary.
- Infection: Antibiotics should be prescribed if cellulitis develops. The patient should be referred for signs and symptoms of sepsis or extensive cellulitis.
- Premature closure of wound edges: Premature closing of the incision site can be caused by premature removal of packing, inadequate probing of the

abscess cavity, or an incision of inadequate size to allow for proper drainage. If the wound edges reunite before adequate drainage, incision and drainage should be repeated.

• Uncontrolled bleeding: Gauze packing acts as an aid to control bleeding. If bleeding persists despite packing, the patient should be referred for medical intervention.

• Recurrence of the abscess: If the abscess recurs, it should be incised and drained as necessary. If the abscess is determined to be chronic, consider referral for resection.

BIBLIOGRAPHY

American Medical Association. (1998). *Physicians' current procedural terminology: CPT.* Chicago: American Medical Association.

Layman, M. (1993). Incision and drainage. In J. Proehl (Ed.), *Adult emergency nursing procedures.* Boston: Jones and Bartlett Publishers, Inc.

Lohr, J. A. (1991). *Pediatric outpatient procedures.* Philadelphia: J. B. Lippincott Company.

Lowe, S. & Saxe, J. M. (1999). *Microscopic procedures for primary care providers.* Philadelphia: Lippincott Williams & Wilkins.

Simon, R. & Brenner, B. (1994). *Emergency procedures and techniques* (3rd ed.). Baltimore: Williams & Wilkins.

The Merck Manual. (1992). *Musculoskeletal abscesses: Felon.* (Online). Available: http://www.merck.com/!!vTjY53WuNvTjYn3oXI/pubs/mmanual/html/mkgfmecd. htm (1998, Sept. 9).

Tobinick, E., Moy, R., & Usatine, R. (1998). Preoperative preparation: Universal precautions, sterilization, and medical evaluation. In R. Usatine, E. Tobinick, R. Moy, & D. Siegel (Eds.), *Skin surgery: A practical guide.* St. Louis: Mosby, Inc.

Usatine, R. (1998). Incision and drainage. In R. Usatine, E. Tobinick, R. Moy, & D. Siegel (Eds.), *Skin surgery: A practical guide.* St. Louis: Mosby, Inc.

chapter 5

Fungal Scraping

CPT Coding:

87220 Tissue examination for fungi (eg, KOH, slide) ($20–$24)

 ## DEFINITIONS

KOH exam is direct microscopic examination of superficial skin scale to determine the presence of fungi for diagnostic confirmation of a fungal infection of the skin. KOH exam may also be used to diagnose fungal infection of the hair and nails. A positive KOH exam confirms the presence of fungi but does not allow for species identification. Fungal cultures identify exact species.

KOH solution (potassium hydroxide solution) is an alkali solution, usually 10%, that dissolves skin keratin and cellular debris but leaves the fungal hyphae and spores intact.

 ALERT: *KOH exam is a test categorized by CLIA as provider-performed microscopy. Nurse practitioners (NPs), physician assistants (PAs), and certified nurse-midwives (CNMs) qualify to perform tests in this category.*

 ## INDICATIONS

• All scaling lesions of the skin should be scraped to rule out a fungal infection.

 ALERT: *All specimen materials should be considered potentially hazardous and should be handled using universal precautions.*

PATIENT EDUCATION

• Reassure patient that collecting the specimen is not painful.

ASSESSMENT

1. Obtain history related to the skin lesion or lesions, such as onset, symptoms, and any treatment or medication applied to the lesion, both prescribed and over-the-counter.
2. Assess the lesion, specifically its location and size. Determine the advancing or leading edge of the lesion for specimen collection.
3. Determine the patient's ability to cooperate and hold still during the procedure.

DEVELOPMENTAL CONSIDERATIONS

Child: It is very important to have child remain still during procedure as the specimen is collected with a #15 scalpel blade. Some means to control the child's movement and hands is very important.

EQUIPMENT

- 70% alcohol
- Gauze square
- Glass slide
- #15 scalpel blade
- KOH solution
- Coverslip
- Heat source (alcohol burner)
- Microscope

Procedure	Special Considerations
Clean skin lesion to be scraped with a gauze square soaked with 70% alcohol to remove any debris or microorganisms on the skin surface. Allow to dry.	Cotton or cotton-tipped swabs should not be used to clean the area, because fibers left behind can be confused with hyphae.
1. Position the patient so that the lesion on the skin is vertical. Place the edge of the glass slide against the skin under the area to be scraped.	
2. Scrape the scale using a #15 scalpel blade from the surface of the skin on the advancing or leading edge of the lesion, and allow the scale to collect on the glass slide positioned below the lesion.	Scale can also be scraped with the edge of another glass slide. The advancing or leading edge of the lesion will provide the best opportunity to obtain a positive specimen.

(procedure continued)

PROCEDURE	SPECIAL CONSIDERATIONS

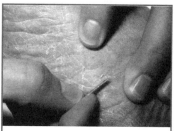

Using #15 blade to obtain specimen

Collect the scrapings and scale together in the middle of the slide.

3. Place no more than two drops of KOH solution on the specimen.

Several strengths of KOH solution are used. A 10% water-based solution is usually used for skin and hair samples; a 20% water-based solution is used for nails.

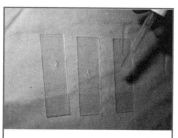

Putting 2 drops KOH solution on specimen

4. Place coverslip over the KOH-soaked specimen

5. Heat specimen for 10 to 20 seconds until it barely bubbles. Do not allow specimen to boil.
Let the KOH slide cool for 10 minutes to allow the KOH to hydrolyze the tissue. Gently press the coverslip to blot off the excess KOH to spread the specimen into a thin layer on the slide. This will appear as a cloudy film under the coverslip.

Heating the specimen hastens the action of the KOH as it dissolves superficial skin cells and lossens the scale. If the specimen boils, the KOH solution can crystallize, making the slide more difficult to interpret.
A KOH solution with a dimethyl sulfoxide (DMSO) base is available that does not require heating to prepare the specimen.

6. Examine the entire specimen under the coverslip under 10× magnification with the condenser diaphragm closed and lowered as far as possible. Light intensity needs to be reduced to enhance the detail of the hyphae. A positive KOH result demonstrates

Blotting off the excess KOH protects the microscope. KOH is a potent alkali.
Microscope objectives can be permanently etched by the KOH solution.
Bright illumination makes hyphae difficult to see. The ease of identifying the hyphae is in-

(procedure continued)

<table>
<tr><td>**PROCEDURE**</td><td>**SPECIAL CONSIDERATIONS**</td></tr>
</table>

the dermatophyte, which stands out as re-fractile, branching, septated hyphae, as shown in next figure.

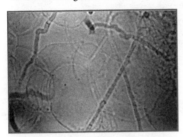

Focus the lens up and down as the specimen is being examined to view it at all levels. The hyphae are embedded in the scale, examine the scale thoroughly.

7. If the KOH is negative and a fungal infection is suspected, collect another specimen to examine. Hyphae are often sparse.

versely related to the amount of light passing through the specimen.

Experience is the key to becoming competent to perform a KOH. Artifacts present a big problem for beginners. Cotton, wool, hairs, fat droplets, and crystallized KOH can confuse the novice.

 ALTERNATIVE PROCEDURES

• KOH preparation for *Candida* infection
• *Candida* infections often have pustules (see below) in addition to scale. If a *Candida* infection is suspected, the specimen is collected from the contents of the pustule and prepared as outlined earlier. A positive KOH for *Candida albicans* demonstrates hyphae or pseudohyphae that are more irregular, shorter, and have numerous branches. You can also often see budding yeasts or blastospores (see figure on p. 36).

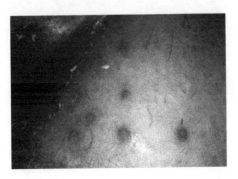

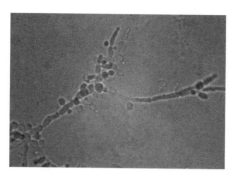

 FOLLOW-UP

- Patient with a demonstrated cutaneous fungal infection should be treated with an antifungal medication.
- Acute, severely inflamed lesions should be referred to a dermatologist for treatment.

BIBLIOGRAPHY

American Medical Association. (1998). *Physicians' current procedural terminology: CPT.* Chicago: American Medical Association.

Arndt, K., Bowers, K., & Chuttane, A. (1995). *Manual of dermatologic therapeutics* (5th ed.). Boston: Little, Brown & Co.

Fitzpatrick, T., Eisen, A., Freedberg, I., & Austin, K. (1997). *Dermatology in general medicine* (4th ed.). New York: McGraw-Hill, Inc.

Healthcare Consultants of America (1998). *1998 Physicians' fee and coding guide.* Augusta, GA.

Lowe, S. & Saxe, J. M. (1999). *Microscopic procedures for primary care providers.* Philadelphia: Lippincott Williams & Wilkins.

Moschella, S. & Hurley, H. (1992). *Dermatology* (3rd ed.). Philadelphia: W. B. Saunders Co.

Orkin, M., Maibach, H., & Dahl, M. (1991). *Dermatology* (1st ed.). Norwalk: Appleton & Lange.

Reeves, J. & Maibach, H. (1998). *Clinical dermatology illustrated* (3rd ed). Philadelphia: F. A. Davis Co.

chapter 6
Herpes Scraping

CPT Coding:

87207 Special stain for inclusion bodies or intracellular parasites (herpes) ($24–$30)

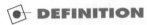 DEFINITION

The Tzanck smear is a cytologic technique used in the diagnosis of vesicular viral infections caused by herpes simplex or the herpes zoster/varicella virus.

 ALERT: *The Tzanck smear is a test categorized by CLIA as provider-performed microscopy. Nurse practitioners (NPs), physician assistants (PAs), and certified nurse-midwives (CNMs) qualify to perform tests in this category.*

INDICATIONS

- A Tzanck smear should be performed on any vesicular lesion in which a herpes infection is suspected.

 ALERT: *All specimen materials should be considered potentially hazardous and should be handled using universal precautions.*

PATIENT EDUCATION

- Discuss potential communicability of herpes lesions with skin-to-skin contact.
- Patients must be told that the herpes virus is infectious to anyone who has not had chicken pox. They should isolate themselves from children and adults who have not been previously infected with chicken pox.

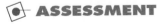 ASSESSMENT

1. Obtain a history related to the skin lesion or lesions, including onset, prodrome symptoms, and any treatment or medication applied to the lesions, both prescribed and over-the-counter.

2. Assess the lesions, specifically their location and distribution. An early lesion with no sign of trauma, manipulation, or infection is the best lesion to choose for specimen collection.

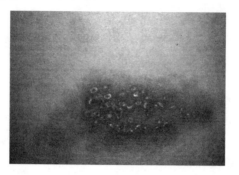

Suspected herpes lesion

3. Determine patient's ability to cooperate and hold still during procedure.

DEVELOPMENTAL CONSIDERATIONS

Child: It is very important to have child remain still during procedure since the specimen is collected with a #15 scalpel blade. Some means to control the child's movement and hands is very important.

EQUIPMENT

- #15 scalpel blade
- Gauze pad
- Glass slide
- 95% ethanol or methanol
- Stain:
  - Wright stain
  - Giemsa stain
  - Toluidine blue stain (0.1% aqueous solution)
  - Or hematoxylin and eosin stain
- Microscope

PROCEDURE	SPECIAL CONSIDERATIONS
1. The blister of the vesicle is removed with the #15 scalpel blade. Excess fluid is absorbed with a gauze pad.	
2. The specimen is collected by gently scraping the base of the vesicle, being careful not to cause any bleeding.	Be gentle. This can hurt.

(procedure continued)

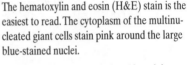

PROCEDURE	SPECIAL CONSIDERATIONS

3. The material collected on the #15 scalpel blade is smeared thinly onto a glass slide and allowed to air dry.

4. If available, fix the tissue by dipping the slide into either ethanol or methanol for 1 to 2 minutes.

5. Stain the slide using one of these stains per the instructions for the stain chosen or available.

6. Examine the entire specimen under 10× magnification to get an appreciation of cell size and staining relationships. Examine the specimen under oil immersion or with 45× magnification to observe morphologic characteristics.

   The presence of multinucleated giant cells and giant epithelial cells yields a positive smear (as shown below).

The hematoxylin and eosin (H&E) stain is the easiest to read. The cytoplasm of the multinucleated giant cells stain pink around the large blue-stained nuclei.

The giant cells can contain 2 to 12 nuclei. Newly infected cells have a single enlarged nucleus. As the infection progresses, cells fuse and become multinucleated.

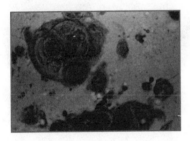

 FOLLOW-UP

- Herpes infections can be treated with antiviral medications. If the infection is severe, the patient may need intravenous (IV) antiviral medication. Consult with a physician or refer the patient to a dermatologist. Refer to physician if the patient is immunosuppressed.

- Early, aggressive treatment for herpes zoster (shingles) often reduces the incidence of post herpetic neuralgia. Consult with a physician or refer the patient to a dermatologist.

- Refer the patient to an ophthalmologist if lesions affect the eye.

- Support groups are available for patients who have genital herpes.

BIBLIOGRAPHY

American Medical Association. (1998). *Physicians' current procedural terminology:* CPT. Chicago: American Medical Association.

Arndt, K., Bowers, K., & Chuttane, A. (1995). *Manual of dermatologic therapeutics* (5th ed.). Boston: Little, Brown & Co.

Fitzpatrick, T., Eisen, A., Freedberg, I., & Austin, K. (1993). *Dermatology in general medicine* (4th ed.). New York: McGraw-Hill, Inc.

Healthcare Consultants of America (1998) *1998 Physicians' fee and coding guide.* Augusta, GA.

Lowe, S. & Saxe, J. M. (1999). *Microscopic procedures for primary care providers.* Philadelphia: Lippincott Williams & Wilkins.

Moschella, S. & Hurley H. (1992). *Dermatology* (3rd ed.). Philadelphia: W.B. Saunders Co.

Orkin, M., Maibach, H., & Dahl, M. (1991). *Dermatology* (1st ed.). Norwalk: Appleton & Lange.

chapter
7

Scabies Scraping

CPT Coding:

87220 Tissue examination for fungi (eg, KOH, slide) ($20–$24)

DEFINITION

Scabies scraping is the direct microscopic examination of superficial skin scrapings of burrows or pustules containing mites, eggs, or fecal pellets of *Sarcoptes scabeii*, the itch mite. The diagnosis is confirmed when any of these elements is identified in the specimen.

Human scabies is a widespread, common skin disease that mimics several other pruritic dermatoses. It is usually transmitted by skin-to-skin contact but can also be spread through towels, linens, and clothing. Intense nocturnal itching is characteristic. Lesions are distributed typically on the hands, in the web space between the fingers, on the sides of the fingers, on the flexor wrist, and on the ulnar border of the hands. The elbows, axillary folds, buttocks, and genitalia are often involved.

Burrow is a unique lesion appearing as a short, wavy, white, threadlike disruption of the skin. Sometimes, the burrow is discolored with feces, eggs, and hatching mites, making them appear as dirty lines.

 ALERT: Scabies scraping is a test categorized by CLIA as provider-performed microscopy. Nurse practitioners (NPs), physician assistants (PAs) and certified nurse-midwives (CNMs) qualify to perform tests in this category.

INDICATIONS

- A scabies scraping should be performed any time a scabies infestation is suspected.
- A scraping should be performed if the patient is being treated for another skin condition and the pruritus continues despite therapy.
- A scraping should be done if the patient has been exposed to scabies and is symptomatic, or when multiple family members complain of a pruritic eruption.

ALERT: *All specimen materials should be considered potentially hazardous and should be handled using universal precautions.*

PATIENT EDUCATION

- Reassure the patient that collecting the specimen will not be very painful.
- Reassure the patient that a scabies infestation is common and can be easily treated once the correct diagnosis has been made.

ASSESSMENT

1. Obtain a history related to the skin lesion(s), including onset, symptoms, and any treatment or medication applied to the lesion, both prescribed and over the counter.
2. Assess for characteristic signs of a scabies infestation, such as nocturnal pruritus or other family members or significant others with similar complaints.
3. Determine the patient's ability to cooperate and hold still during procedure.

DEVELOPMENTAL CONSIDERATIONS

Child: It is very important to have child remain still during procedure as the specimen is collected with a #15 scalpel blade. Some means to control the child's movement and hands is very important.

EQUIPMENT

- Light source, magnifier, otoscope
- Mineral oil
- Fountain pen, or blue or green marker
- Alcohol
- #15 scalpel blade
- Glass slide
- Coverslip
- Microscope

PROCEDURE	SPECIAL CONSIDERATIONS
1. Burrows can be seen better by using a light and a magnifier, like an otoscope.	Several techniques enhance burrows, allowing involved areas to be localized and specimens collected more effectively. There may be as few as 10 living mites in a full-blown infestation.

(procedure continued)

| PROCEDURE | SPECIAL CONSIDERATIONS |

2a. Mineral oil is applied over suspicious areas. Mineral oil changes the refractory index of the stratum corneum and allows better visibility of the burrows.

Mineral oil enhancement is a technique that is particularly useful over elbows and dry scaly areas.

Mineral oil is an excellent vehicle to use to collect specimens because it keeps the mites alive, motile and it does not dissolve the feces. Mineral oil also provides a high-yield specimen because the debris obtained scraping adheres to the oil.

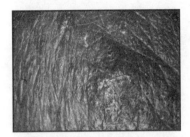

2b. The suspicious area is rubbed with the fountain pen or marker. The marked area is cleaned off with alcohol. The retained ink clearly demonstrates the location and depth of the burrow.

The burrow ink technique is a quick method to identify potentially high yield lesions. Marker colors other than blue or green obscure the findings.

The burrow ink technique also helps the clinician know how vigorously to scrape the lesion. Scraping should be done until the inked area is gone.

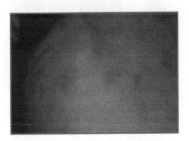

(procedure continued) ———————————————————————————————

| PROCEDURE | SPECIAL CONSIDERATIONS |

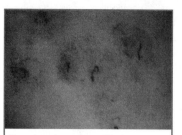

Knee after using marker, making burrows
more prominent.

3. Once located, the best way to collect the specimen is to apply mineral oil to the area or to the scalpel blade and shave or vigorously scrape the lesion. The material collected is placed on a glass slide, and a coverslip is placed on top of the specimen.

As scraping is done, the blade is held perpendicular to the skin. It is important to scrape vigorously 6 to 7 times to obtain an adequate specimen.

Shavings should be obtained from several sites to increase the chances of obtaining a positive scraping.

The adult mite can be found beyond the area of inflammation of the burrow. The greatest degree of inflammation is at the oldest end of the burrow.

4. Clean off the patient's skin where the specimens were obtained.

5. Examine the entire specimen under the coverslip with 10× magnification objective. Identification of mites, eggs, or feces in the specimen confirms the diagnosis of scabies.

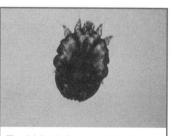

The adult female *Sarcoptes scabiei* mite.
(Courtesy of Stephen E. Estes, MD)

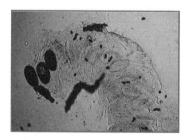

Illustrations 4 and 6 courtesy of Stephen E. Estes, MD.

FOLLOW-UP

- The patient with a demonstrated scabies infestation should be treated with a scabicide.
- Patient education should include proper application technique, and the treatment of asymptomatic family members and significant others, if indicated, as well as environmental control measures.

BIBLIOGRAPHY

American Medical Association. (1998). *Physicians' current procedural terminology: CPT.* Chicago: American Medical Association.

Fitzpatrick, T., Eisen, A., Freedberg, I., & Austin, K. (1993). *Dermatology in general medicine* (4th ed.). New York: McGraw-Hill, Inc.

Healthcare Consultants of America (1999). *1999 Physicians' fee and coding guide.* Augusta, GA.

Lowe, S. & Saxe, J. M. (1999). *Microscopic procedures for primary care providers.* Philadelphia: Lippincott Williams & Wilkins.

Moschella, S. & Hurley H. (1992). *Dermatology* (3rd ed.). Philadelphia: W. B. Saunders Co.

Orkin, M., Maibach, H., & Dahl, M. (1991). *Dermatology* (1st ed). Norwalk, CT: Appleton & Lange.

Reeves, J. & Maibach, H. (1998). *Clinical dermatology Illustrated* (3rd ed). Philadelphia: F. A. Davis Co.

chapter 8

Skin Lesion Removal

CPT Coding:

10060 Incision and drainage of abscess (simple or single lesion) (also includes cyst removal) ($91–$108)

10120 Incision and removal of foreign body, subcutaneous tissue, simple ($97–$114)

10160 Puncture aspiration of abscess, hematoma, bulla, or cyst ($81–$98)

11055–11057 Paring or cutting of benign hyperkeratotic lesions (corns, calluses)

11300–11313 Shaving of skin lesions (dermal or epidermal lesions) ($48–$60)

11300 Single lesion, trunk, arms, or legs <0.5 cm ($81–$99)

11301 Lesion 0.6 cm to 1.0 cm ($104–$127)

11302 Lesion 1.1 cm to 2.0 cm ($132–$159)

11303 Lesion >2.0 cm ($180–$219)

11305 Single lesion, scalp, hands, neck, feet, or genitalia < 0.5 cm ($88–$109)

11306 Lesion 0.6 to 1.0 cm ($116–$139)

11307 Lesion 1.1 to 2.0 cm ($142–$172)

11308 Lesion >2.0 cm ($195–$237)

11310 Lesion, single, face, ears, eyelids, nose, lips, or mucous membrane <0.5 cm ($104–$128)

11311–11313 Dependent on size ($135–$261)

11400–11471 Excision of benign skin lesions (usually requires closure)

11400 Excision, trunk, arms, or legs <0.5 cm ($104–$132)

11401 Lesion 0.6 to 1.0 cm ($140–$169)

11402 Lesion 1.1 to 2.0 cm ($179–$218)

11403–11406 Lesions from 2.1 to >4.0 cm ($236–$492)

11420–11426 Lesions on scalp, neck, hands, feet, or genitalia ranging in size from 0.5 cm to >4.0 cm ($117–$593)

11440–11446 Lesions on face, ears, eyelids, lips, or mucous membranes ranging in size from 0.5 cm to >4.0 cm ($147–$655)

17000–17250 Destruction of benign skin lesions

17000 Destruction by any method, 1st lesion ($65–$81) (includes common or plantar warts)

17003 2nd through 14th lesions each ($24–$31)

17004 15 or more lesions ($330–$455)

17106 Destruction of cutaneous vascular proliferative lesions <10 sq cm ($480–$598)

17110 Destruction of flat warts or molluscum contagiosum, milia, 1 to 14 lesions ($70–$86)

17111 >15 lesions ($99–$128)

11600–11606 Excision of malignant skin lesions on trunk, arms, or legs ranging in size from 0.5 cm to 4.0 cm ($173–$608)

DEFINITIONS

- An elliptical excision is a procedure that removes the full-thickness dermis in the shape of an ellipse for pathology that extends to the subcutaneous fat.
- A shave excision is a tissue-sparing procedure that leaves most of the dermis. Samples a wide area without excessive depth.
- A punch biopsy is the introduction of curette throughout the dermis to remove lesions less than 5 mm in diameter.
- Snipping is removal with scissors.
- Skin tags (acrochordons) are pedunculated papilloma that occur on eyelids, neck, axillae, and groin.
- Destruction is ablation of benign, premalignant, or malignant tissues by any method, with or without curettement, including local anesthesia, and not usually requiring closure. Methods that may be used include electrosurgery, cryosurgery, laser, and chemical treatment. Lesions include condylomata, papillomata, molluscum contagiosum, herpetic lesions, warts, or other benign, premalignant (eg, actinic keratoses) or malignant lesions.
- Cryosurgery is the destruction of tissue by freezing.

INDICATIONS

- To make a definitive diagnosis that usually includes pathology examination.
- To cure the lesion through excision.
- Removal of a lesion for cosmetic reasons.

TYPES OF REMOVAL

Type of removal	Indications
Elliptical excision	Removal of suspicious or miscellaneous skin lesion by surgical cutting. Specimen is submitted for pathologic analysis, which confirms diagnosis. Also can treat and cure lesion or be done for cosmetic reasons.
Shave excision	Preferred for removal of elevated benign or epidermal lesions, ie, suspected actinic keratosis, basal cell, or squamous cell. Limited to the superficial dermis or epidermis.
Punch biopsy	Preferred for all inflammatory conditions. May be used for full-thickness skin examination of lesions less than 5 mm in diameter.

table continued

table continued

Type of removal	Indications
Snipping	Removal of small skin tags with scissors for cosmetic reasons or if skin tags irritated or bleeding, or both.
Cryosurgery	Minimal scar formation, less time needed than conventional surgery for a variety of skin lesions. May cause skin pigment changes in patients with darker skin.
Cautery and curettement	Indicated for basal cell carcinoma, with cure rates of approximately 92% to 95%.

◉ PATIENT EDUCATION

- Patient should sign a surgery permit.
- Obtain the patient's current medical history including allergies, especially those to local anesthetic and povidone-iodine (Betadine) solutions. This includes a family history of malignant hyperthermia (ester-type local anesthesia agents are preferred if there is a positive family history of malignant hyperthermia).
- Obtain baseline vital signs.
- Inform the patient that a local anesthetic is not necessary for skin tags smaller than 1 cm.
- All of the above-mentioned procedures with the exception of snipping require a sterile procedure. Therefore, it is necessary to explain to the patient what will occur throughout the procedure to reassure and relax the patient, allowing for better pain control.
- Postoperative complications should be reviewed, that is, bleeding, temperature, infection, and scarring.
- Discuss the healing time and the anticipated results of procedure.
- Let the patient know that all excised skin lesions are sent to the pathology department for a definitive diagnosis.

◉ ASSESSMENT

1. Conduct history and physical appropriate to lesion.
2. Determine how long the lesion has existed, what treatments have been tried, and the results.
3. Note if previous excision has been attempted.
4. Describe the lesion according to its characteristics, pattern of arrangement, location, and distribution.
5. Be sure to measure and record all dimensions; consider photography of lesion.

◉ DEVELOPMENTAL CONSIDERATIONS

Child: Warts, moles, and molluscum contagiosum are seen in children.
Elderly: Common skin lesions in the elderly include

- Cherry angiomas: number increase with age (>30)

- Seborrheic keratoses: pigmented, raised lesions
- Actinic keratoses: premalignant lesions resulting from excessive sun exposure, usually occurring on the dorsal surface of the hands, arms, neck, and face
- Skin tags: increase in number with aging
- Cutaneous horns: small, hard projections of the epidermis
- Senile lentigines: "age spots" that occur in sun-exposed areas

ELLIPTICAL EXCISION

- The goal is to leave a straight scar less apparent than the original lesion.

Equipment
- Laceration tray equipped with sterile field, sterile drapes, sterile 4 × 4 gauzes
- Sterile normal saline
- Sterile gloves
- #15 scalpel blades
- Suture material: see Chapter 14: Lacerations
- Postoperative dressing material: Steri Strips
- Sterile instruments to include
  - Scalpel handle
  - Needle holder
  - Adson forceps with and without teeth
  - Tenotomy scissors
  - Small straight sharp scissors
  - Skin hooks
  - Mosquito hemostat
  - Anesthesia material: see Chapter 12: Local Anesthesia for Lacerations
  - Prep solution
  - Marking pen

PROCEDURE	SPECIAL CONSIDERATIONS
Position patient to obtain full exposure of lesion.	Make sure to draw the outline of the planned excision before administering anesthetic, since the anesthetic may distort the lesion and surrounding skin.
Premark the lesion—the incision lines should be parallel to the skin tension lines.	

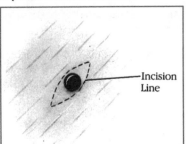

Incision Line

(procedure continued) ————————————————————————————

PROCEDURE	**SPECIAL CONSIDERATIONS**
Anesthetize the area using a field block. Allow blanching of skin indicating effect of agent.	
Using sterile technique, prep the skin on and around the lesion with Betadine paint, starting at the center of lesion and moving in a circular method around the lesion. Do not cross back over the wound area.	
Place sterile drapes around lesion.	
Make the elliptical incision around lesion.	About 3× as long as it is wide: The corner of the elipse should be approximately 30 degrees.
Grasp the dermis of the lesion with the forceps with teeth and excise the tissue within the incision.	
Excise from one end to center, then from opposite end to center.	
Pull the lesion and its contents out en bloc.	
Remove any remaining lesion wall.	It may be necessary to undermine the wound edges to avoid undue tension on suture line.
Using a scissors, undermine the subcutaneous plane beneath the dermis to allow the skin to glide together.	

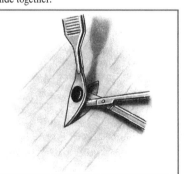

Close the skin opening with appropriate suture technique. If incision is deep, it is necessary to close in layers to minimize dead space and hematoma formation.	An absorbable suture such as Vicryl is recommended.
Final closure is done with nylon suture using interrupted sutures. Test tension of knot by tugging on suture and pulling knot across wound.	
Clean incision with normal saline. Then apply Steri-Strips.	

(procedure continued)

PROCEDURE	SPECIAL CONSIDERATIONS
Provide patient with patient education handout and appropriate follow-up appointment. Send lesion for pathology examination.	

Illustrations from Lohr, J. A., (1991). Pediatric outpatient procedures. Philadelphia: J. B. Lippincott Company.

Follow-up

- Remove sutures according to protocol depending on site of excision (see Chapter 14: Lacerations)
- Inform patient of biopsy results and instruct on any further treatment if necessary, such as referral to plastic surgeon. Refer the patient to a plastic surgeon when additional excision is needed or if the excision is in a cosmetically important area or if the patient requests it.
- Manage infection of surgical incision, if necessary.

SHAVE EXCISION

Equipment

- Laceration tray equipped with sterile field, sterile drapes, sterile 4×4 gauzes
- Sterile instruments to include
  - Needle holder
  - Adson forceps with and without teeth
  - Tenotomy scissors
  - Small straight sharp scissors
  - Scalpel handle
  - Anesthesia material (see Chapter 12: Local Anesthesia)
  - Prep solution
  - Sterile normal saline
  - Sterile gloves
  - #10 and #15 scalpel blades
  - Hot temp cautery or Monsel's solution
  - Postoperative dressing material: polymyxin B sulfate (Polysporin) (PSO) ointment and an adhesive bandage

PROCEDURE	SPECIAL CONSIDERATIONS
Position patient to obtain full exposure of lesion. Anesthetize area using field block. Allow blanching of skin, indicating effect of agent. Using sterile technique, prep the skin in and around the lesion with Betadine paint, starting at the center of lesion and moving in a cir-	**If a melanoma is suspected, a shave biopsy is contraindicated.** The depth of the lesion is important in determining prognosis for melanoma lesions. Shave biopsy used for obviously benign intradermal or compound nevi, epithelial tags, and small basal cell carcinoma.

(procedure continued) ———————————————————————————————————

PROCEDURE	**SPECIAL CONSIDERATIONS**

cular method around the lesion.
Place sterile drapes around the lesion.

Grasp the lesion with the Adson forceps with teeth producing firm counter-traction on the skin. Shave with blade. The entry angle of the obliquely held blade determines the depth of tissue removal.

The blade held nearly parallel to the skin surface produces a shallow shave. A 30- to 45-degree angle results in a thicker specimen.

Cauterize bleeding capillaries with hot temp cautery or apply Monsel's solution.

Monsel's solution decreases bleeding.

Clean the wound with normal saline. Then apply PSO and adhesive bandage.

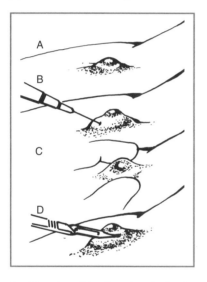

Provide patient with patient education handout and appropriate follow-up appointment.
Send lesion for pathology report.

Follow-up
- Inform the patient of pathology results. Instruct patient on any further treatment, if necessary.

PUNCH BIOPSY

Equipment
- Sterile field, sterile fenestrated drape, and sterile 4 × 4 gauzes

• Sterile instruments to include
  – Adson forceps with teeth
  – 2-mm punch
  – Sterile gloves
  – Anesthesia material: Refer to Chapter 12: Local Anesthesia
  – Prep solution
  – Sterile normal saline
  – Postoperative dressing material: Polysporin ointment and an adhesive
    bandage

PROCEDURE	SPECIAL CONSIDERATIONS
Position patient to obtain full exposure of lesion.	**Punch biopsies are not appropriate for eyelids, lips, or penile lesions.**
Anesthetize the area using direct local infiltration.	

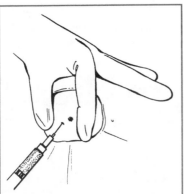

Stabilize tissue. Infiltrate local anesthetic. (Salom, T., Cutler, B., and Wheeler, H. [1988]. *Atlas of Bedside Procedures*, (2nd ed.). Boston: Little, Brown and Company.)

Using sterile technique, prep the skin on and around the lesion with prep solution, starting at the center of lesion and moving in a circular method around the lesion.	Use the most recently developed lesion for punch biopsy because it is most likely to yield a diagnosis.
Place fenestrated drape over lesion.	
Gently insert 2-mm punch into area of lesion of greatest concern. Turn biopsy punch in one direction only. The punch should carry through the dermis. Withdraw and remove biopsy delicately with Adson's forceps. The punch biopsy should have a short tail of fatty tissue.	Apply tension to area perpendicular to skin tension lines. This helps to make the lesion more of an elliptical lesion, which is a more cosmetically pleasing lesion.

(procedure continued)

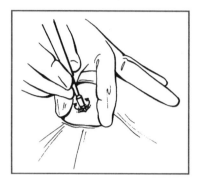

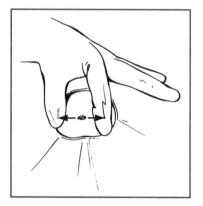

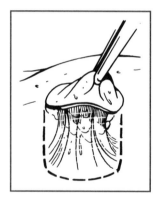

There is a definite distinguishable feel between soft, friable tumor tissue and gritty, firm, healthy dermis.

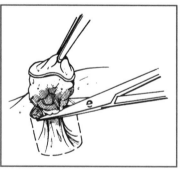

(procedure continued)

PROCEDURE	SPECIAL CONSIDERATIONS
Apply hemostasis. Clean wound with normal saline. They apply PSO and adhesive bandage.	Punch biopsies of <3 mm do not usually need to be sutured closed.
Provide patient with patient education handout and appropriate follow-up appointment. Send biopsy for pathology examination.	

Follow-up

- Inform patient of biopsy result and instruct on further treatment if necessary, that is, referral (if further excision is needed, refer patient to a plastic surgeon).

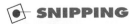

SNIPPING

Equipment

- Sterile Adson forceps with teeth
- Sterile sharp straight scissors
- Silver nitrate sticks, hot-temperature cautery, or Monsel's solution (ferric subsulfate)
- Postoperative dressing material:
  - PSO and adhesive bandage.

PROCEDURE	SPECIAL CONSIDERATIONS
Position patient to obtain full exposure of tags.	Monsel's solution can be applied before snipping to help decrease bleeding.
Grasp skin tag with forceps to position tag on its apex. Snip with scissors.	
Use hot temp cautery, Monsel's solution, or silver nitrate sticks to stop bleeding if necessary. Apply PSO and adhesive bandage.	

(procedure continued)

PROCEDURE	SPECIAL CONSIDERATIONS

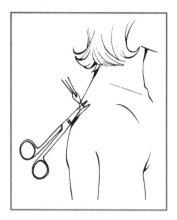

Follow-up
• No follow-up is necessary unless infection occurs.
• Signs and symptoms include redness, pain, swelling, and fever.

CAUTERY AND CURETTEMENT

Equipment
• Dermal curette
• Cautery
• Prep solution
• Gauze dressing

PROCEDURE	SPECIAL CONSIDERATIONS
Anesthetize the lesion using local anesthesia. Prep lesion using povidone-iodine (Betadine), chlorhexidine gluconate (Hibiclens), or other antiseptic.	This procedure works best on lesions ≤3 cm in size.
Scoop out the lesion using a large dermal curette, scraping the bottom of the lesion until a gritty sensation is encountered.	The gritty feeling is felt when normal tissue is scraped.

(procedure continued)

| PROCEDURE | SPECIAL CONSIDERATIONS |

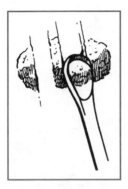

Cauterize the entire base.

Cauterizing the entire base is necessary to eliminate any remaining cells and to help control bleeding.

Repeat the curettement and cautery again.

A 3rd round of curettement (using a smaller dermal curette) and cautery is completed.

Do not pass through the entire dermis.

Place PSO and a dressing over the lesion.

Follow-up
- Patients should wash the area 3 to 4 times a day and apply an antibiotic ointment.
- Close observation is essential because 50% of patients develop new basal cell cancers within 5 years.

CRYOSURGERY

Equipment
- Nitrous oxide through cryoprobe unit or liquid nitrogen
- K-Y jelly
- Cotton-tipped applicators
- Second and minute timer

| PROCEDURE | SPECIAL CONSIDERATIONS |

Use either the cryoprobe unit or liquid nitrogen.

If using liquid nitrogen, pour liquid into a cup. A styrofoam cup works well. The spray comes with a changeable nozzle that can be adapted to the shape of the lesion. The nozzle should be held close to the skin. Less freeze time is needed for spray liquid nitrogen.

(procedure continued)

PROCEDURE	SPECIAL CONSIDERATIONS

Apply the cryoprobe or cotton-tipped applicator to the lesion. Freeze the lesion until the ice ball extends 2 to 3 mm beyond the edge of the lesion. This is evident by the whitish discoloration of the lesion.

The duration of the freeze is important. A general rule of thumb is 1 minute for skin (adjusted as needed for each patient). The more pressure that is applied to the swab the more the depth of penetration.

Identify the patient's response to the freezing (sensitive, supersensitive, normal, resistant).

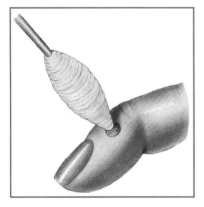

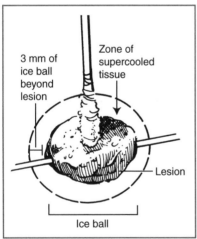

Illustration 1 from Lohr, J. A., (1991). Pediatric outpatient procedures. Philadelphia: J. B. Lippincott Company.

Specific Procedures for Cryosurgery Based on Type of Lesion

PROCEDURE	TYPE OF LESIONS
Full-thickness freeze	Benign and premalignant lesions: Actinic keraqtoses: freeze 1 to $1\frac{1}{2}$ minutes Vascular lesions: freeze, thaw, refreeze technique: $1\frac{1}{2}$ minutes. Wait 5 to 7 minutes then refreeze.
Full-thickness destructive freeze	Basal cell carcinoma (must have biopsy (punch) before treatment). Freeze for 1 to $1\frac{1}{2}$ minutes until freeze is 5 to 8 mm beyond the lesion. Document the time and extent of the freeze. Wait 5 to 7 minutes for thaw and then repeat the freeze. **Do not use for melanoma or squamous cell carcinoma lesions.**
Specific types of lesions	Molluscum: 30 sec to $1\frac{1}{2}$ minutes. Prepare lesions with water-soluble gel. Avoid freezing normal skin. Verruca: approx. 1 to $1\frac{1}{2}$ minutes Plantar warts: (after débridement): 40 sec Condyloma: 45 sec
Lesions NOT recommended for cryosurgery	Recurrent basal cell cancer Where hair loss is critical Where pigment changes may occur Lower extremities where circulation is poor (especially in diabetic patient) Basal cell cancers in nasolabial fold (more extensive and recur frequently) Port wine stain (use a laser)

Follow-up
- Instruct the patient to protect the healing crust to decrease the chance of scar formation.
- Dressings are usually not needed after treatment.
- Let the patient know that the treated area is first pale and then red. Later, a blister will form over the whole lesion. After a few days, the blister will dry up and a scab will form, which lasts 1 to 2 weeks.
- If a lesion is not removed after three treatments, the patient should be referred to dermatology or plastic surgeon for more definitive treatment.

Appropriate Removal Method
Based on Type of Lesion

• A biopsy should be taken of all nonhealing, changing, or enlarging skin lesions. The only lesion for which a pathologic examination is not strongly recommended is skin tags; all others should be sent for analysis.

Type of lesion	Removal Method
Skin tag	Snipping or shave biopsy
Basal cell carcinoma	Punch biopsy, then treat with curettement and cautery for lesion <1 cm Lesions >1 cm, lesions in more aggressive locations, sclerosing type lesions, or lesions with ill-defined border: elliptical excision
Squamous cell carcinoma	Deep-punch biopsy, then elliptical excision
Dermatofibroma	Punch biopsy, then excision. Cryosurgery can be tried, but dermatofibromas are usually resistant.
Keratocanthoma	Cryotherapy, excision, curettement and cautery
Actinic keratoses	Retinoic acid, punch biopsy, shave biopsy, elliptical excision, cryotherapy
Seborrheic keratoses	Shave excision, cryotherapy (only use if absolutely sure of diagnosis or after biopsy), electrosurgery
Lentigo	Cryotherapy
Lipomas	Elliptical excision
Melanoma	Use ABCDE mnemonic to help identify melanomas: 　　Asymmetry 　　Border irregularity 　　Color variation 　　Diameter >6 mm 　　Elevation above skin surface 　　Punch or elliptical excision. Use the area that is the most atypical in color or inflammed. **Never use shave excision.**
Molluscum contagiousum	Curettement with dermal curette, cryotherapy
Acquired nevi	If malignancy suspected, do full-thickness elliptical excision before removal. Otherwise shave biopsy can be used with raised or pedunculated lesions.
Sebaceous cysts	Elliptical excision
Telangiectasis	Cherry hemagiomas: cautery Spider veins: sclerotherapy
Common and plantar warts	Cryotherapy, watchful waiting (many warts will resolve spontaneously)

BIBLIOGRAPHY

(1998). Tackling warts on the hands and feet. *Drug Therapy Bulletin, 36*(3), 22–24.

American Medical Association. (1998). *Physicians' current procedural terminology:* CPT. Chicago: American Medical Association.

Alguire, P. & Mathes, B. (1998). Skin biopsy techniques for the internist. *Journal of General Internal Medicine, 13*(1), 46–54.

Arpey, C. (1998). Biopsy of the skin. Thoughtful selection of technique improves yield. *Postgraduate Medicine, 103*(3), 179–182, 185–189, 193–194.

Barrett, B. M. (1982). *Manual of patient care in plastic surgery.* Boston: Little, Brown and Co.

Barron, J. N. & Saad, M. N. (Eds). (1980). *Operative plastic and reconstructive surgery* (Vol. 2) Edinburgh: Churchill Livingstone.

Boriskin, M. I. (1994). Primary care management of wounds. *Nurse Practitioner, 19*(11), 38.

Edmunds, M. W. & Mayhew, M. S. (1996). *Procedures for primary care practitioners.* St. Louis: Mosby.

Healthcare Consultants of America. (1998). *1998 Physicians' fee and coding guide.* Augusta, GA.

Hughes, N. (1986). Basic techniques of excision and wound closure. In T. Barclay & D. Kernahan (Eds), *Rob and Smith's operative surgery: plastic surgery* (4th ed.), 33–57. Boston: Butterworths.

Leslie, T. (1997). Skin biopsy: How to do it. *British Journal of Hospital Medicine, 58*(7), 341–342.

Lohr, J. (1991). *Pediatric outpatient procedures.* Philadelphia: J. B. Lippincott.

Lowe, S. & Saxe, J. M. (1999). *Microscopic procedures for primary care providers.* Philadelphia: Lippincott Williams & Wilkins.

Pfenninger, J. L. & Fowler, G. C. (1994). *Procedures for primary care physicians.* St. Louis: Mosby.

Plastic Surgery Educational Foundation. (1987). *Plastic and reconstructive surgery: Essentials for students* (3rd ed.). Chicago: Author

Plastic Surgery Educational Foundation. (1991). *Everyday wounds: A guide for the primary care physician.* Chicago: Author

Rivellini, D. (1993). Local and regional anesthesia. Nursing Implications. *Nursing Clinics of North America,* 28(3), 547.

Salm, T., Cutler, B., & Wheeler, H. (1988). *Atlas of bedside procedures* (2nd ed., p. 467). Boston: Little, Brown and Company.

Simon, R. & Brenner, B. (1994). *Emergency procedures and techniques.* Baltimore: Williams & Wilkins.

Trott, A. T. (1997). *Wounds and lacerations: Emergency care and closure* (2nd ed.). St. Louis: Mosby.

Zouboulis, C. (1998). Cryosurgery in dermatology. *European Journal of Dermatology,* 8(7), 466–474.

chapter
9
Corn and Callus Management

CPT Coding:

> 11055 Débridement of lesion with or without cautery ($48–$60)
> 11056 Débridement of lesions (2–4) with or without cautery ($62–$80)
> 11057 Débridement of lesions (>5) with or without chemicals ($82–$104)

DEFINITION

In the medical field, calluses are referred to as tylomas. These lesions are localized keratoses that are formed when intermittent pressure from outside persists with solid resistance within. Tylomas are usually located over bony prominences.

CORNS: THREE TYPES

- Heloma durum is a hard corn that is usually located dorsally on hammer toes and bunions. Occasionally, it is located on dorsal surface of hands.
- Heloma molle is a soft corn that is usually located in interspaces of toes over bony prominences.
- Intractable plantar keratoses (IPKs) are condensed, usually enucleated lesions on plantar surface of feet beneath bony prominences.

ETIOLOGY

- All of these lesions are caused most generally by friction and pressure.
- Other intrinsic causes include verruca, epidermal inclusion cysts, cicatrix or scar, foreign body granuloma, pocokeratosis punctate, and hereditary dermatoses.

PATIENT EDUCATION

- Inform the patient of the need to débride the lesion to prevent further breakdown of skin and possible ulcer formation.
- In rare cases, deep IPKs may require the use of a local anesthetic before débridement.
- If lesions get progressively worse or show any signs of infection, refer the patient (especially a diabetic) to a podiatrist.

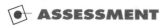 ASSESSMENT

1. A complete medical history is necessary.
2. A history of the lesion or lesions must be obtained. When was it noticed initially? What were the previous treatments? What makes it better? What aggravates lesion?

 ALERT: If patient has a history of peripheral vascular disease, diabetes, peripheral neuropathies, or systemic disease affecting lower extremities, consult a podiatrist.

Lesions	Equipment
Plantar tyloma or callus (< 2 cm × 2 cm)	#15 Blade and scalpel handle
Plantar tyloma or callus (> 2 cm × 2cm)	#10 or #15 Blade and scalpel handle
Heloma molle (interspaces)	#11 or #15 Blade and scalpel handle
Heloma durum (hard corns)	#10 or #15 Blade and scalpel handle
Intractable plantar keratoses	#11 or #15 Blade and scalpel handle

3. Determine whether the lesions were previously infected or ever ulcerated.
4. Determine the cooperative ability of patient. Is he or she scared of being cut with a blade? If the patient is a child, use caution due to the unpredictability of children's behavior.
5. Check if patient has a dorsalis pedis pulse and a posterior tibial pulse.

 ALERT: Always débride lesions away from the practitioner's hands or body.

Procedure	Special Considerations
Débride or shave parallel to skin surface.	May use padding after treatment to disperse weight-bearing pressure.

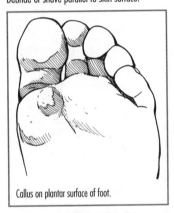

Callus on plantar surface of foot.

Procedure	Special Considerations
Débride or shave parallel to skin surface.	Again, may disperse pressure with padding.
Débride in circular motion if necessary.	Caution due to thin skin.
Débride parallel to skin surface.	May have to soften lesion with soapy warm water.

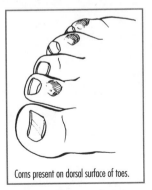

Corns present on dorsal surface of toes.

Procedure	Special Considerations
Enucleate core with circular motion.	May have to excise through epidermis.

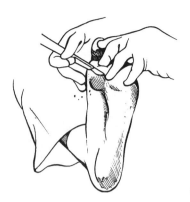

Always debride away from practitioner's body or hands.

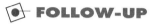

FOLLOW-UP

• Patients with good lower extremity vascularity can have lesions débrided routinely.

• P.V.D. patients and diabetics should follow-up with a podiatrist.

• Other medical problems affecting the lower extremities must each be evaluated individually by the nurse practitioner, and a judgment of the treatment must be made accordingly.

BIBLIOGRAPHY

American Medical Association. (1998). *Physicians' current procedural terminology: CPT.* Chicago: American Medical Association.

Burch, G. E. & Winsor, R. Diffusion of water through dead plantar, palmar and torsal human skin and through toenails.

Healthcare Consultants (1998). *1998 Physicians' fee and coding guide.* Augusta, GA.

Lapidus, P.W. (1966). Orthopaedic skin lesions of the soles and toes. *Clinical Orthopaedics,* 45, 87–100.

Lowe, S. & Saxe, J. M. (1999). *Microscopic procedures for primary care providers.* Philadelphia: Lippincott Williams & Wilkins.

Port, M. (1980). Podiatric dermatology: Nail disorders. Dermatology, 10, 10–22.

chapter 10

Fishhook Removal

CPT Coding:

10120 Removal of subcutaneous foreign body, simple ($97–$114)
10121 Incisional removal, foreign body, complex ($284–$338)

⊙ INDICATIONS

• The patient presents with a fish hook that he or she has been unable to remove.

> **ALERT:** Do not try to remove hook from the eye, where the removal might endanger the globe, nerves, or arteries.

⊙ PATIENT EDUCATION

• Reassure the patient that removal will be painless once the area has been anesthetized.
• Emphasize the need for tetanus prophylaxis if more than 5 years has elapsed since the last tetanus inoculation.
• Instruct the patient in infection precautions and wound care, and warn of signs and symptoms of infection.
• Antibiotic and appropriate medication for pain management: Usually a nonsteroidal anti-inflammatory agent (NSAID) is sufficient.

⊙ ASSESSMENT

1. Obtain a history related to episode: How long ago did it happen and initial measures taken.
2. Assess for signs of infection, such as redness, discharge, and swelling.
3. Assess the patient's neurovascular status; make sure there are no vascular or neurologic deficits.
4. Verify immunization status: tetanus.

⊙ DEVELOPMENTAL CONSIDERATIONS

Child: It is very important to have child remain still during procedure to prevent further injury. Use of papoose board or other means to control movement and hands is very important.

⟨●⟩ EQUIPMENT

- Lidocaine or bupivacaine (Marcaine); appropriate syringe and needle (See Ch. 12)
- Large hemostat
- Heavy-duty wire cutters
- Disinfectant and dressing

PROCEDURE	SPECIAL CONSIDERATIONS
Prep with povidone-iodine (Betadine) solution or chlorhexidine (Hibiciens) before the procedure. Infiltrate anesthetic at the entrance and future exit site.	Do not use anesthetic with epinephrine on fingers, toes, nose. (Generally, epinephrine should not be required).
Grasp end of hook, and rotate hook pushing point through skin at site previously anesthetized (as if completing its passage through tissue).	**Ensure you do not cause further damage to nerves or blood vessels.**
a. Cut barb off, and rotate hook back out entrance wound.	Triple hooks require very heavy duty wire cutters.

If you cut off the eye end of a hook (which is necessary with double barbed hooks and frequently with triple hooks), be sure that you leave enough room to be able to push the point of hook through the skin or you can lose hook trying to rotate it out, necessitating excision of the hook.

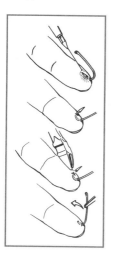

b. With a double-barbed hook or sometimes with triple hooks, you will need to cut off the eye of the hook. Rotate tip through, then grasp tip and continue to rotate hook, removing it through exit wound.

(procedure continued)

| PROCEDURE | SPECIAL CONSIDERATIONS |

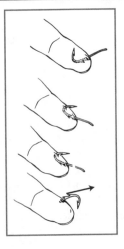

Clean and dress the wound.

These puncture wounds are considered dirty wounds and prophylaxis with appropriate antibiotics is indicated. Dicloxacillin, cephalosporin, and amoxicillin (Augmentin) are good choices. Consider intramuscular antibiotic for patients you may not be able to follow up or who may be noncompliant.)

Illustrations from Lohr, Jacob A. (1991). Pediatric outpatient procedures. Philadelphia: J.B. Lippincott Company.

ALTERNATIVE PROCEDURES

- If hook is in a position that you believe is not appropriate for removal, as noted earlier (such as near the eye or other structure you would rather not puncture), then you should not push the hook through (as mentioned earlier). Instead, you may go along the inside edge of hook with an 18-gauge needle and cover the barb as noted in illustration so the hook is "housed" by the lumen of the needle, then just back the hook out.
- This is much harder to do than you might imagine from description and the illustration. This procedure may end up causing as much or more skin damage with the 18-gauge needle than just pushing hook through.
- A method described by Cooke (1961) is to use a long piece of sewing thread or silk. The thread is place around the curve of the hook, with the other end wrapped around the remover's finger or hand. The end of the

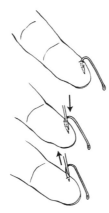

hook is then depressed, while the other hand makes the thread taut. A
quick jerk is then applied to dislodge the hook. The involved area should
be held flatly against a firm surface during the procedure.

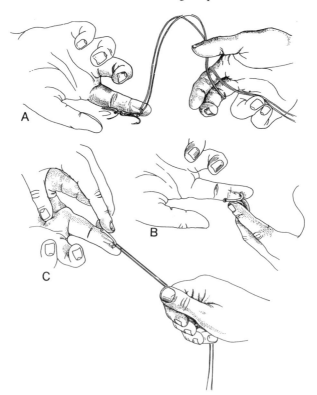

A: Silk suture material or a string is placed around the curve of the fishhook. *B:* The involved digit is then held firmly against a flat
surface and the shank is depressed until resistance is met. *C:* While the shank is depressed and the string is held taut, a quick jerk
is applied to dislodge the needle. (Simon, R. & Brenner, B. [1994]. *Emergency procedures and techniques,* [3rd ed]. Baltimore:
Williams & Wilkins.)

- This method is said to require no anesthetic and causes no additional puncture wound.

⊕ FOLLOW-UP

- Depending on the amount of trauma sustained and the area involved, it may be appropriate to have the patient return in 24 to 48 hours, and certainly at first sign of any infections.

BIBLIOGRAPHY

Cooke, T. (1961). How to remove fish-hooks with a bit of string. *Medical Journal of Australia, 48,* 815.

Healthcare Consultants of America. (1998). *1998 Physicians' fee and coding guide.* Augusta, GA.

Pfenninger, J. & Fowler, G. (1994). *Procedures for primary care physicians.* St. Louis: Mosby–Year Book, Inc.

chapter
11

Hair Tourniquet

CPT Coding:
• N/A

 DEFINITION

Hair or thread fibers stick to infant clothing and occasionally become tightly wrapped around the child's digits or genitals. The offending fibers may be difficult to visualize, and parents often do not seek treatment until signs of distal ischemia appear. If these fibers are left in place, automatic amputation may eventually occur.

 INDICATIONS

• Hair or thread wrapped around digit or genitals.

ASSESSMENT

1. Thoroughly assess the affected digit for evidence of tissue ischemia.
2. Also, inspect other digits and the genitals of male children for other hair tourniquets.

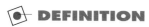

PROCEDURE	**SPECIAL CONSIDERATIONS**
Occasionally, the fiber can be grasped with toothless forceps or a small hemostat and unwrapped. More commonly, the fibers cannot be identified and are deeply embedded in swollen tissue.	
A #11 blade can be used to cut constricting bands. A regional nerve block may need to be performed. Often, multiple hairs are involved. Because the bands may be quite deep, the incision should avoid known neurovascular tracts (Rudnitsky & Barnett, 1998).	It may be difficult to identify individual hairs that are deeply embedded in a swollen digit and even more difficult to assess the success of one's interventions.

EQUIPMENT

- Toothless forceps
- Hemostat
- #11 scalpel blade
- Hair removal product (Nair, Neet)

ALTERNATIVE PROCEDURE

- Another method found to work occasionally is the application of hair removal products (Nair, Neet) directly to the site, using a cotton-tipped applicator. There have been few studies regarding the use of these products, but clinical experience has seen some success. It is essential to place the solution deep into the fissure, using the applicator. After a waiting period of 10 to 15 minutes, the distal tissue is re-evaluated for improvement in color and perfusion. If no change has occurred, a more invasive technique may be indicated. Refer the patient to the emergency department for a hand surgeon or hand plastics surgeon consultation if attempts to remove the hair tourniquet are unsuccessful.

FOLLOW-UP

- Generally, conservative wound care is sufficient once the band has been removed. Application of an antibiotic ointment may enhance healing and allow easier removal of serous drainage from the circumferential laceration.
- Clinical reassessment in 24 hours will indicate whether any constricting bands remain.

BIBLIOGRAPHY

Rudnitsky, G. & Barnett, R. (1998) Soft tissue foreign body removal; hair-thread tourniquet. In J. Roberts & J. Hedges (Eds.). *Clinical procedures in emergency medicine* (3rd ed., pp. 632–633). Philadelphia: W. B. Saunders Co.

chapter 12

Local Anesthesia for Lacerations

CPT Coding:
Not applicable; included in specific procedure

 DEFINITION

Local Anesthesia: Temporary loss of sensation due to the prevention of the generation and conduction of nerve impulses in a specific part of the body. Use of local anesthesia makes it possible to perform procedures on an outpatient basis, providing patient comfort and cooperation.

 TYPES OF LOCAL ANESTHESIA

- Topical anesthesia: Sensory blockade of nerve endings by placement of agent directly on tissue where anesthesia desired, usually without use of a needle.
- Local anesthesia: Sensory blockade of subcutaneous nerve endings by injection of agent at site where anesthesia desired.
- Digital nerve block: Sensory blockade achieved by injection of agent near the nerve branch supplying sensation to particular area, desensitizing all adjacent tissue.

 INDICATIONS

- Local anesthesia is indicated for minor procedures and emergency wound or laceration repair.

Anesthesia type	Advantages	Disadvantages
Topical	It is useful for superficial lesions or uncomplicated lacerations, especially in children. It is more effective in lacerations 5 cm or smaller on the face and scalp. A variety of solutions can be used, such as tetracaine, adrenalin, cocaine, and lidocaine. One mixture includes tetracaine (0.5%), and epinephrine	Cannot be used on fingers, toes, nose, pinna of ear, penis, or mucous membranes. It is not as effective on trunk or proximal extremities.

table continued

Anesthesia type	Advantages	Disadvantages
	(1:2000 concentration), and cocaine (11.8%). Onset is 5 to 15 minutes, lasting 20 to 30 minutes. Approximately 2 to 5 mL of solution is used.	This composition yields and average dose of cocaine of 590 mg/5 mL and an average dose of tetracaine 25 mg/5 mL.
	Lidocaine 4% can be used as a topical anesthetic agent for large wounds and wrapped firmly with Kerlix for 10 minutes.	
Local	It is effective in minor suturing procedures.	
	Direct infiltration is used in minimally contaminated lacerations in anatomically uncomplicated areas.	
	Field block is used in grossly contaminated wounds and lesion removal. It provides for less tissue damage at the wound site.	
Digital nerve block	It is recommended for lacerations distal to the level of the midproximal phalanx of fingers or toes.	
	It is used for nail removal, paronychia drainage, or repair of lacerations of digits.	

PATIENT EDUCATION

• Explain procedure and purpose to minimize pain.
• Emphasize the importance of not moving.

ASSESSMENT

1. See the more detailed assessment needed based on the specific procedure to be done.
2. Obtain a history of allergies to anesthesia products. Ask if the patient has ever had rashes, urticaria, wheezing, or anaphylaxis in the past related to anesthesia. Also ask about a history of familial malignant hyperthermia. If a positive history is obtained, the ester-type local anesthesia agents (procaine, chloroprocaine, and tetracaine) are preferred.
3. Obtain history of medications that the patient is presently taking.

DEVELOPMENTAL CONSIDERATIONS

Child: Having parents present during the procedure may be calming to small children. Additional anesthesia may be necessary for smaller children. Older children may prefer an explanation of what is to occur.

Adequate restraint is necessary to prevent movement during the anesthesia procedure.

 ## ANESTHETIC SOLUTIONS

• There are three anesthetic solutions commonly used for local infiltration and simple nerve block.

Anesthetic agent	Comments
Lidocaine (xylocaine 1% and 2%, with or without epinephrine)	Lidocaine is most commonly used owing to its rapid onset of action and tissue-spreading properties with direct infiltration. It works in approximately 4 to 10 minutes when used in a block, lasting 30 to 120 minutes. With epinephrine, the block lasts 60 to 240 minutes. ALERT: Toxic limit of lidocaine is 7 mg/kg/hr. This represents one 50-mL bottle of 1% xylocaine per hour for an average of 70-kg person.
Mepivacaine (Carbocain 1% and 2%)	Immediate onset of action when it is used as an infiltrating agent. Mepivacaine has a slower onset of action when it is used as a blocking agent (6–10 minutes) and somewhat longer duration of action than lidocaine (lasts 90–180 minutes when used as a block)
Bupivacaine (Marcaine 0.25% and 0.5%)	Bupivacaine has a slower onset of action yet a longer duration of action (8–12 minutes onset for block, lasting 240–480 minutes).
Epinephrine added to anesthetic agents, usually lidocaine (such as Lidocaine 1% with epinephrine)	The use of epinephrine along with local anesthesia decreases bleeding, reduces systemic absorption, and prolongs the duration of action.

 ALERT: *Vasoconstrictive agents (epinephrine) should not be used on the nose, ear, penis, or ends of digits. Patients with peripheral vascular disease have an exaggerated vasoconstriction response to these agents.*

 ## TOPICAL ANESTHESIA

Equipment
• 3 to 5 mL anesthetic solution
• 2 × 2 gauze
• Disposable gloves
• Gauze, if needed to wrap around location

Place a saturated 2 × 2 gauze in or around laceration for a minimum of 20 minutes. Apply gentle, manual pressure over sponge.

Patients or parents can assist with process by applying pressure. Make sure a glove is worn to apply pressure because the solution will be absorbed by the person applying the pressure.

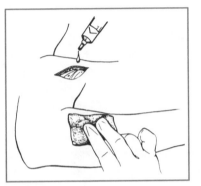

Maximum dose of solution is 2 to 5 mL. Anesthesia is reached when zone of blanching is observed around wound.

Supplemental infiltration may be required to achieve complete anesthesia. Be sure to warn parents that this may be required.

LOCAL ANESTHESIA

Equipment
- Anesthetic solution
- 5 mL syringe needles: 25, 27, or 30 gauge, $1/2$ to $1^1/2$ inch in length
- Gloves

DIRECT WOUND INFILTRATION

Draw up anesthetic solution into syringe.

The plane of anesthesia for local skin infiltration is immediately beneath the dermis at the junction of the superficial fascia (subcutaneous tissue).

Place a few drops of anesthetic in the wound, then insert the needle through open wound parallel to and just below the dermis. Inject a small bolus of anesthesia solution, withdraw and inject another bolus at adjacent site until

(procedure continued) ———————————————————————————————

PROCEDURE	**SPECIAL CONSIDERATIONS**

all edges and corners of wound are anesthe-
sized.

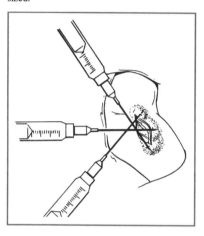

Test for sensation before proceeding.	Prick the distal portion of the digit with the injection needle to test the effectiveness of anesthesia.

FIELD BLOCK

Equipment
- Anesthetic solution
- 5-mL syringe needles: 25, 27, or 30 gauge, $\frac{1}{2}$ to $1\frac{1}{2}$ inches in length
- Gloves

PROCEDURE	**SPECIAL CONSIDERATIONS**

The plane of anesthesia is immediately beneath the dermis at the junction of the superficial fascia (subcutaneous tissue).

Insert needle through intact skin at one end of the wound. Injections are made during advance and withdrawal of the needle. Reinsert needle at distal end of first track where skin is becoming anesthetized.	If anesthesia is for removal of lesion, try not to distort the anatomy of the lesion.

(procedure continued)

| PROCEDURE | SPECIAL CONSIDERATIONS |

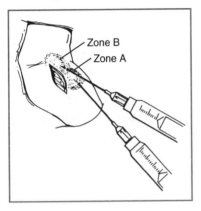

Repeat on all sides of wound until complete infiltration achieved. Test for sensation before proceeding.

DIGITAL NERVE BLOCK (FINGER AND TOE BLOCK)

Equipment
- Anesthetic solution
- 5-mL syringe needles: 25, 27, or 30 gauge
- Gloves $\frac{1}{2}$ to $1\frac{1}{2}$ inches in length

DIGITAL TECHNIQUE

| PROCEDURE | SPECIAL CONSIDERATIONS |

Anesthesia solutions include lidocaine 1% and 2% plain or carbocaine 1% plain.

Insert needle into dorsolateral aspect of proximal phalanx in portion of web space just distal to the MCP joint. Advance at a 90-degree angle toward plantar digital nerve.

All four digital nerves (two palmar and two dorsal) must be blocked to achieve complete digital anesthesia.

ALERT: Epinephrine (a vasoconstrictor) is contraindicated in fingers and toes.

(procedure continued)

PROCEDURE	SPECIAL CONSIDERATIONS

Palpate needle with support of index finger under plantar surface and withdraw slightly. Deliver 0.5 mL of anesthetic. Again withdraw needle slightly, and redirect toward volar surface of digit. Deliver 1 mL of anesthetic. Repeat procedure on opposite side of digit.

Place a $\frac{1}{2}$ ring of anesthetic around digit by injecting over the bone and under the bone in the same subcutaneous plane.

Swelling should be palpated as the anesthetic is deposited into the web space. If no swelling is evident, the anesthetic has probably moved dorsal to the ligaments and will not be adequately anesthetized (Simon & Brenner, 1994).

Do not completely encircle digit or use too much anesthetic because of tourniquet effect or
One to two milliliters of anesthetic agent should be sufficient.

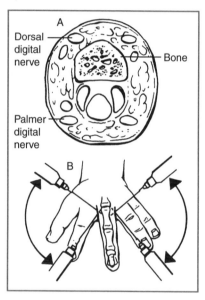

A
Dorsal digital nerve
Bone
Palmer digital nerve
B

Thumb: The needle should be inserted at the level of the most proximal thumb crease, approximately 2 to 3 mm deep, along either side of the thumb flexor tendon. Use the same insertion site for both injections.

Inject 1 to 2 mL of 2% lidocaine. Palpate the subcutaneous fullness of anesthetic.

(procedure continued)

PROCEDURE	SPECIAL CONSIDERATIONS

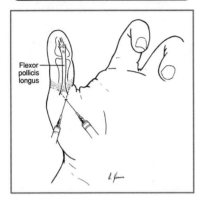

Flexor
pollicis
longus

Test for sensation before proceeding.   As above

MCP, metacarpophalangeal. (Illustration 2 from Simon, R. & Brenner, B. [1994]. Emergency procedures and techniques, [3rd Ed]. Baltimore: Williams & Wilkins.)

GREAT TOE

Equipment
- A 1½-inch 25-gauge needle with 10-mL syringe
- 1% lidocaine WITHOUT epinephrine

PROCEDURE	SPECIAL CONSIDERATIONS

Insert injection A at the anterior lateral portion of the toe, directed medially in subcutaneous tissue. Redirect the needle posteriorly through the same puncture site, and instill anesthetic in this area.

Insert injection B along the anterior medial portion of the great toe, and instill the anesthetic posteriorly as shown.

The base of the toe must be blocked circumferentially.

(procedure continued)

PROCEDURE	SPECIAL CONSIDERATIONS

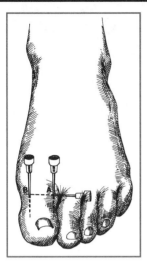

For last injection, introduce the needle to the base of the toe over the volar surface. Direct the anesthetic medially.

This block takes 5 to 10 minutes to work.

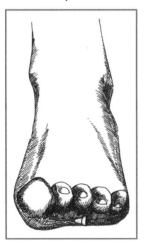

Illustrations from Simon, R. & Brenner, B. [1994]. Emergency procedures and techniques, [3rd Ed]. Baltimore: Williams & Wilkins.)

TOE BLOCK (OTHER THAN THE GREAT TOE)

Equipment
• As mentioned earlier

PROCEDURE	SPECIAL CONSIDERATIONS
For second to fifth toes, insert needle mid-dorsal aspect of the proximal phalanx. Deliver anesthetic on one side of toe, withdraw slowly, and pass down opposite side using a single needle stick.	Approximately 2 mL of anesthetic is needed along each side of the toes.

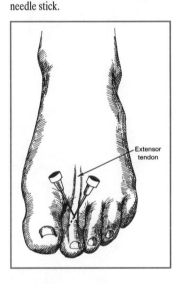

Test for sensation before proceeding.

BIBLIOGRAPHY

American Medical Association. (1998). *Physicians' current procedureal terminology: CPT.* Chicago, AMA.

Barrett, B. M. (1982). *Manual of patient care in plastic surgery.* Boston: Little, Brown and Co.

Barron, J. N. & Saad, M. N. (Eds.). (1980). *Operative plastic and reconstructive surgery* (Vol. 2). Edinburgh: Churchill Livingstone.

Boriskin, M. I.(1994). Primary care management of wounds. *Nurse Practitioner,* 19(11), 38.

Edmunds, M. W. & Mayhew, M. S. (1996). *Procedures for primary care practitioners.* St. Louis: Mosby.

Healthcare Consultants of America. (1998). *1998 Physicians' fee and coding guide.* Augusta, GA.

Hughes, N. (1991). Basic techniques of excision and wound closure. In T. Barclay & D. Kernahan (Eds.): *Rob and Smith's operative surgery: Plastic surgery* (4th ed.). Boston: Butterworths.

Lowe, S. & Saxe, J. M. (1999). *Microscopic procedures for primary care providers.* Philadelphia: Lippincott Williams & Wilkins.

Pfenninger, J. L. & Fowler, G. C. (1994). *Procedures for primary care physicians.* St. Louis: Mosby.

Plastic Surgery Educational Foundation. (1987). *Plastic and reconstructive surgery: Essentials for students* (3rd ed.). Chicago: Author.

Plastic Surgery Educational Foundation. (1991). *Everyday wounds: A guide for the primary care physician.* Chicago.

Rivellini, D. (1993). Local and regional anesthesia. Nursing Implications, *Nursing Clinic of North America 28*(3), 547.

Simon R. & B. Brenner. (1994). *Emergency procedures and techniques.* Baltimore: Williams & Wilkins.

Trott, A. T.(1997). *Wounds and lacerations: Emergency care and closure* (2nd ed.). St. Louis, Mosby.

chapter
13

Subungual Hematoma

CPT Coding:

11740 Evacuation of subungual hematoma ($62–$75)

 DEFINITION

A subungual hematoma is a collection of blood between the nail and the nail bed of a finger or toe. The hematoma results from trauma to the digit. The blood is under pressure and usually causes throbbing pain.

 INDICATIONS

Patient complains of pain under nail that is usually throbbing and continuous.

 ALERT: There is controversy as to whether a subungual hematoma release should be performed when there is a fracture present. The current recommendation is that the benefit of pain relief outweighs the small chance of infection.

 PATIENT EDUCATION

- Tell the patient that there may be a slight sting at the moment the paper clip or cautery unit penetrates the nail.
- Reassure the patient that the discomfort should be momentary.
- After the procedure, watch for signs of infection such as increased swelling, pain, erythema, purulent drainage, or red streaks extending from the finger to the hand, and unusual warmth of finger or hand.
- Inform the patient that because the nail has separated from the bed, the nail may be lost as a new one grows back up under the traumatized nail. If the nail matrix was damaged, the new nail may be irregular or distorted.

 ASSESSMENT

1. History of trauma with swelling and throbbing pain in tip of the finger or toe. Dark blue-black discoloration from the base of the nail. It is not usually necessary to release a hematoma if it covers less than a third of the nail bed.
2. Perform an x-ray study, if necessary, for possible tuft fracture.

3. If any open wound occurred with the trauma, check the patient's tetanus status. If it has been more than 10 years since the patient's last booster, give tetanus-diptheria (T-d) 0.5 mL IM.

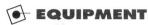 EQUIPMENT

- Soap, water, and gauze pads
- Towel
- Goggles and gloves
- Straightened paper clip and lighter or disposable cautery unit
- Adhesive bandages

PROCEDURE	SPECIAL CONSIDERATIONS
1. Gently wash nail and allow to dry.	
2. Rest the digit on towel on firm surface. Place gauze pads beside the digit.	
3. Don goggles and gloves.	Use goggles and gloves in accordance with blood and body fluids precautions.
4. Hold tip of paper clip in flame of lighter until it is glowing red. If using a cautery unit, remove cap.	If disposable cautery unit is used, there may be an additional charge to the patient ($10–$15).

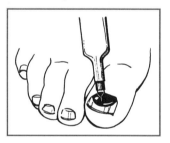

5. Stabilize the digit at joint.	Inform patient that there may be a momentary sting when the paper clip penetrates the nail but that the pooled blood under the nail will prevent the occurrence of a burn.
6. Apply the glowing tip of paper clip or apply cautery unit to the center of the hematoma with just enough pressure to penetrate the nail.	A sizzle and spurt of blood will occur when the nail is penetrated. Pain relief is usually obtained quickly after procedure as pressure decreases.

(procedure continued)

PROCEDURE	SPECIAL CONSIDERATIONS

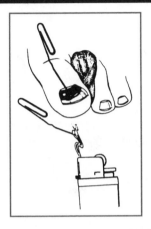

7. Absorb blood with gauze pad as it drains through hole in nail.

8. Apply an adhesive bandage.

Slight pressure to the nail or palmar surface of digit will help express additional blood.

Advise patient that warm soapy soaks may promote further drainage. DO NOT apply antibiotic ointment, which could prevent drainage.

 FOLLOW-UP

• Instruct the patient to contact his or her health care provider if any sign of infection develops.

BIBLIOGRAPHY

American Medical Association. (1998). *Physicians' current procedural terminology: CPT.* Chicago: American Medical Association.

Healthcare Consultants of America. (1998). *1998 Physicians' fee and coding guide.* Atlanta, GA.

Lowe, S. & Saxe, J. M. (1999). *Microscopic procedures for primary care providers.* Philadelphia: Lippincott Williams & Wilkins.

Simon, R. & Brenner, B. (1994). *Emergency procedures and techniques* (3rd ed). Baltimore: Williams & Wilkins.

chapter 14
Lacerations

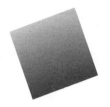

CPT Coding:
Based on three factors: type of closure, site of the repair, and length of the wound (measured in centimeters), summed if more than one wound is closed.

12001 Simple repair of superficial wounds of scalp, neck, axillae, external genitalia, trunk, and/or extremities, 2.5 cm or less ($115–$140)

12002 2.6 to 7.5 cm ($142–$175)

12004 0.76 to 12.5 cm ($183–$226)

12005 12.6 to 20.0 cm ($267–$321)

12006 20.1 to 30.0 cm ($324–$390)

12007 >30.0 cm N/A

12011 Simple repair of face, ears, eyelid, nose, lips, and/or mucous membranes, 2.5 cm or less ($151–$181)

12013 2.6 to 5.0 cm ($189–$226)

12014 5.1 to 7.5 cm ($232–$280)

12015 7.6 to 12.5 cm ($341–$407)

12016 12.6 to 20.0 cm ($432–$517)

12017 20.1 to 30.0 cm ($590–$710)

12031 Layer closure of wounds of scalp, axillae, trunk, and/or extremities 2.5 cm or less ($163–$193)

12032 2.6 to 7.5 cm ($234–$284)

12034 7.6 to 12.5 cm ($302–$365)

12051 Layer closure of face, ears, eyelids, nose, lips, and/or mucous membranes, <2.5 cm ($208–$244)

12052 2.6 to 5.0 cm ($294–$353)

Consult CPT manual for additional codes

◉ DEFINITIONS

- A laceration is a wound produced by the tearing of body tissue.
- A suture is thread used to sew the body tissues together.
- A simple repair involves a superficial wound (primarily the epidermis or dermis or subcutaneous tissues without significant involvement of deeper structures). It requires a simple one-layer closure (American Medical Association [AMA], 1999).
- An intermediate repair, in addition to a simple repair, requires layered closure of one or more layers of the deeper layers of subcutaneous tissue and superficial (nonmuscle) fascia. Single-layer closure of heavily contaminated

wounds that have required extensive cleaning or removal of particulate matter also constitutes intermediate repair (AMA, 1999).

 INDICATIONS

• Suturing simple lacerations stops bleeding, prevents infection, preserves function, and restores appearance.
• It is optimal to close a wound within 4 to 8 hours; however, the health care provider may delay up to 24 hours.

 PATIENT EDUCATION

• Discuss wound and suture care (see postoperative instructions in the discussion of follow-up).
• Teach signs and symptoms of infection, that is, redness, increased pain, swelling, fever, and bleeding.
• Instruct the patient to elevate the injured extremity above the level of the heart.
• Teach the patient daily wound care according to suture care protocol.
• Remove sutures within recommended time frame to decrease scarring from suture.
• Review postoperative massage and use of sunscreen protection according to suture care protocol.
• Let the patient know that a foreign body may not be located, so subsequent referral and removal may be needed.

ASSESSMENT

1. Obtain the patient's history to determine the mechanism of injury, time of occurrence, location of injury, associated injuries, and tetanus immunization status.
2. Administer tetanus based on the following schedule:

History of Adsorbed Tetanus Toxoid (doses)	Clean Minor Wounds Td*	Clean Minor Wounds TIG (250 U)	All Other Wounds[†] Td	All Other Wounds[†] TIG (250 U)
Unknown or <3	Yes	No	Yes	Yes
≥3[‡]	No[§]	No	No[‖]	No

*For children <7 years of age, DTP is preferred to tetanus toxoid; for persons ≥7 years of age, Td is preferred to tetanus toxoid

[†] Such as, but not limited to, wounds contaminated with dirt, feces, soil and saliva; and puncture wounds, avulsions, and wounds resulting from missiles, crushing, burns, and frostbite

[‡] If only three doses of fluid toxoid has been received, then a fourth dose of toxoid, preferably an adsorbed toxoid, should be given

[§] Yes, if >10 years since last dose

[‖] Yes, if >5 years since last dose

(MMWR, 40 [RR-10]; 1-50. 1991).

ALERT: *Do not give diphtheria, pertussis, and tetanus (DPT) vaccine to children older than 7 years of age.*

3. Obtain medical history including preexisting medical conditions and allergies.

DEVELOPMENTAL CONSIDERATIONS

Child: In children, lacerations are a traumatic event for both the child and the parent. Take the extra time needed to explain what is going to happen to the child. In children younger than 2 years of age, it may not be possible to explain so that the child understands, given the trauma of the event. Children need to hold still or be restrained to facilitate the best closure possible.
Elderly: Elderly patients have dry skin. The epidermis begins to thin and flatten, and the dermis is less elastic with less elastin and collagen fibers than in younger adults. Healing may be decreased in the elderly due to poorer circulation.

PRINCIPLES OF WOUND CLOSURE

• Layer matching: Match each layer of the wound edge to its counterpart, that is, superficial fascia to superficial fascia, dermis to dermis, and epidermis to epidermis.

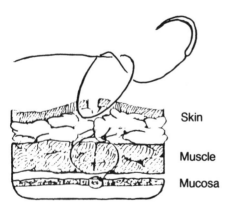

Skin

Muscle

Mucosa

Layer by layer closure. (Simon, R. & Brenner, B. [1994]. *Emergency procedures and techniques*, [3rd ed]. Baltimore: Williams & Wilkins.)

• Closure of dead space: This procedure is necessary to avoid accumulation of blood or serum, which can act as a natural culture medium for organisms and which, in turn, can lead to infection.

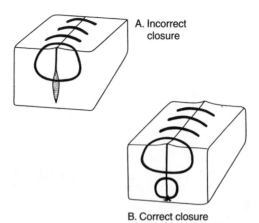

A. Incorrect
closure

B. Correct closure

Closure of the dead space with buried sutures. The least number of sutures necessary to close a subcutaneous space should be used. (Simon, R. & Brenner, B. [1994]. *Emergency procedures and techniques*, (3rd ed). Baltimore: Williams & Wilkins.)

• Proper knot-tying technique: The common knot is the surgeon's knot, in which the double first throw offers better knot security. There is less slippage of suture material as the wound is pulled together.
• Wound edge eversion: Slightly raised wound edge above the plane of normal skin is needed because the wound edge will flatten with healing.

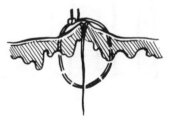

Proper wound edge eversion. Wound edge unversion leads to pitting or depression of the scar.

EQUIPMENT

• Laceration tray equipped with sterile field, sterile drapes, and sterile 4 × 4 gauzes
• Sterile instruments to include
  – Scalpel handle
  – Needle holder
  – Adson forceps with or without teeth

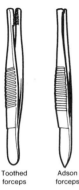

Toothed   Adson   Toothed forceps and Adson forceps. (Simon, R. & Brenner, B. [1994]. *Emergency procedures and*
forceps   forceps   *techniques,* (3rd ed). Baltimore: Williams & Wilkins.)

– Tenotomy scissors
– Small straight sharp scissors
– Skin hooks
– Mosquito hemostat
– Anesthesia material: Refer to Chapter 12: Local Anesthesia
– Prep solution
– Sterile normal saline
– Sterile gloves
– #15 scalpel blade

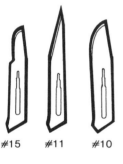

Various blades. A #15 blade is used for fine precision work, a #10 for larger incisions,
and #11 for stab incision. (Simon, R. & Brenner, B. [1994]. *Emergency procedures*
#15   #11   #10   *and techniques,* (3rd ed). Baltimore: Wlliams & Wilkins.)

– Suture material
– Postoperative dressing material: Steri-Strips

SUTURE MATERIAL

• Suture material can be divided into two large categories: absorbable and
  nonabsorbable.
• Absorbable suture is used for layer closure of deep lacerations. It is eventually metabolized by the body in approximately 60 days. Vicryl is an example
  of absorbable suture.
• Nonabsorbable sutures are required for superficial lacerations. There are

two basic kinds of nonabsorbable sutures—braided and monofilament. Braided sutures tie more easily, whereas monofilament sutures are less inflammatory. Silk is an example of braided suture material. Nylon (Ethilon) is the most common monofilament.

• Suture size is indicated by the number of 0s (for example, 00 [2-0]). The more 0s, the smaller the size of the suture and the weaker the suture. It is best to use the smallest size suture as possible, that is, 5-0 and 6-0.

Body Area	Recommended Suture Size: Skin	Recommended Suture Size: Subcutaneous
Face	5-0 or 6-0	4-0 or 5-0
Extremities	4-0 or 5-0	3-0 or 4-0
Scalp	4-0	

From Simon, R. & Brenner, B. (1994). Emergency procedures and techniques. (3rd ed., p. 293). Baltimore, Williams & Wilkins.

Suture	Tensile Strength	Wick Action	Infection	Reactivity	Uses
Absorbable					
Chromic gut (natural)	##	#	##	###	Oral mucosa
Polyglycolic acid (PGA) (dexon) Vicryl (braided)	#	##	#	##	For subcutaneous closure, fascia (not for prolonged hold)
Polyglyconate (Maxon) (Monofilament)	####	N/A	N/A	#	Subcutaneous closure less reactive and stronger than PGA and polyglactin
Nonabsorbable					
Nylon (monofilament)	###	0	0–#	#	Strong, poor knot-holding ability, requires six knots, used in skin closure
Polypropylene (Prolene) monofilament	###	#	0–#	#	Strong, easier to tie and holds knot better than nylon, requires only three knots, used for skin

table continued

table continued

Suture	Tensile Strength	Wick Action	Infection	Reactivity	Uses
Silk (braided)	###	####	####	####	Knots well, easy to sew, more tissue reaction, increased potential for infection, not usually used in skin unless removed in 2 to 3 days
Dacron (Mersilene)	###	##	#	##	Easy to tie, knots well, like silk but only 2% with inflammation at site, used for skin.
Polybutester (Novafil) (monofilament)	####	Unknown		#	Handles well, expands and contracts with changes in tissue edema

From Trott, A. (1997). Wounds and lacerations: Emergency care and closure, (2nd ed., p. 113). St Louis: Mosby.

→ ####: weakest to strongest

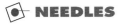 **NEEDLES**

- There are two types of needles: cutting and tapered. Cutting needles are used when one is penetrating through tough tissue such as skin or fascia. A tapered needle is used in vascular work and fine mucosal closures. An ordinary cutting needle is used for the skin and dermis. Usually a 3/8 s curvature is adequate. FS means "for skin," whereas "cutting" is usually used on thicker skin. "P" denotes plastic needles, which are commonly used on the face. The larger the number, the smaller the needle size within a series (for example, FS-1 is larger than FS-3).

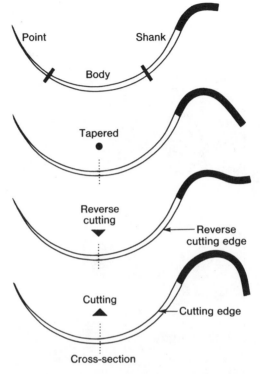

Needles used in suturing. (Simon, R. & Brenner, B. [1994]. *Emergency procedures and techniques,* (3rd ed). Baltimore: Williams & Wilkins.)

 ## WOUND CLOSURE AND TYING TECHNIQUES: ADVANTAGES AND DISADVANTAGES

Closure/Tying Technique	Advantages	Disadvantages
Simple interrupted	Permits good eversion of the wound edges. Is commonly used and can be applied rapidly.	Proper technique to provide eversion of edges requires practice to master. Eversion is not as good in difficult wounds as with other techniques. Does not relieve extrinsic tension from the wound edges.

table continued

table continued

Closure/Tying Technique	Advantages	Disadvantages

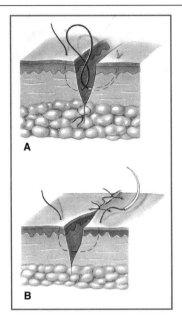

| Continuous over-and-over | Can be applied rapidly to close multiple lacerations and large wounds. | Apposition of the wound edges and eversion is more difficult. Inclusion cysts may form. |

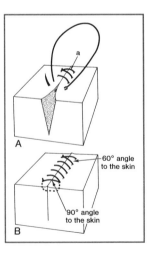

table continued

Closure/Tying Technique	Advantages	Disadvantages
Continuous single-lock stitch	Can be applied rapidly. Apposition of the wound edges is more complete than with continuous over-and-over stitch. Less epitheliazation of the tracts.	Apposition of the wound edges is not as perfect as with the simple interrupted unless the procedure is mastered well.

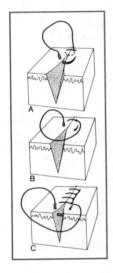

Vertical mattress stitch	Unsurpassed in its ability to provide eversion of the wound edges and perfect apposition. Relieves tension from the skin edges.	Takes time to apply. Produces more cross marks.

table continued

Closure/Tying Technique	Advantages	Disadvantages

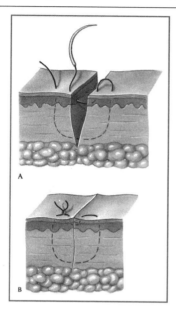

Closure/Tying Technique	Advantages	Disadvantages
Horizontal mattress switch	Reinforces the subcutaneous tissue. Relieves extrinsic tension from the wound edges more effectively than does the vertical mattress.	Does not provide as good apposition of the wound edges as the vertical mattress.

table continued

Closure/Tying Technique	Advantages	Disadvantages

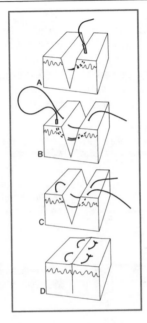

Continuous mattress | Can be rapidly placed to approximate large lacerations in cosmetically unimportant areas. | Does not provide good apposition of the wound edges or eversion.

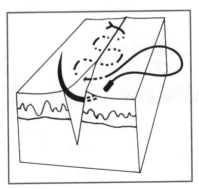

table continued

Closure/Tying Technique	Advantages	Disadvantages
Staples	Provide for good approximation of wound edges. They do not come in contact with skin surface and do not leave suture marks when removed. Easier to place than sutures. Can be rapidly placed to close wound. Best used on back, arms, thighs, or head in wounds that are linear and clean.	Have a damaging effect on local tissue defenses. Stapled wounds are more susceptible to infection than taped wounds. More expensive to use. Does not permit eversion of the wound edges. Patients may have aversion to sight of staples in the wound.
Skin tape (Steri-Strips)	Does not require local anesthesia to apply. Useful on superficial wounds and when patient is frightened of needle. Steri-Strips can be applied quickly.	Can only be used when wound in not widely separated. Does not work well in some areas: axilla, palms, soles. Should not be used when there is much moisture, oil, or over flexor surfaces of joints. Does not provide for eversion of wound edges. Children might remove the tape before healing of the wound. Cannot be used in wounds that are under significant tension when closed.

Adapted from Simon R., & Brenner, B. (1994). Emergency procedures and techniques (3rd ed., p. 327). Baltimore: Williams & Wilkins.

SUTURING PROCEDURE

PROCEDURE	SPECIAL CONSIDERATIONS
Anesthetize wound using direct local infiltration.	Topical anesthesia is an option in children (TAC: tetracaine, adrenalin, and cocaine) for minor lacerations. It cannot be used for lacerations of the pinna of the ear, digits, or penis due to compromise of vascular integrity. Mucous membranes accelerate the absorption, so TAC cannot be used in lacerations of the mouth, eyes, etc. The TAC is applied with a saturated sterile 2×2 gauze pad applied with firm pressure for a minimum of 10 minutes.

(procedure continued)

PROCEDURE	SPECIAL CONSIDERATIONS

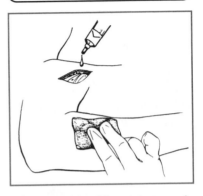

Examine wound for foreign bodies, deep tissue layer damage, nerve, tendon, or blood vessel involvement.

Wound prep: Mechanically cleanse the wound with saline using 4 × 4 sponges. Prep with anesthetic in a circular motion, beginning at center of wound and moving away to periphery without crossing back over the actual wound area. Cleanse until skin is visibly free from contamination.

Irrigate with sterile saline using a 35-mm syringe with a large-bore cannula (16–18 gauge). Prep wound until clean to the eye.

Ground-in particles of dirt must be removed. If they are left in place, they will be embedded in the wound, leaving a tattoo.

Iodophors are the best agents for cleansing with little tissue toxicity or damage. Alcohol cleans the skin but is not an effective antiseptic. Hydrogen peroxide is a weak disinfectant but is toxic to tissues in open wounds. Hibiclens is a solution that is not toxic to tissue; it may be the agent of choice by some providers. *Animal bites:* Controversy exists as to whether or not to close wound. Clean and débride area. Irrigate thoroughly. Close with either Steri-Strips or loose sutures. *Human bites:* Head or face: cleansed, débrided, irrigated, and closed loosely. Place on antibiotics. Other locations: dependent on location and depth of wound.

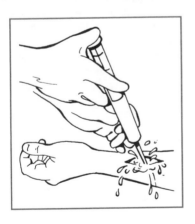

Hair removal should be performed only when the hair will interfere with wound closure. Cutting the hair with scissors is recommended

Never shave the eyebrows.

(procedure continued)

PROCEDURE	SPECIAL CONSIDERATIONS
Débridement may be needed when preparing a traumatic wound for closure because it removes bacteria and devitalizes tissue.	Facial wounds require little débridement due to high vascularity. Lower extremities may need débridement due to less blood flow. When a wound is in nondemonstrative area and is parallel to wrinkle lines, an elliptical excision is preferred (see Chapter 8: Skin Lesion Removal).
Foreign bodies in wound: removal is dependent on mechanism of injury, type of foreign body, physical exam findings, and ability to locate the foreign body.	Wood and other vegetative material need to be removed immediately because of likelihood of infection. Other materials, such as innocuous metal foreign bodies are sometimes left embedded in soft tissue. Do not spend more than 1 hour trying to remove a foreign body with local anesthetic.
	Plain x-ray films may be helpful to see the location of the foreign body. Almost all glass in soft tissues can be detected by x-ray. Vegetative material: thorns, wood splinter, or cactus spines are not usually visualized. Ask the x-ray technician to use an underpenetrated technique to increase the likelihood of finding the foreign body on x-rays.
Apply sterile drapes.	Use of fenestrated drape may be helpful to create a sterile field upon which to work.
Close the wound. The simple interrupted everting stitch is the most commonly used stitch for closure. Angle the needle away from the wound edge slightly when first piercing the skin. Introduce the suture needle at a 90-degree angle to the epidermis. Come out of the wound for the second grasping. Pierce each side of the wound at the same depth with each stitch so that the wound edges meet exactly.	This is sometimes called the wide-based "u" or "pear" stitch. The purpose of the "pear" stitch is to produce eversion of the wound edges, placing dermis against dermis. Natural contraction of the wound will eventually produce a flat wound.
	Use the least number of sutures needed to bring the skin edges together without causing increased skin tension at the wound edges.

(procedure continued)

| PROCEDURE | SPECIAL CONSIDERATIONS |

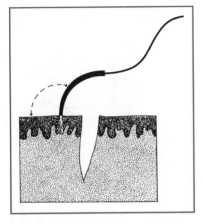

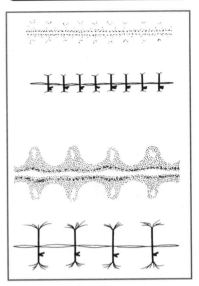

Débridement or cutting may be needed to make sure the edges are well approximated.

Whenever possible the skin should be incised parallel, never perpendicular, to the normal tension lines and relaxed skin tension lines to produce the most inconspicuous scars

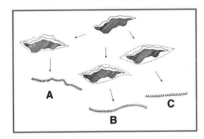

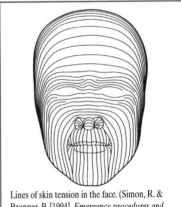

Lines of skin tension in the face. (Simon, R. & Brenner, B. [1994]. *Emergency procedures and techniques,* [3rd ed]. Baltimore: Williams & Wilkins.)

(procedure continued)

PROCEDURE

SPECIAL CONSIDERATIONS

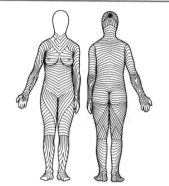

Skin tension lines. In the male, the semicircular lines over the deltoid region extend down over the breasts, producing curved radial lines as opposed to the horizontal lines demonstrated above in the female. (Simon, R. & Brenner, B. [1994]. *Emergency procedures and techniques,* [3rd ed]. Baltimore: Williams & Wilkins.)

(procedure continued) ───

| PROCEDURE | SPECIAL CONSIDERATIONS |

Tie the knot with the instrument tie.

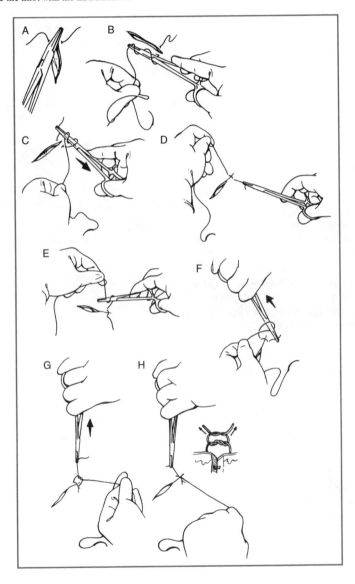

(procedure continued) ——

PROCEDURE

SPECIAL CONSIDERATIONS

Test the tension of the knot by tugging on the suture and pulling the knot across the wound.

Methods to reduce blood flow into the wound may be helpful to increase visualization of the wound. Blood pressure cuffs pumped up to systolic B/P can help control bleeding. In digit, use a Penrose drain to help decrease the bleeding.

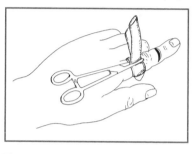

Layer closure may be required for deep wounds or wound under tension. The "buried stitch" is used for this procedure, using absorbable suture. This is a subcutaneous suture with an inverted knot. Begin at the bottom of the wound, come up through the lower dermis, go across the incision, down through the dermis to the base again, and tie.

The purpose of layer closure is to seal potential dead space and take the tension off the skin surface, thus avoiding suture marks.

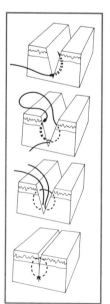

(procedure continued)

PROCEDURE	SPECIAL CONSIDERATIONS
Wash suture line with sterile normal saline. Apply adhesive Steri-Strips as a reinforcement to sutures.	
Applying Steri-Strips: make sure skin has been cleansed with alcohol or acetone. Tincture of benzoin applied only to where the Steri-Strip is to be attached to the skin assists in improving adhesion between the skin and strip.	Cleansing with alcohol or acetone removes skin oils and improves the contact of the tape with the skin. Cleanse even after using idophor. Steri-Strips are useful when the edges of the wound are cleanly incised and come together naturally without tension.
Provide patient with patient education handout and appropriate follow-up appointment.	

Illustration 9 from Simon, R. & Brenner, B. (1994). Emergency procedures and techniques, (3rd ed). Baltimore: Williams & Wilkins.

ALTERNATIVE PROCEDURE

• Dermabond (2-octylcyanoacrylate) is a new method to close skin wounds that does not require anesthesia or sutures. This method was recently approved by the Food and Drug Administration (FDA). With this method, closure and cosmetic appearance seem to be equal to those of the traditional method of wound closure. The approximate cost is $25 for a very small tube, and on-site instruction is required by the manufacturer before implementation of the technique.

FOLLOW-UP

SUTURE CARE
PLEASE FOLLOW ONLY THOSE INSTRUCTIONS THAT ARE MARKED

_____ Keep Steri-Strips dry for 48 hours, then you may shower, pat dry or blow dry with cool hair dryer. Change Steri-Strips if they fall off.

_____ If clear plastic dressing is used, you may shower over plastic.
 _____ Remove plastic in 2 days, leave it off, shower as normal.
 _____ Leave plastic on until next office visit.

_____ If your sutures have been left open to the air, clean as follows:
 ——— Wash the surface line gently with warm water twice a day starting 24 to 48 hours from the time of injury.
 _____ Then apply Polysporin ointment to the suture line. DO NOT allow excess ointment to build up on wound.
 ——— Leave sutures open to air; do not apply ointment.

_____ If the wound is on the hand, arm, or leg, keep the extremity elevated as much as possible.

_____ If you have been placed on antibiotics, take them untill they are completely gone.

_____ Make appointment to have your sutures checked in _____ days.

_____ Call *IMMEDIATELY* if you notice any of the following:
1. Bleeding within 12 hours after surgery, such as the dressing becomes soaked with blood and continues to bleed.
2. Increased redness and heat around the wound.
3. Temperature higher than 101°F.
4. Increased pain, swelling, foul odor, or drainage from the wound after 48 hours.
5. Rash or blistering.

_____ After 2 weeks, when healed, wear sun protection (#15 or #30 sunscreen or higher) whenever out in the sun for 1 year.

POTENTIAL COMPLICATIONS

- Bleeding and hematoma formation
- Infection
- Skin necrosis
- Wound dehiscence
- Hypertrophic scarring
- Keloid formation

WHEN TO REFER

- The patient asks for a plastic surgeon.
- There is a high likelihood of a complication or an unfavorable result.
- The patient's wound involves more than one type of tissue, that is, tendon/nerve damage, facial wounds, infected wound.

Suture Location	Recommended Suture Removal
Scalp	6 to 8 days
Face or ear	4 to 5 days
Chest/abdomen/hand	8 to 10 days
Arm or leg	7 to 10 days (additional 2–3 days are needed over extensor joints)
Fingertip	10 to 12 days
Back or foot	12 to 14 days

SUTURE REMOVAL

CPT Coding:
Suture removal is considered a part of the suture insertion process and is not billed separately.

Definition
• Suture removal is removal of nonabsorbable sutures from a wound. The optimal time for suture removal depends on a number of various factors. Such factors include location of the wound, the rate of wound healing, and the amount of tension on the wound.

Indications
• Removal of sutures before scarring from the sutures develops.
• Removal of sutures before an infection develops.

 ALERT: Removing sutures too early may result in wound dehiscence and widening of the scar.

Patient Education
• Reassure the patient that removal of sutures is important to prevent an infection and additional scarring by the sutures.
• Reassure the patient that removal of sutures should not be painful.
• Inform the patient that after removal of sutures, the scar may increase in width over the next 3 to 5 weeks. The use of skin tape to support the wound can help minimize the increase in scar size as well as reopening of the wound.
• Emphasize to the patient that exposure to sunlight will cause the scar to redden more than the surrounding skin. Emphasize the use of a sunscreen containing para-amino benzoic acid (PABA) if prolonged exposure is expected.
• Emphasize to the patient that care of the wound after suture removal is necessary to prevent further complications. The patient should be instructed to keep the injury site clean and protected so the wound does not reopen.

ASSESSMENT

1. Obtain a history related to wound, such as the location and when sutures were inserted.
2. Assess for any signs of infection (redness, swelling, discharge).
3. Determine the patient's ability to hold still during the procedure. The use of a papoose board may be necessary to ensure that a child will remain still during the procedure.

Developmental Considerations

Child: Additional time may be needed to reassure and explain the procedure adequately. Distraction during the procedure is helpful.

Equipment

- Povidone-iodine (Betadine) or Betadine swabs
- Gauze
- Warm water
- Scissors or a #11 scalpel blade
- Clamps or forceps
- Skin tape or Steri-Strips

PROCEDURES	SPECIAL CONSIDERATIONS
Remove any crusts on the wound surface or surrounding the sutures with warm water and gauze.	
Cleanse area with povidone-iodine (Betadine) and gauze or with betadine swabs.	Hibiclens can also be used to cleanse the area.
Grasp suture above the knot with hemostat, pulling it taut, and cutting the suture between the knot and skin close to the skin surface with scissors (standard or iris) or a #11 scalpel blade.	This technique prevents passage of the contaminated outer portion of the suture back through the skin. Make sure that there is a tail left to grasp to pull the suture out of the skin. Do not leave any portion of the suture in the skin. A #11 scalpel blade should be used for removal of fine sutures.

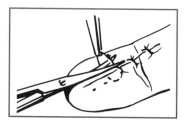

After cutting the suture, pull it gently through the suture tract.	Removal of every other suture helps determine whether or not the wound has tensile strength to prevent reopening. If the wound is gapping, then sutures may need to remain in place for an additional 1 to 3 days. If the wound separates it usually occurs on the 3rd to 5th days after insertion and is most likely due to infection.
After sutures are removed, determine whether or not wound needs further cleaning or use of skin tape (Steri-Strips).	The use of skin tape may be beneficial if extra support is needed; for example, if the wound is over a joint.

Alternative Procedure

• Staples may be used as a means for skin closure. A special removal instrument is needed to remove the staples. If the staples are placed in the emergency room, most patients are given a kit for staple removal. The feet of the instrument are placed under the central portion of the staple. The hand grip is then squeezed, which lifts the portion of the staple out of the skin for easy removal.

Follow-up

• Encourage the patient to keep the wound clean to prevent infection.
• Encourage the patient to protect the wound so it does not reopen.
• Encourage the patient to return to the office if complications occur.

BIBLIOGRAPHY

American Medical Association (AMA). (1998). *Physicians current procedural terminology : CPT.* Chicago: AMA.

Barrett, B. M. (1982). *Manual of patient care in plastic surgery.* Boston: Little, Brown and Co.

Barron, J. N. & Saad, M. N. (Eds.). (1980). *Operative plastic and reconstructive surgery* (Vol. 2). Edinburgh: Churchill Livingstone.

Boriskin, M. I. (1994). Primary care management of wounds. *Nurse Practitioner, 19*(11), 38.

Edmunds, M. W. & Mayhew, M. S. (1996). *Procedures for primary care practitioners.* St. Louis: Mosby.

Healthcare Consultants of America. (1998). *1998 Physicians' fee and coding guide.* Augusta, GA.

Hollander, J., Singer, A., & Valentine, S. (1998). Comparison of wound care practices in pediatric and adult lacerations repaired in the emergency department. *Pediatric Emergency Care, 14*(1), 15–18.

Hughes, N. (1991). Basic techniques of excision and wound closure. In T. Barclay & D. Kernahan (Eds.), *Rob and Smith's operative surgery: Plastic surgery* (4th ed.). Boston: Butterworths.

Liebelt, E. L. (1997). Current concepts in laceration repair. *Current Opinion in Pediatrics, 9*(5) 459–564.

Lohr, J. (1991). *Pediatric outpatient procedures.* Philadelphia: J. B. Lippincott.

Lowe, S. & Saxe, J. M. (1999). *Microscopic procedures for primary care providers.* Philadelphia: Lippincott Williams & Wilkins.

Pfenninger, J. L. & Fowler, G. C. (1994). *Procedures for primary care physicians.* St. Louis: Mosby.

Plastic Surgery Educational Foundation. (1987). *Plastic and reconstructive surgery: Essentials for students* (3rd ed.). Chicago: Author.

Plastic Surgery Educational Foundation. (1991). *Everyday wounds: A guide for the primary care physician.* Chicago.

Rivellini, D. (1993). Local and regional anesthesia. *Nursing Implications. Nursing Clinics of North America 28*(3), 547.

Roberts, J. R. & Hedges, J. R. (1992). *Clinical procedures in emergency medicine* (3rd ed.). Philadelphia: W. B. Saunders.

Sabiston, D. C. (1997). *Textbook of surgery: The biological basis of modern surgical repair* (50th ed.). Philadelphia: W. B. Saunders.

Shafi, S. & Gilbert, J. (1998). Minor pediatric injuries. *Pediatric Clinics of North America, 45*(4), 831–851.

Simon, R. & Brenner, B. (1994). *Emergency procedures and techniques* (3rd ed.). Baltimore: Williams & Wilkins.

Singer, A. J., Hollander, J. E., Valentine, S. M., Turque, T. W., McCuskey, C. F., & Quinn,

J. V. (1998). Prospective, randomized, controlled trial of tissue adhesive (2-octyl-cyanoacrylate) vs standard wound closure techniques for laceration repair. Stony Brook Octylcyanoacrylate Study Group. *Academy of Emergency Medicine, 5*(2), 94–99 .

Trott, A. T. (1997). *Wounds and Lacerations: Emergency care and closure* (ed 2.). St. Louis: Mosby.

Usgaocar, R. (1998). Lessening the pain of suture removal. *Plastic Reconstructive Surgery, 102*(1), 268.

chapter
15
Tick Removal

CPT Coding:

10120 Removal of subcutaneous foreign body, simple ($94–$111)
10121 Incisional removal, foreign body, complex ($278–$332)

DEFINITION

A tick is any of various arachnids of the super family *Ixodidae*, related to mites but larger. An adult tick has an oval, nonsegmented body with a movable head through which it draws blood from humans or other animals after burrowing under the skin.

INDICATIONS

Tick removal is required any time a tick is embedded to decrease the likelihood of transmission of tick-borne pathogens.

PATIENT EDUCATION

• Reassure the patient that the removal of the tick is important to reduce the likelihood of transmission of tick-borne pathogens.
• Many patients have great anxiety over subsequent tick-borne diseases following removal of the tick. These include Lyme disease, Rocky Mountain spotted fever, tularemia, and ascending paralysis (also known as tick paralysis). Theoretically, a tick infected with Lyme disease must remain attached for 24 hours to transmit the disease, and even then, only 10% to 20% of bites from infected ticks will result in transmission (Su, 1997).
• Use of oil to smother or a hot match to get the tick to release itself is not recommended. Using these techniques causes the tick to regurgitate into the site and may promote disease transmission.

ASSESSMENT

1. Obtain a thorough history ascertaining probable exposure time, such as recent walk in wooded or grassy areas, contact with pets or livestock, gardening, and so on.
2. Assess the area surrounding the tick for erythema, edema, or discharge.
3. Assess the tick itself to determine how far the parasite has burrowed into the skin (ie, mandibles only, entire head segment).

4. Determine patient's ability to cooperate and hold still during the removal procedure.

 DEVELOPMENTAL CONSIDERATIONS

Infant & Child: It is very important to have the infant or child hold still during the removal procedure. Use of a papoose board may be indicated to prevent injury of the infant or child during the procedure (see Chapter 50: Child Restraints). Encourage parents to talk to their child in a calm manner throughout the procedure to minimize the anxiety of both the parent and the child.

◉ **EQUIPMENT**

• Hemostats or tweezers
• Gloves
• Povidone-iodine
• Punch biopsy instrument

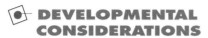

PROCEDURE	SPECIAL CONSIDERATIONS
Wash hands thoroughly. Put on gloves.	
Expose area surrounding tick. One may use saline or petroleum jelly to flatten hair and keep it out of the working area. Clean the surrounding area with povidone-iodine solution.	
Using hemostats or tweezers, grasp the tick as close to the skin as possible and apply steady even traction upward and perpendicular to the skin.	Twisting the tick in a counterclockwise direction may facilitate removal because ticks screw themselves into the skin in a clockwise direction.

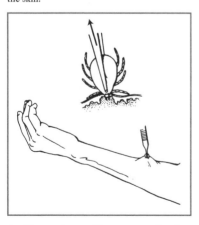

Avoid squeezing, crushing, or puncturing the tick during removal.

Tick fluids may contain infectious agents.

(procedure continued)

PROCEDURE	SPECIAL CONSIDERATIONS

If mouth parts are left behind after removal of the body, excision under local anesthetic is needed to prevent local infection.

If there are retained tick pieces remaining, use lidocaine to infiltrate the area around the bite.

Locate the punch biopsy instrument so that tick is within the punch biopsy radius.

Stretch the skin on either side of the instrument.

Push the instrument downward using moderate pressure through the epidermis and dermis; a decrease in resistance will be felt at this time.

Apply pressure to contain bleeding or close with suture. Apply bandage.

Submit the tissue for histologic study.

FOLLOW-UP

- Discuss signs and symptoms of tick-borne diseases with patient. Prophylactic antibiotic therapy is seldom used (Rudnitsky & Barnett, 1998).
- Follow-up is indicated if symptoms of a tick-borne illness or infection develop.
- Encourage frequent checking for ticks following outdoor activities or close contact with pets. Use of protective measures when outside in tick environs.
- Wear long pants tucked into socks and a long-sleeved shirt tucked in at the waist.
- Wear light-colored clothes when in a tick environment so ticks are easily detected.
- Use an insect repellent (diethyltoluamide [DEET]) that is safe for all ages.
- Avoid tick-infested areas from May through August.

BIBLIOGRAPHY

American Medical Association. (1998). *Physicians' current procedural terminology: CPT.* Chicago: American Medical Association.

Lowe, S. & Saxe, J. M. (1999). *Microscopic procedures for primary care providers.* Philadelphia: Lippincott Williams & Wilkins.

Rudnitsky, G. & Barnett, R. (1998) Tick removal. In J. Roberts & J. Hedges (Eds.). *Clinical procedures in emergency medicine* (3rd ed., 631–632). Philadelphia: W. B. Saunders Co.

Su, E. (1997). Tick removal. In R. Dieckmann, D. Fiser, & S. Selbst (Eds.), *Illustrated textbook of pediatric emergency & critical care procedures* (720–722). St. Louis: Mosby–Year Book, Inc.

chapter 16
Toenail Removal Procedures

CPT Coding:

11730 Avulsion of nail plate, partial or complete ($101–$124)
11732 Avulsion, each additional plate ($55–$68)

DEFINITIONS

Partial nail removal is excision of either nail border (alleviates acute pressure).
Complete nail removal is excision of the complete nail.
Partial or complete matrixectomy is permanent removal of either border or the entire nail.

INDICATIONS

- Remove nail (partial or complete) if patient has recurrent nail border infections (more than 3 per year).
- Remove nail if it is loose (usually due to trauma).
- Remove nail if it is dystrophic (deformed) and causing chronic pain.

 ALERT: Although nail removals are often performed to decompress the area of infection, permanent nail removals (matrixectomies) should be avoided if the patient has an infection. The trauma inflicted to the toe could exacerbate an infection.

PATIENT EDUCATION

- Inform the patient of the necessity of the procedure to alleviate pressure to the nail border to facilitate healing.
- Inform patient of consequences if the procedure is not performed (recurrent infections, cellulitis, amputations, and so on).
- Always have the patient sign an informed consent form for matrixectomies (permanent surgical procedure) by patient or person with power of attorney. With children, have the child's legal guardian sign.
- Patient must be aware of postoperative care (soaks, antibiotics, dressing, and so on) and be willing to comply.

☉ ASSESSMENT

1. Obtain a complete medical history and history of condition initiating the nail procedure.
2. Determine whether the patient is capable of having the procedure performed in the office. Rarely, underlying medical conditions require hospitalization (for example, an elderly patient with diabetes, peripheral vascular disease, and cellulitis).
3. If an infection is present, one must gauge its level. Moderate to severe cellulitis may prevent a local anesthetic from being effective due to altered pH.
4. Preoperative complete blood count with differential should be performed on all patients undergoing a matrixectomy.
5. Diabetics should have fasting blood sugar levels checked.
6. Determine level of cooperation from patient.

 ALERT: Need to have knowledge of general anatomy of nail and vascularity of toes.

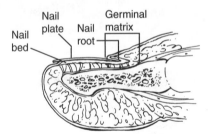

Normal nail anatomy.

☉ EQUIPMENT

- Sterile drapes
- 3- or 5-mL syringe with 25-gauge needle (1 or $1^{1}/_{2}$ inch); 1% or 2% lidocaine for local anesthesia
- Gauze, peroxide, normal saline for flushing
- Straight spatula or Freer elevator, English anvil nail splitter, hemostat (needle-nosed straight), or Kelly clamp
- Curette (small)
- Antibiotic cream or povidone-iodine (Betadine) with nonadherent bandage

PROCEDURE	**SPECIAL CONSIDERATIONS**

Digital Block

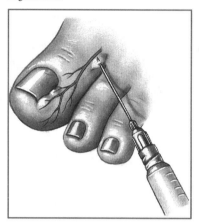

Use of epinephrine is not recommended owing to lasting effects of blood coagulability and stasis in digits.

One may or may not use rubber tubing around digit for tourniquet.

Test for anesthesia effects before performing procedure.

Prep digit with povidone-iodine (Betadine).

Goal is to be as clean as possible, even though nails are technically considered dirty.

PROCEDURE	**SPECIAL CONSIDERATIONS**

Partial nail avulsion (slant back):

No anesthesia usually is required.

1. Free corner with straight spatula.

2. Cut slanted portion of nail with English anvil.

Used to decompress an acute paronychia.

3. Remove with hemostat or Kelly clamp.

Use gauze to absorb any drainage.

(procedure continued)

PROCEDURE	**SPECIAL CONSIDERATIONS**

Partial nail avulsion (straight back):

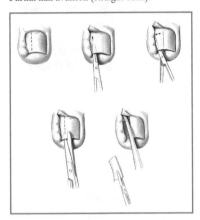

Same procedure as slant back, except cut (2–4 mm slice) from nail edge to matrix (not including matrix).

Patient may need local anesthesia unless nail has previously separated from nail bed.

Used to decompress more severe paronychia.

Use gauze to absorb any drainage.

PROCEDURE	**SPECIAL CONSIDERATIONS**

Complete nail avulsion (entire nail):

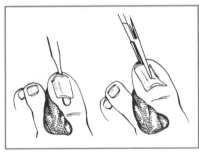

Free entire nail with straight spatula.

Cut nail in half with English anvil.

Remove entire nail with hemostat or Kelly clamp.

Local anesthesia is required unless nail has previously separated from nail bed. Procedure is indicated for severe infection at both borders, trauma to nail, or previously ineffective partial nail avulsions. Lidocaine is teratogenic and should not be used on a pregnant patient.

Use betadine bandage with nonadherent bandage, or antibiotic cream may be used 3–5 days with dressing.

PROCEDURE	SPECIAL CONSIDERATIONS
Matrixectomies (partial straight back of entire nail)	Partial indicated for more than three or four paronychias on one nail border. Complete matrixectomy is indicated for chronically deformed nail or chronic infections on both medial and lateral borders. Local digital block necessary; many patients prefer partial matrixectomies at both borders instead of removal of entire nail.

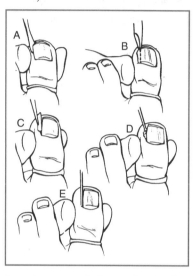

	Be careful not to get phenol on skin (it will mildly burn). Phenol is teratogenic.
Same steps are required as mentioned earlier except push through matrix with straight spatula.	Use betadine bandage with nonadherent bandage, or antibiotic cream may be used 3–5 days with dressing.
Cut and remove nail.	
Use curette to remove remaining matrix cells.	
Use phenol soaked cotton-tipped swabs for 30 seconds; roll at matrix area.	
Pour alcohol over matrix for 10 to 15 seconds	
Repeat phenol and alcohol.	

 FOLLOW-UP

- Patient will need antibiotics if infection is present or if he or she is diabetic.
- If bandages are used, they must be kept clean and dry, and they must be changed daily.
- Have patient return to the office in 3 to 5 days to monitor for infection and compliance.

BIBLIOGRAPHY

American Medical Association. (1998). *Physicians' current procedural terminology: CPT.* Chicago: American Medical Association.

Andrew, T. A. (1982). Ingrown toenails, an evaluation of two treatment. (Letter to the Editor.) *British Medical Journal, 284,* 118.

Dangle, J. C. (1981). The history, development and current status of nail matrix phenolisation. *Chiropodist, 36,* 315–324.

Frost, L. A. (1976). Surgical correction of ingrown nails. (Letter to the Editor.) *Journal of Foot Surgery,* 15, 37–38.

Frost, L. A. (1962). Surgical correction for the incurvated nail. *Current Medical Digest, 29,* 119–121.

Gallocher, J. (1977). The phenol alcohol method of nail matrix sterilization. *New Zealand Medical Journal, 86,* 140–141.

Papidus, P. W. (1972). The ingrown toenail. *Bulletin/Hospital of Joint Diseases, 33,* 181–192.

Murray, W. R. & Bedi, B. S. (1975). The surgical management of ingrowing toenail. *British Journal of Surgery, 62,* 409–412.

Nyman, S. P. (1956). The phenol alcohol technique for toenail excision. *Journal of the New Jersey Chiropodists Society, 5,* 2–4.

Yale, J. F. (1974). Phenol-alcohol technique for correction of infected ingrown toenail. *Journal of the American Podiatry Association, 64,* 46.

chapter 17

Ingrown Toenail Infection

CPT Coding:

11730 Avulsion of nail, partial or complete ($101–$124)
11732 Avulsion, each additional plate ($55–$68)

 DEFINITION

- In the medical literature, ingrown toenail infections are referred to as paronychias. These lesions are most always bacterial infections involving the surrounding soft tissue and skin. Rarely, fungal infections cause paronychias.

 INDICATIONS

- Skin and soft tissue infections secondary to all or part of an intruding nail plate
- Tight shoegear (repetitive microtrauma)
- Blunt trauma to nail
- Congenital defect of nail
- Subungual bone tumors of underlying distal phalanx resulting in deformed nail plate
- Subungual exostosis of distal phalanx resulting in deformed nail plate
- Onychomycosis (fungal nail) resulting in thickened, ingrown nail plate
- Systemic diseases can contribute to the severity of paronychia (eg, diabetes, peripheral vascular disease, scleroderma, etc.)

 PATIENT EDUCATION

- Inform patients of complications, such as cellutitis, bone infection, bacteria, gangrene, amputation of involved toe, or more proximal amputation, if the condition is left untreated.
- Stress the importance of compliance of patient in following treatment instructions at home (daily soaks in Epsom salts, antibiotics, dressings, etc.).

ALERT: Be sure to inquire about allergies to antibiotics, local anesthetics, povidone-iodine (Betadine), etc.

Type of Nail Infection	Procedure	Special Considerations
1. Stage I—Mild	1. Partial nail avulsion on affected side. 2. Epsom salt soaks × 2 to 3 days. 3. Keep toe clean and dry.	1. If diabetic or PVD, may need antibiotic 2 to 3 days.
1. Stage II—Moderate	1. Partial nail avulsion on affected side. 2. 3 to 5 days oral antibiotics. 3. Epsom salt soaks 3 to 5 days. 4. Keep toe clean and dry (If draining, use gauze daily to bandage.).	1. Take culture if patient has diabetes, PVD, or if lesion has odor. 2. If diabetic or PVD, follow up with a podiatrist. 3. May need pain medication.

Stage II.

TYPE OF NAIL INFECTION	PROCEDURE	SPECIAL CONSIDERATIONS
1. Stage III—Severe	1. If tolerable, decompress by avulsing nail on affected side.	1. Owing to infection, pH alteration prevents local anestheic from being effective.
	2. Oral antibiotics 7 to 10 days.	2. Pain medication likely needed.
	3. Epsom salt soaks.	3. Check patient's vital signs.
	4. Keep toe bandaged.	
	5. If diabetic or PVD, patient should see a podiatrist immediately or may need to be admitted to hospital for IV antibiotics and local daily care.	
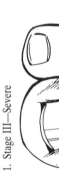 Stage III.		
1. Stage IV—Ascending cellutis or gangrene	1. Check vital signs.	1. Should always perform x-ray study to rule out gas in tissue (medical emergency).
	2. Admit to hospital for IV antibiotics and local care.	
	3. If diabetic or PVD, send to emergency room immediately.	
	4. Cover affected area with dressing.	

ASSESSMENT

1. Obtain a complete medical history and history of the involved ingrown nail (duration, onset, fevers, previous treatment).
2. Evaluate the lesion clinically. Is there erythema, cellulitis, abscess, drainage, anaerobic odor, or damage to the nail?
3. Differentiate between paronychia and other rare similar pathologies such as frostbite, periungual warts, fibromas, myxoid cysts, noninfected pyogenic granulomas, glomus tumor, nevus, keratoacanthoma, melanoma, soft tissue tumors, and Raynaud's disease.
4. If nail removal (partial or complete) is necessary, assess patient's cooperative ability (see table on pages 123 and 124).

 FOLLOW-UP

- On follow-up visits, the patient may need complete nail removal if nail has been deformed or traumatized. This procedure should be done only when infection is resolved.
- If on the initial visit the nail is considerably loose, then it is best to remove it.
- The nail bed is very sensitive. If the nail is removed, then use a nonadhesive bandage.
- If a patient has more than two to three nail infections per year or if the patient requests, permanent nail removal (partial or complete) may need to be done.
- All nail procedures are discussed in Chapter 16.
- First-generation cephalosporins are the drug of choice for paronychias. If the patient is a diabetic and paronychia is Stage II or worse, use a broad-spectrum oral antibiotic, such as amoxicillin (Augmentin). If the patient is allergic to penicillin, use clindamycin or erythromycin. If a culture taken, treat infection appropriately according to identified organism.
- If green drainage is present (indicating Pseudomonas infection), then one may use ciprofloxacin (Cipro) or some of the newer quinolones.
- If the lesion is a rare fungal paronychia (most always caused by *Candida albicans*), use a drying agent such as Betadine on a bandage. One can also soak the nail for 15 minutes daily with 1 part Betadine to 3 parts sterile saline. Oral antifungal agents may or may not need to be used.
- Don't forget pain medication if an aggressive nail procedure is performed or Stage II or greater infection is present.

BIBLIOGRAPHY

American Medical Association. (1998). *Physicians' current procedural terminology: CPT.* Chicago: American Medical Association.
Baran, R., Bureau, H., & Syag, J. (1979). Congenital malalignment of the big toenail. *Clinical and Experimental Dermatology, 4,* 350–360.
Brearley, R. (1958) Treatment of ingrown toenails. *Lancet, 2,* 12.
Healthcare Consultants of America. (1998). *1998 Physicians' fee and coding guide.* Augusta, GA.

Kipell, H. P., Winokur, J., & Thompson, W. A. (1968). Surgical relief for ingrown toenail. *Current Podiatry, 17,* 20.

Lowe, S. & Saxe, J. M. (1999). *Microscopic procedures for primary care providers.* Philadelphia: Lippincott Williams & Wilkins.

Mogensen, P. (1971). Ingrowing toenail. *Acta Orthopaedica Scandinavica, 42,* 94–101.

Murray, W. R. & Robb, J. E. (1979). Gutter treatment for ingrowing toenails (letter to the editor). *British Medical Journal, 2,* 391.

Samman, P. D. (1978). Great toe nail dystrophy. *Clinical and Experimental Dermatology, 3,* 81–82.

Townsend, A. C. & Scott, P. J. (1966). Ingrowing toenail and onychogryposis. *Journal of Bone and Joint Surgery, 48B,* 354–358.

Wallace, W. A., Milne, D. D., & Andrew, T. (1979). Gutter treatment for ingrowing toenails. *British Journal of Medicine, 2,* 168–171.

chapter 18
Unna Boot

CPT Coding:

29580 Unna boot ($63–$74)
29700 Removal of Unna boot ($63–$75)

DEFINITION

• An Unna boot is a gauze wrap impregnated with zinc oxide, gelatin, and glycerin that is wrapped snugly around the leg, followed by an Ace bandage. Some Unna boots contain calamine lotion.

INDICATIONS

• To minimize edema associated with venous ulcerations
• To treat venous stasis ulcers
• To provide compression therapy for patients unable to apply compression stockings
• For lymphatic edema
• For acute ankle sprain with severe swelling when non-weight bearing and immobilization is needed
• When a soft immobilizer is needed, such as in acute and chronic tendonitis

 ALERT: An Unna boot is contraindicated in patients with arterial disease; weeping, friable skin surrounding the ulcer; ulcer infection; known sensitivity reactions to zinc oxide; acute sprains with fractures; or active phlebitis.

PATIENT EDUCATION

• Explain that some type of long-term compression therapy will be required.
• If the patient has home health nurses, the boot may be changed in the patient's home.
• Unna boots should be changed once or twice a week depending on the amount of ulcer exudate.
• If an ulcer is present, a dressing may be required under the Unna boot.
• Reinforce that there may be an unpleasant odor when the boot is changed.
• Report any pain or significant toe changes such as swelling, loss of feeling, or blue or purple discoloration.

- Elevate the legs during the day. Six-inch blocks under the foot of the bed are recommended.

ASSESSMENT

1. Determine the patient's willingness to wear the boot.
2. Confirm the diagnosis of venous ulcers (as opposed to arterial ulcers).
3. Assess the location of the ulcer: Venous ulcers are located below the knee and above the ankle, usually on the medial or lateral aspect of the leg.
4. Assess pain: Pain associated with venous ulcers usually occurs when the legs are maintained in a dependent position.
5. Assess for presence of leg edema, associated with venous ulceration.
6. Assess for fibrosis and chronic brown discoloration of the skin on the lower extremities (hemosiderin deposits), which are characteristic of venous disease.
7. Palpate the posterior tibial and dorsalis pedis pulses. In the presence of a palpable pulse, arterial blood flow is present.
8. Calculate the ankle-brachial index (ABI). An index greater than 0.8 is needed to indicate venous disease.
9. To calculate the ABI, obtain by Doppler the systolic brachial blood pressure (both arms) and the posterior tibial blood pressure (both ankles). Using the highest brachial and posterior tibial pressures, divide the brachial pressure by the posterior tibial pressure.

For example:

Left arm 130/80
Right arm 134/84
Left posterior tibial 150/84
Right posterior tibial 146/82
Divide 134/150 = .89 (ABI)

USE OF THE UNNA BOOT WITH NO ULCER PRESENT

Equipment
- Doppler stethoscope
- Normal saline
- Gauze 4 × 4
- Alcohol-free lotion
- Unna boot
- Ace or Coban wrap

PROCEDURE	SPECIAL CONSIDERATIONS
Calculate ABI. Requires an ABI greater than 0.8 to apply Unna boot.	Less than 0.8 ABI indicates the presence of arterial disease.
Clean the foot and leg and pat dry. Apply lotion to intact skin. Leave no lotion residue on the skin.	Lotion keeps the skin soft and moist.

(procedure continued)

PROCEDURE	SPECIAL CONSIDERATIONS

The boot can be applied directly to the skin, or a snug layer of Kerlex or Kling can be placed over the area first.

Hold the foot at approximately a 30-degree angle. Beginning at the base of the toes, wrap the Unna boot in a circular fashion, overlapping by approximately 50% from the toes to 1 to 2 inches below the knees.

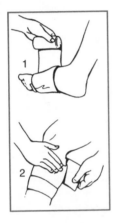

Apply the boot to the leg with greatest pressure at the ankle and lower third of the leg.

No skin should be visible

Progressively diminish pressure on the remainder of the leg. Cover the entire heel. Keep the foot at a 90-degree angle to the leg.

Clip and smooth the Unna boot where necessary to provide a wrinkle-free smooth wrap.

Apply the Ace or Coban wrap from base of toes to below the knees.

Protects the patient's clothing and applies additional compression.

(procedure continued) ───

| **PROCEDURE** | **SPECIAL CONSIDERATIONS** |

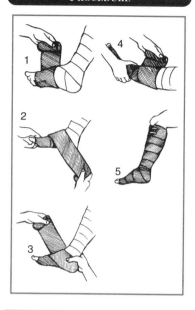

───

 USE OF THE UNNA BOOT WITH ULCER

───

| **PROCEDURE** | **SPECIAL CONSIDERATIONS** |

Débridement should be carried out first, if indicated.

Then clean ulcer gently with normal saline. Apply a hydrocolloid or foam wound dressing to the ulcer, if present.

Dressing should be at least 1 inch larger than ulcer.

The dressing should absorb wound fluid and not injure adjacent tissues.

The ulcer should be free of necrotic tissue.

- Small ulcers with little drainage can be managed by the Unna boot. Large ulcers require additional dressing to absorb moisture and provide a moist wound-healing environment that is essential for healing.

ALTERNATIVE PROCEDURES

- The following options can be used instead of the Unna boot. These methods supply compression, which is an essential component of the therapy. The dressings are for local ulcer care.
- Compression stockings providing 30 to 40 mmHg pressure at the ankle can be used.
- Intermittent pneumatic compression
- New skin subtitute. A newly approved bioengineered two-layered skin substitute (Apligraf, Organogenisis Inc.) has been shown to improve healing of skin ulcers in venous stasis. It is indicated for use with ulcers that have not healed with conventional therapy.

FOLLOW-UP

- Initial follow-up should be performed in 4 days.
- An offensive odor and appearance of purulent exudate **may** be present at the time of dressing change. Assess the ulcer after cleaning.
- Improvement is expected immediately, with dissolution of the wound exudate, resolution of edema, and the appearance of granulation tissue, followed by epithelialization.
- Complete healing takes from 1 week to several months.
- Subsequent follow-up is dependent on the appearance of the wound and in what environment the boot is changed.
- If the Unna boot is applied in the office, it should be changed every 4 to 7 days
- If the boot is applied in the patient's home, evaluation of treatment should be performed every 2 to 4 weeks by the primary care provider.
- Patients who show no improvement should be referred to a vascular surgeon in 2 to 4 weeks.
- When the ulcer has fully epithelialized and any palpation tenderness has resolved, the patient should be fitted with a compression stocking that provides 30 to 40 mmHg ankle compression. Knee length–graded compression stockings are sufficient for most patients.

BIBLIOGRAPHY

American Medical Association. (1998). *Physicians' current procedural terminology: CPT.* Chicago: American Medical Association.

Bryant, R. (1992). *Acute and chronic wounds: Nursing management.* St. Louis: Mosby.

Burton, C. (1993). Treatment of leg ulcers. *Dermatologic Clinics 11*(2), 315–323.

Cahall, E. & Spence, R. (1994). Nursing management of venous ulceration. *Journal of Vascular Nursing, 12,*(2), 48–56.

Cordts, R., Hanrahan, L., Rodriguiz, A., Woodson, J., LaMorte, W., & Menzoian, J. (1992). A prospective, randomized trial of Unna boots vesus Duoderm CGF hydroactive dressing plus compression in the management of venous leg ulcers. *Journal of Vascular Surgery, 15*(3), 480–486.

Jarrett, F. (1990). Leg ulcers of vascular etiology. *Clinics in Dermatology, 8*(3/4), 40–48.

Lowe, S. & Saxe, J. M. (1999). *Microscopic procedures for primary care providers.* Philadelphia: Lippincott Williams & Wilkins.

Phillips, T. & Dover, J. (1991). Leg ulcers. *Journal of the American Academy of Dermatology, 25*(6), 965–989.

Richelson, C. (1990). Leg ulcers. *Journal of Enterostomal Therapy, 17*(5), 217–219.

chapter 19

Screening Audiometry

CPT Coding:

92551 Pure tone audiogram ($25–$30)

 DEFINITIONS

- **Audiometers** produce pure tones of varying frequency and intensity to screen for hearing loss. Measurements are made by air conduction, in which the sound is transmitted through headphones into the ear.
- **Frequency** is measured as Hertz (Hz), or cycles per second, and is perceived as pitch. Human hearing ranges from approximately 20 to 20,000 Hz. Speech frequency is in the range of 500 to 4000 Hz.
- **Intensity** is measured in decibels (dB) and is perceived as loudness.
- **Conductive hearing loss** results from a dysfunction of the middle ear, with impairment of the passage of sound vibrations to the middle ear. Conductive hearing loss is usually correctable.
- **Sensory hearing loss** results from the deterioration of the cochlea, usually due to the loss of hair cells from the organ of Corti. Causes of sensory hearing loss include noise trauma, aging, and otoxicity. Sensory loss is usually not correctable.
- **Neural hearing loss** results from lesions of the 8th cranial nerve, auditory nuclei, or auditory cortex. It is the least common cause of hearing loss. Causes of neural hearing loss include multiple sclerosis, neuroma, and cerebrovascular disease.

Categories of hearing loss are shown in Table 19-1 and Figure 19-1.

Avg Threshold (dB)	Hearing Loss	Causes	What Can Be Heard
0 to 25	Normal		All speech sounds
26 to 40	Mild	Serous otitis, perforation, tympanosclerosis, sensorineural loss	Hears only some of speech sounds, the louder voice sounds
41 to 65	Moderate	Chronic otitis, middle ear anomoly, sensorineural loss	Misses most speech sounds in normal conversation

table continued

table continued

Avg Threshold (dB)	Hearing Loss	Causes	What Can Be Heard
66 to 90	Severe	Sensorineural loss or mixed loss	Hears no speech sound of normal conversatio
91+	Profound	Sensorineural loss or mixed	Hears no speech or other sounds

Adapted from Northern, J. & Downs, M. (1984). Hearing in children, Baltimore: Williams & Wilkins.

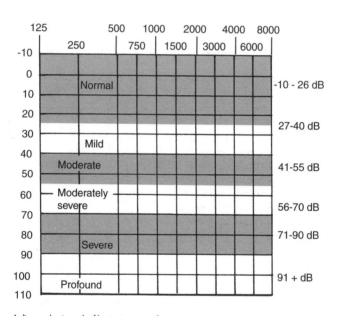

Audiogram showing scale of hearing impairment frequency in Hz.

⊙- INDICATIONS

- Identification of hearing loss
- Screening for hearing loss
- Conducted when a person or child has speech or language delays or difficulties
- Conducted as part of evaluation for a number of conditions (attention deficit–hyperactivity disorder, recurrent otitis media, etc.)
- Conducted as part of a routine physical examination
- Conducted as part of a Department of Transportation physical examination for drivers

PATIENT EDUCATION

- Discuss the purpose of the audiometry examination, as well as the need for possible referral and more elaborate testing, depending on findings.
- Describe how the test will be conducted and give a practice tone.
- Emphasize the importance of conducting the test in a quiet room. Other people in the room need to remain quiet or leave the room (especially small children). Other distracters in the room should also be removed, if possible.
- The procedure does not cause pain or discomfort.
- Discuss ways to assist with hearing:
  - Face people when talking
  - Obtain the attention of the person before speaking
  - Use gestures
  - Speak at a moderate pace
  - Use adequate lighting
  - Decrease background noise
  - Use of TDD phone

 RESOURCES FOR HEARING LOSS

- American Speech-Language-Hearing Association: (1-800-638-8255)
- National Institute on Deafness and Other Communication Disorders: (1-800-241-1044)
- Self-Help for Hard of Hearing People: (301-657-2248) www.shhh.org
- The Ear Foundation: www.theearfound.com
- National Information Center on Deafness: www.gallaudet.edu/~nicd
- The Hearing Alliance: www.hearingalliance.com/~hearnow

 ASSESSMENT

Conduct a complete history related to hearing problems:

1. History of present illness: Determine whether or not the patient has any of the following:
   Difficulty hearing spoken words
   Difficulty hearing only in noisy environments
   Use of hearing aids
   Complaints of nausea and vomiting, tinnitus, vertigo, otalgia, otorrhea, facial weakness
   Sense of fullness in the ears
   Loss of equilibrium
   Involvement of one or both ears
   Onset gradual or sudden
   Fluctuation in hearing since hearing loss began
2. Past medical history: Ask about history of ear infections, increased cerumen production, hypertension, mumps, head trauma, diabetes, hypothyroidism, syphilis, neurologic problems, or prematurity.

3. Medications: Ask about the use of
   Acetylsalicylic acid
   Antibiotics, aminoglycosides
   Diuretics
   Quinine
4. Family history: Ask about a family history of hearing loss.
5. Social history: Ask about environmental exposures to loud noises and the use of protective measures or ear plugs. Also, ask about exposure to loud music.
6. Conduct a complete physical examination related to the ear:
   Evaluate: External canal, tympanic membrane (TM), check for TM movement with pneumatic otoscopy
   Neuro: Check sensation of face and facial movement
   May consider doing tympanogram for evaluation of TM function

◉ DEVELOPMENTAL CONSIDERATIONS

Child: Children 4 years of age and older can be tested with the audioscope. Children younger than 4 years of age are not able to follow instructions and are not as successful in completing the test owing to the interactive nature of the exam.

Development of hearing abilities in children:
- 0 to 3 months: respond to noise
- 3 to 5 months: turns to noise
- 6 to 10 months: responds to name
- 10 to 15 months: imitates simple words

Elderly: Elderly persons have a progressive hearing loss, mainly in the high frequencies, due to aging (presbycusis). It may be increased due to genetic predisposition. This loss of hearing is more evident in noisy environs when the individual is unable to hear well and has poorer speech discrimination abilities.

◉ EQUIPMENT

- Audioscope
- Quiet room

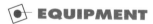

PROCEDURE	**SPECIAL CONSIDERATIONS**
The patient should be seated during the procedure. A small child can be seated on the parent's lap.	Have the small child face a blank wall to decrease distractions. Very young or uncooperative children should be referred to an audiologist.
Check to make sure the lens is centered in the instrument.	

(procedure continued)

| PROCEDURE | SPECIAL CONSIDERATIONS |

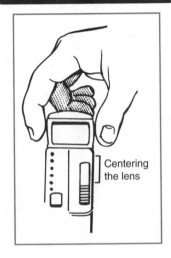

Centering the lens

Select a small, medium, or large ear speculum. Twist the speculum clockwise onto the instrument.

Turn the audioscope on. Select the desired screening level. The READY indicator will become illuminated, indicating the instrument is ready to use.

Use the largest speculum that will fit comfortably in the ear canal. A snug fit is needed to ensure an acoustic seal of the speculum in the ear canal.

Select the decibel level based on the following:

20 dB	School-aged child
25 dB	Standard screening level for adults and in noisy situations when 20 dB cannot be used
40 dB	May be used to assess hearing impairment in people older than 65

(procedure continued) ─────────────────────────────────────

PROCEDURE ────── ⟨ SPECIAL CONSIDERATIONS ⟩

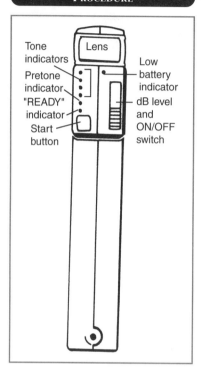

Tone indicators

Lens

Pretone indicator

"READY" indicator

Start button

Low battery indicator

dB level and ON/OFF switch

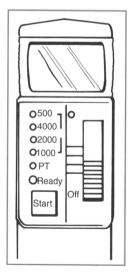

500
4000
2000
1000
PT
Ready
Start
Off

(procedure continued)

PROCEDURE	SPECIAL CONSIDERATIONS

Instruct the patient that a loud tone or beep will be heard. The patient is to respond every time a tone is heard. Responses include saying "yes" or using gross motor movements.

Very young children seem to respond better using a verbal response.

Seniors seem to respond better using a gross motor response (raising a hand, waving a paper towel).

Retract the patient's pinna with the thumb and index finger. Gently pull it slightly up and back. Insert the speculum into the canal.

In children, pull back more than up.

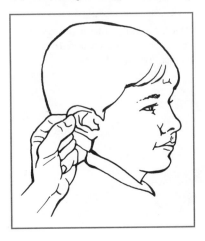

(procedure continued)

PROCEDURE	SPECIAL CONSIDERATIONS
Position the speculum so that a portion of the TM can be visualized.	If the canal is significantly occluded by cerumen, the ear should be cleaned before performing the test.
Press the start button. The green light will go out, and the tone indicators will indicate the tone that is being conducted.	Once a decibel level is chosen, the sequence of sounds presented in that decibel range are 500, 1000, 2000, and 4000.
	A pretone sound is delivered before the screening so the patient can hear a test tone louder than the test tones.
Observe for each tone indicator and the patient's response. Repeat the test in the opposite ear.	If the test is disrupted due to patient movement or noise, the test can be restarted by pressing the start button again.

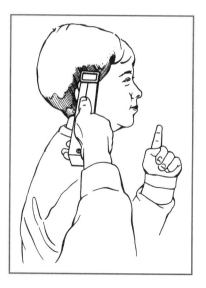

If there is a failure at one or more frequencies in either ear, instruct the patient and screen again. Failure at one or more frequencies constitutes failure.

A second failure indicates that the patient should be referred to an audiologist for further testing.

Turn the instrument off. Complete the screening results form and include it in the patient's chart.

(procedure continued)

| PROCEDURE | SPECIAL CONSIDERATIONS |

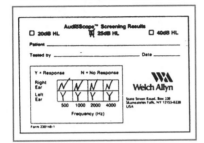

Photos courtesy of Welch Allyn. Illustration 7 from Lohr, Jacob A., (1991). Pediatric outpatient procedures. Philadelphia: J.B. Lippincott Company.

 ALTERNATIVE PROCEDURE

Other tests are available to determine whether or not the person needs to be referred for further testing. These tests are used for screening only. The Weber and the Rinne are most helpful in differentiating conductive hearing loss from sensorineural hearing loss.

- Whisper test
- Rinne and Weber test

Audiometric studies are conducted in a soundproof room. Pure tone thresholds in decibels are obtained over the ranges of 250 to 8000 Hz for both air and bone conduction. Play audiometry is used with children $2^1/_2$ to 5 years old. Visual reinforcement audiometry is used for children 5 to 6 months to $2^1/_2$ years of age. Behavioral observation audiometry is used for children younger than 5 months of age.

 FOLLOW-UP

- Patients with middle ear effusion should be retested after the effusion has resolved. If the effusion persists for more than 2 or 3 months, the patient should be referred to an ear, nose, and throat (ENT) specialist for a more complete evaluation.
- Very young or uncooperative children should be referred to an audiologist.
- Failure at a second screening test indicates the need for further testing, and the patient should be referred to an audiologist or otolaryngologist.
- Children at high risk for hearing loss should be referred to a pediatric audiologist by 3 months of age.

BIBLIOGRAPHY

American Medical Association. (1998). *Physicians' current procedural terminology: CPT.* Chicago: American Medical Association.

Arnold, J. (1996). The ear. In W. Nelson (Ed.). *Nelson textbook of pediatrics* (1808–1827). Philadelphia: W. B. Saunders.

Deloian, B. (1997). Screening tests. In J. Fox (Ed.). *Primary Health Care of Children* (148–157). St. Louis: Mosby.

Hayden, G. & Lambert, P. (1991). Ear, nose and throat procedures. In J. Lohr (Ed.). *Pediatric outpatient procedures*. Philadelphia: J. B. Lippincott.

Healthcare Consultants of America. (1998). *1998 Physician's fee and coding guide*. Augusta, GA.

Jacker, R. & Kaplan, M. (1998). Ear, nose, throat. In L. Tierney, S. McPhee & M. Papadakis (Eds.). *Current medical diagnosis and treatment* (pp. 214–216). Stamford, CT: Appleton & Lange.

Jerger, J. (1995). Hearing Impairment in older adults: New concepts. *Journal of the American Geriatric Society, 43,* 928.

Lowe, S. & Saxe, J. M. (1999). *Microscopic procedures for primary care providers*. Philadelphia: Lippincott Williams & Wilkins.

Mitchell, G. (1994). Otologic devices. *Emergency Clinics of North America, 12,* 787.

Northern, J. & Downs, M. (1984). *Hearing in Children*. Baltimore: Williams & Wilkins.

chapter
20
Avulsed Tooth/Tooth Fractures

CPT Coding:

N/A

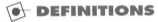 **DEFINITIONS**

A tooth fracture includes seven different types of tooth injury, including dislocations of the teeth.

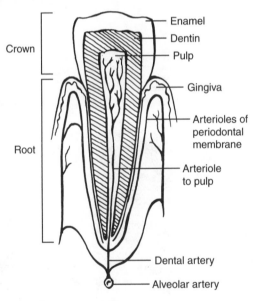

Normal anatomy of tooth including blood supply. (Lohr, Jacob A. [1991]. *Pediatric outpatient procedures*. Philadelphia: J.B. Lippincott Company.)

- **Crown fractures** are incomplete fractures of the teeth, without separation of the fragments.
- **Type I fractures** are enamel-only fractures. Patients may complain of increased sensitivity and rough tooth edges.

- **Type II fractures** involve the dentin. These injuries are very sensitive to cold and touch.
- **Type III fractures** involve the pulp of the tooth. This is usually identified by drops of blood on the surface of the tooth or visualization of exposed pulp. A type III fracture is usually very painful. The more exposed the pulp is, the more painful the tooth and the more contaminated the pulp becomes. The pulp will appear as a pinkish blush in a normal tooth. The teeth are very sensitive to cold and manipulation.
- **Root fractures** involve the root of the tooth, including horizontal fractures of the neck of the tooth, and fractures of the middle third of the tooth. A vertical fracture is usually not restorable.

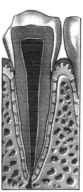

Class I
Coronal Fracture

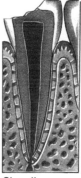

Class II
Coronal Fracture

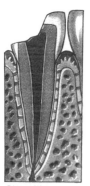

Class III
Coronal Fracture

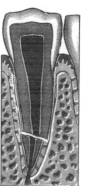

Root Fracture

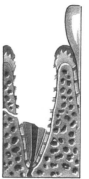

Root Fracture
and Avulsion

Replacement or reduction of a displaced tooth. Basic types of fractures of teeth. (Lohr, Jacob A. [1991]. *Pediatric outpatient procedures*. Philadelphia: J.B. Lippincott Company.)

- **Displacement injuries:**
  - **Tooth concussion** does not involve the supporting structures and there is no mobility of the tooth.

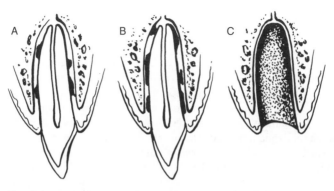

Effects of trauma to tooth. Slightly concussed tooth (A); Moderately concussed tooth (B); and avulsed tooth (C). (Pfenninger, J., Fowler, G. [1994]. *Procedures for primary care physicians.* Mosby—Year Book, Inc.)

- **Subluxation** involves minor tooth mobility, but there is no displacement from the original position.
- **Luxation** involves physical displacement of the tooth ranging from minor to major displacement.
- **Avulsion** is total dislocation of the tooth from its normal position in the socket. Tooth avulsion is generally caused by traumatic injury to the mouth.

INDICATIONS

- Replacement of an tooth removed completely from its socket.
- Determine appropriate treatment based on the degree of tooth damage.

PATIENT EDUCATION

- Inform the patient that any tooth that sustains trauma may undergo devitalization.
- The blood flow may be disrupted, causing death of the tooth.
- Dental follow-up care is essential.

ASSESSMENT

Determine how the tooth trauma occurred: When, where, how? Was there loss of consciousness or neurologic damage (amnesia, headache)?

1. Complete a thorough but brief past medical history, with specific information obtained relating to medical conditions, mitral valve prolapse, other valve problems or prostheses, altered immune status, and heart condition.
2. Assess for other injuries besides tooth trauma such as intraoral lacerations.
3. Conduct a thorough assessment of the tooth socket.
4. Carefully look at the oral soft tissue for embedded tooth fragments of the lip and tongue.
5. Consider an x-ray study of the area, if possible.
6. Determine the patient's tetanus status.

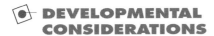

DEVELOPMENTAL CONSIDERATIONS

Child: Avulsion of a primary tooth requires no specific treatment beyond dental evaluation for other associated injuries, local wound care, and mild analgesics. Avulsion of a permanent tooth requires replacement of the tooth, preferably within 30 minutes. The prognosis of successful tooth replacement is time dependent; delays of more than 30 minutes often result in complete loss of the tooth and of periodontal ligament viability. The goal of treatment of an avulsed tooth is rapid replacement of the tooth into the original socket to preserve key tooth attachments.

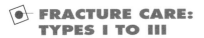

FRACTURE CARE: TYPES I TO III

Equipment
- Saline
- Cotton roll
- 2 × 2 gauze pads
- Dycal and applicator
- Emery board
- Periodontal mirror
- Clear nail polish or copalite (tooth varnish)

PROCEDURE	SPECIAL CONSIDERATIONS
Smooth the rough edges of the tooth with an emery board. Cover the tooth with clear nail polish if the patient is sensitive to cold.	**Type I** tooth fractures do not damage the tooth pulp.
Rinse the tooth with warm saline and dry with air or cotton. Cover the area with a thin coat of Dycal followed by several layers of clear nail polish or Copalite. Use the emery board to smooth the edges of tooth gently as needed.	If the fracture is a **type II** fracture, the goal is to protect dentin tubules from exposure and to eliminate any sharp edges of the tooth.
Clean and dry the tooth surface and apply Dycal. Follow with several coats of tooth varnish to help keep the Dycal in place and to protect the tooth. If a large amount of pulp is visible and more than 2 hours have elapsed since the tooth was displaced, a root canal will be required. Smooth the edges of the tooth.	**Type III** fracture Mild to moderate analgesia will be needed by the patient.

◉ DISPLACEMENT INJURIES

Equipment
- 5-mL syringe
- 1% lidocaine (xylocaine)
- 18-gauge needle
- 23-gauge $1\frac{1}{2}$-inch needle
- Tooth preservation solution
- Wire
- Gauze pads

PROCEDURE	SPECIAL CONSIDERATIONS

Handle the tooth by the crown only, using sterile gauze, and immerse it as soon as possible into a preservative solution ("Save a Tooth") or milk. The "Save a Tooth" solution markedly extends the 30-minute replantation window up to at least 6 and possibly 24 hours.

The third place for safekeeping of the tooth is in the patient's mouth. This is less than ideal due to the hypotonic state and bacterial contamination.

Patients with peridontitis, gross caries, or fractures in the avulsed tooth should not have the tooth replaced.

Socket preparation requires first anesthetizing the area with a dental nerve block. After anesthetizing the socket, suction any clots from the socket and irrigate the socket with normal saline.

Clean dirt from the tooth using only gentle irrigation or agitation using a tooth-preservation solution or saline. Avoid scrubbing the tooth because it may remove any adherent bone spicules on the root of the tooth. Do not touch the tooth root.

Once the socket has been prepared, orient the tooth and gently place it into the socket. Apply firm pressure on the tooth using your finger to place it back into the proper position. If the tooth does not fit back into the proper position, remove it and inspect the socket for possible obstruction.

A dental x-ray can be taken to see that the tooth is well fitted into the socket.

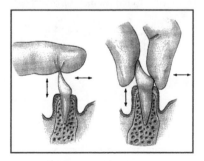

(procedure continued)

PROCEDURES	**SPECIAL CONSIDERATIONS**
The use of a splint to help hold the teeth in position is recommended for 7 to 14 days.	The use of a loop technique may provide temporary splinting for a partially avulsed tooth until the patient is seen by the dentist.

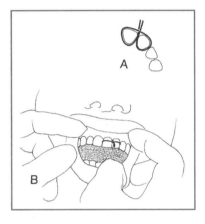

Illustration 1 from Lohr, Jacob A., (1991). Pediatric outpatient procedures. Philadelphia: J.B. Lippincott Company.

ALTERNATIVE PROCEDURES

• A variety of methods are available to secure loose teeth.
• Use of a loop technique to splint a partially avulsed tooth is helpful to secure the tooth until the patient sees a dentist.

FOLLOW-UP

• After replantation, immediately refer the patient to a dentist or orthodontist.
• The average life span of an implanted tooth is 5 to 10 years.
• Antibiotics should always be prescribed after replanting teeth. For example, Pen Vee K, 1-g dose, then 500 mg QID for 4 to 6 days may be given.
• *Child:* 15–56 mg/kg/day in 3–6 divided doses.
• Administer tetanus toxoid if no booster has been documented within 5 years.

POSTAVULSION BLEEDING

• Bleeding may be seen after a tooth avulsion or extraction. Suction the fossa of the tooth of all clots and irrigate with warm saline. Use a 2 × 2 gauze pad to apply compression directly to the socket by having the patient bite down firmly for 20 minutes. This technique usually stops the bleeding. If not, use Oxygel in the socket and apply pressure again for 20 more minutes.

BIBLIOGRAPHY

American Medical Association. (1998). *Physicians' current procedural terminology: CPT.* Chicago: American Medical Association.

Healthcare Consultants of America. (1998). *1998 Physicians' fee and coding guide.* August, GA.

Lowe, S. & Saxe, J. M. (1999). *Microscopic procedures for primary care providers.* Philadelphia: Lippincott Williams & Wilkins.

Simon, R. & Brenner, B. (1994). *Emergency procedures and techniques* (3rd ed.). Baltimore: Williams & Wilkins.

Sweeney, R. (1997). Tooth stabilization and replantation. In R. Dieckmann, D. Fiser, & S. Selbst (Eds.). *Illustrated textbook of pediatric emergency & critical care procedures* (pp. 738–741). St. Louis: Mosby–Year Book, Inc.

chapter 21

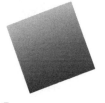

Cerumen Removal

CPT Coding:

69210 Removal of impacted cerumen (separate procedure), one or both ears ($45–$57)

 DEFINITIONS

- **Cerumen:** the waxlike, soft-brown secretion found in the external canal of the ear.
- **Impacted cerumen:** The apocrine and sebaceous glands lining the external auditory canal (EAC) excrete cerumen, which then comes out the auditory meatus. Cerumen repels water, has documented antimicrobial activity, and forms a protective barrier against infection. Cerumen often becomes impacted, causing complaints of "clogged" ear, hearing impairment, and dizziness. Symptomatic impaction is an indication for removal, although symptoms are rare until complete obstruction is present. Usually, cerumen obstructs visualization of the tympanic membrane and needs to be evacuated as part of the evaluation of a febrile child or the patient complaining of ear pain (Manthey & Harrison, 1998).

 INDICATIONS

- Removal of impacted cerumen causing decreased ability to hear, infection, or pain
- Need for cerumen to be removed so that the tympanic membrane can be visualized

 PATIENT EDUCATION

- Reassure the patient that removal of the cerumen is necessary in the thorough evaluation of the ear or to cleanse the canal of debris so topical antibiotics can work adequately.

 ASSESSMENT:

1. Obtain a thorough history of the presenting problem.
2. Evaluate the ear for the presence of pain, drainage, or erythema.
3. Assess the mastoid bone for tenderness.

DEVELOPMENTAL CONSIDERATIONS

Infant and Child: It is very important to have the infant or child hold still during the examination and removal procedure. Use of a papoose board may be indicated to prevent injury during the procedure. Encourage parents to talk to their child in a calm manner throughout the procedure to minimize the anxiety of both the parent and the child (see Chapter 50: Child Restraint).

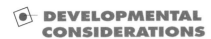 EQUIPMENT

- Otoscope
- Ceruminolytic agent, such as trolamine polypeptide oleate-condensate (Cerumenex) or carbamide peroxide 6.5% (Debrox)
- Benzocaine (Auralgan)
- Aluminum sulfate (Buro-Sol)
- C Tagli swab
- Ear loops or cerumen spoon
- Sterile water

PROCEDURE	SPECIAL CONSIDERATIONS
Use a ceruminolytic before removal of cerumen to soften hardened or impacted cerumen. Although many products are available to assist in this procedure, a 5% or 10% solution of sodium bicarbonate disintegrates cerumen much more quickly and efficiently compared with commercially prepared ceruminolytics (Manthey & Harrison, 1998). Colace (available in liquid form) is also useful.	Ceruminolytic agents may take 2 to 3 days to work. Have patient use 2 gtts in affected ear for 2 to 3 days and then return for irrigation or disimpaction.
Manual extraction: This procedure is more advantageous and it is usually quicker. Harder or larger amounts of cerumen can be removed under direct visualization. Either the diagnostic or operating head of the otoscope or an ear speculum may be placed in the auditory meatus to serve as a protective port through which instruments are passed and manipulated.	To prevent startling or agitating an already anxious patient, allow the patient to experience the sensation of the otoscope or speculum in the canal for a few moments before inserting the extraction instrument.

(procedure continued)

PROCEDURE	SPECIAL CONSIDERATIONS

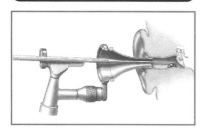

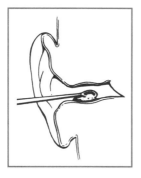

Gently lift the cerumen off the canal wall using loops and then pass hooks or loops around the cerumen and withdraw the cerumen slowly as shown in figure above. Keep both hands in contact with the patient's head because any sudden movement may cause trauma to the canal or the TM (Manthey & Harrison, 1998).

Complications most often occur when contact is made with the external canal. These complications include lacerations, perforation of the tympanic membrane, and hematomas.

 ALTERNATIVE PROCEDURE

• Ear irrigation (see Chapter 23)

 FOLLOW-UP

• Generally, once cerumen is removed, the patient's symptoms subside. Follow-up is indicated when there is suspicion of otitis media or tympanic perforation.
• If cerumen is lodged against the tympanic membrane and removal is unsuccessful, refer the patient to an otolaryngologist for removal.

BIBLIOGRAPHY

American Medical Association. (1998). *Physicians' current procedural terminology: CPT.* Chicago: American Medical Association.

Healthcare Consultants of America. (1998). *1998 Physicians' fee and coding guide,* Augusta, GA.

Manthey, D. & Harrison, B. (1998) Cerumen removal. In J. Roberts & J. Hedges (Eds.). *Clinical procedures in emergency medicine* (3rd ed., pp. 1128–1130). Philadelphia: W. B. Saunders.

chapter
22
Corneal Abrasion

CPT Coding:

65220 Removal of corneal foreign body (FB), without slit lamp ($91–$110)
65222 Removal of corneal FB, with slip lamp ($110–$133)

 DEFINITION

• A corneal abrasion is an abrasion or scratch in the cornea of the eye. Most corneal abrasions are very painful, and the patient may present with severe anxiety and fear from the feelings of visual loss. The central cornea is the least protected by the lids and is easily injured by scratching or foreign bodies.

 INDICATIONS

• If the patient complains of eye pain, tearing, or redness of eye, an examination should be performed for a corneal abrasion or injury.
• A history of a foreign body in the eye or the eye being scratched.

 PATIENT EDUCATION

• Reassure the patient of the need to evaluate the eye thoroughly.
• Pain can be treated with topical anesthetic agents.
• Keep the infant's nails trimmed to avoid eye injuries.

 ASSESSMENT

1. Obtain a thorough history of the events leading up to the injury.
2. Evaluate visual acuity of both eyes.
3. Evaluate cardinal fields of vision.

 **DEVELOPMENTAL
CONSIDERATIONS**

Infants: Infants, especially newborns, may present with inconsolable crying and should be evaluated for possible corneal injuries. Many infants have long fingernails and inadvertently scratch their cornea.
Child: Children are also prone to corneal injuries secondary to foreign bodies in the eye. Children are less likely to protect their own eyes or those of their playmates during play. Activities that increase the risk of foreign

body invasion and subsequent corneal injury include throwing sand and rocks (Sacchetti & Harris, 1997). Be suspicious if the child complains of photophobia.

EQUIPMENT

- Topical anesthetic, such as proparacaine 0.5%
- Gloves
- Fluorescein strips
- Wood's lamp
- Sterile cotton-tipped applicators
- Slit lamp
- Antibiotic ointment, such as erythromycin ophthalmologic ointment
- Eye patch and tape

PROCEDURE	SPECIAL CONSIDERATIONS

Wash hands thoroughly.

Put on gloves.

The first step is the examination of the eye itself. Apply traction to the upper and lower lids, exposing as much of the eye as possible. Evert both eye lids to examine the eye completely.

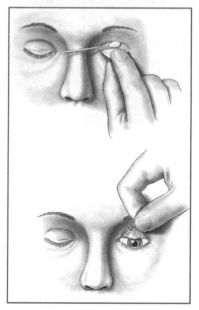

(procedure continued)

PROCEDURE	SPECIAL CONSIDERATIONS

Have the patient look slowly in all directions. Examine the intactness of the globe. The presence of erythema or microhemorrhages may indicate trauma or foreign bodies.

1 to 2 drops of topical anesthetic should be instilled into the lower conjunctival sac. After a few minutes, fluorescein is applied to the inside of the lower lid. The fluorescein is grasped by the nonorange end, and the orange end is wetted with one drop of saline. The wetted strip is then placed gently onto the inside of the patient's lower lid. The strip is withdrawn and the patient is instructed to blink. The patient's blinking spreads the fluorescein over the eye.

The topical anesthetic may be applied initially before any exam is performed. It may be needed before the visual acuity exam so the patient is able to keep the eye open.

Alert: Never prescribe a topical anesthetic for home use—they retard healing.

A Wood's lamp, the blue filter of a slit lamp, or a penlight with a blue filter should be used to examine the eye in a darkened room. Check for areas of bright green fluorescence on the corneal and conjunctival surfaces.

A slit lamp facilitates the eye exam. It provides a magnified view of the anterior chambers giving depth to the view (see Chapter 27: Foreign Body: Eye for explicit directions)

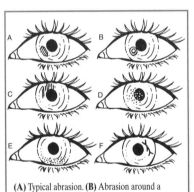

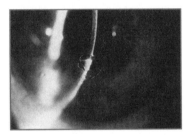

(**A**) Typical abrasion. (**B**) Abrasion around a corneal foreign body. (**C**) Abrasion from a conjunctival foreign body under the upper lid. (**D**) Abrasion from excessive wearing of a contact lens. (**E**) Ultraviolet exposure. (**F**) Herpetic dendritic keratitis.

The margins of the abrasions are usually sharp and linear if seen in the first 24 hours. Circular defects are seen about embedded foreign bodies and may persist for up to 48 hours after removal of a superficial foreign object. Deeply embedded objects may be as-

Alert: Any patient with acute visual loss, chemical burns (irrigate first) and penetrating eye trauma should be referred to an opthalmologist immediately.

(procedure continued)

PROCEDURE	SPECIAL CONSIDERATIONS

sociated with defects persisting for more than 48 hours.

Objects under the lid often produce *vertical linear lesions* on the upper surface of the cornea. When vertical lesions are noted, *a search for a retained FB under the upper lid should be conducted.*

Corneal abrasions usually occur in the central cornea because of the limited protection of the patient's closing eyelids.

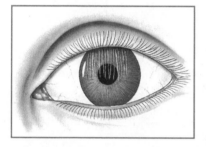

Any area of corneal staining with an infiltrate or opacification beneath or around the lesion should alert the practitioner to the possibility of a viral, bacterial, or fungal keratitis. Many *Pseudomonas* organisms fluoresce when exposed to ultraviolet light. The presence of fluorescence before the instillation of fluorescein in the red eye should suggest the possibility of a pseudomonal infection (Manthey & Harrison, 1998).

Urgent ophthalmologic consultation should be obtained so that cultures of the possible etiologic agents can be procured and treatment initiated (Manthey & Harrison, 1998).

Following the removal of the foreign body, an antibiotic ointment is applied to the interior surface of the lower lid. Good choices include gentamycin (which provides good gram negative coverage) or sulfacetamide 10% (which produces few hypersensitivity reactions).

At present, there is much controversy over the issue of patching the eye and the practice is not recommended.

The purpose of patching is to reduce pain, decrease eye movement, and hasten healing. Recent studies indicate that patching may not be helpful and, in fact, may be more harmful due to the possibility of organism growth.

Contact lenses wearers should never wear a patch owing to the potential of growth of *Pseudomonas*.

Illustrations 1 and 4 from Lohr, Jacob A. (1991). Pediatric outpatient procedures. Philadelphia: J.B. Lippincott Company

📵 FOLLOW-UP

- Instruct the patient to follow up in 24 hours. The majority of superficial abrasions heal within this length of time without complication.
- If healing has not taken place, refer the patient to an ophthalmologist.

BIBLIOGRAPHY

American Medical Association. (1998). *Physicians' current procedural terminology: CPT.* Chicago: American Medical Association.

Hulbert, M. (1991). Efficacy of eye pad in corneal healing after corneal foreign body removal. *Lancet, 337,* 643.

Jacoby, D. (1998). A 26 year old woman with eye pain and tearing. In D. Robinson (Ed.). *Clinical decision making for nurse practitioners.* Philadelphia: Lippincott Williams & Wilkins.

Jampal, H. (1995). Patching for corneal abrasion. *Journal of American Medical Association, 274*(19), 1504.

Kaiser, P. & Pineda, R. (1997). A study of topical nonsteroidal anti-inflammatory drops and no pressure patching in the treatment of corneal abrasions. *Ophthalmology, 104*(8), 1353–1359.

Kirkpatrick, J., Hoh, H., & Cook, S. (1993). No eye pad for corneal abrasion. *Eye, 7,* 468–471.

Lowe, S. & Saxe, J. M. (1999). *Microscopic procedures for primary care providers.* Philadelphia: Lippincott Williams & Wilkins.

Manthey, D. & Harrison, B. (1998). Corneal abrasion. In J. Roberts & J. Hedges (Eds.). *Clinical procedures in emergency medicine* (3rd ed., pp. 1096–1100, 1112–1115). Philadelphia: W. B. Saunders.

Patterson, J., Fetzer, D., Krall, J., Wright, E., & Heller, M. (1996). Eye patch treatment for the pain of corneal abrasions. *Southern Medical Journal, 89*(2), 227–229.

Poole, S. (1996). Corneal abrasions in infants. *Pediatric Emergency Care, 11*(1), 25–26.

Sacchetti, A. & Harris, R. (1997). Eye injuries. In R. Dieckmann, D. Fiser, & S. Selbst (Eds.). *Illustrated textbook of pediatric emergency & critical care procedures* (pp. 724–726). St. Louis: Mosby–Year Book, Inc.

chapter
23
Ear Irrigation

CPT Coding:

   69210 Removal of impacted cerumen (separate procedures), one or both
   ears ($45–57)

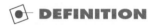 DEFINITION

• Ear irrigation is defined as the cleansing of the canal by flushing with water
or other fluids.

INDICATIONS

• Irrigation of the external ear canal is indicated for the removal of cerumen
or foreign bodies in the canal.

PATIENT EDUCATION

• Reassure the patient that removal of the foreign body is necessary.
• Many patients may display great anxiety related to the foreign body. This is
particularly true if a live insect is in the external canal. The movement of
the insect can cause great pain and anxiety in the patient. Reassure these
patients that it is necessary to evaluate the ear thoroughly and then remove
the foreign body.
• Reassure the patient that irrigation is painless and simple to perform.
• The patient does not have to hold still completely during the procedure.
• Encourage the patient to use a half-and-half mixture of isopropyl alcohol
and hydrogen peroxide prophylactically (2 gtts 2 times per week) to help
prevent cerumen impactions

ASSESSMENT

1. Obtain a thorough history of the situation: When the foreign body was noticed, how long has it been present, and what other removal methods have
been tried?
2. Evaluate the ear canal to determine the causative agent (eg, sand, insect,
beads, small toy pieces).

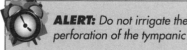

ALERT: Do not irrigate the ear if the patient is known to have a
perforation of the tympanic membrane.

DEVELOPMENTAL CONSIDERATIONS

Child: Toddlers are the high-risk age group for foreign bodies in the ear.

EQUIPMENT

- 18- or 20-g angiocath
- 10-mL syringe
- Otoscope
- Emesis basin
- Towels or chux

PROCEDURE	SPECIAL CONSIDERATIONS
The patient should be in a sitting position, with towels or Chux (water-resistant covering) placed over his/her shoulders.	Warn the patient that he or she may get wet even though all precautions are taken to keep him or her dry.
Place an emesis basin against the neck, directly below the ear to be irrigated.	An assistant, the patient, or family member may be asked to hold the basin.

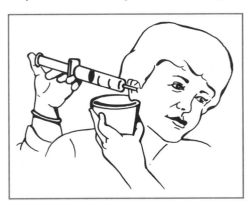

A plastic catheter from a 18- to 20-g IV needle is of adequate size for most ear canals. Attach the plastic catheter to a 20-mL syringe. A solution of warm water is then drawn up into the syringe. The tip of the catheter is placed into the external ear canal only as far as the cartilage bone junction. Water is then injected into the ear canal above the impaction or foreign body.

Use only the plastic portion and discard the needle in a sharps container.

A butterfly needle can also be used once the wings and needle are cut off.

Warm water is used to avoid caloric stimulation that results in nausea and vomiting. **Stop the irrigation if the patient experiences any sudden nausea and vomiting, tinnitus, vertigo, pain, or hearing loss.**

(procedure continued)

PROCEDURE	SPECIAL CONSIDERATIONS

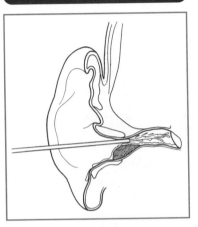

It may also be helpful to put traction on the pinna to straighten out the canal for more efficient irrigation.

The irrigation should be continued until the cerumen or foreign body is washed out of the ear. Re-evaluate the external canal and tympanic membrane for signs of infection or trauma after all of the cerumen is removed.

It may be helpful to manually try to extract some of the cerumen periodically to help the process along.

Several drops of isopropyl alcohol can be instilled in the ear canal to assist with evaporation of any remaining irrigation fluid. Topical Cortisporin drops may be soothing to the external canal if it is irritated.

Make sure that the tympanic membrane is intact before the instillation of alcohol.

Illustration 2 from Roberts, J. & Hedges, J. (Eds.) Clinical procedures in emergency medicine. (3rd Ed.). Philadelphia: W.B. Saunders Co.

ALTERNATIVE PROCEDURES

- Oral jet irrigators (Water Pik) have been used to irrigate the external ear canal. Caution should be taken to use only the lowest power setting and to direct the stream toward the canal wall and not the tympanic membrane to prevent tympanic membrane rupture.

FOLLOW-UP

- Once the foreign body is successfully removed from the ear canal, a thorough otoscopic examination of the ear should be conducted to look for evidence of trauma, perforation of the tympanic membrane, or small fragments of the foreign body. If there is evidence of trauma to the canal walls, a small amount of antibiotic drops can be instilled into the external canal (Manthey & Harrison, 1998).

• If the tympanic membrane is perforated, prescribe antibiotics for otitis media and refer the patient to an otolaryngologist for follow-up and possible tympanic membrane grafting.

BIBLIOGRAPHY

American Medical Association. (1998). *Physicians' current procedural terminology: CPT.* Chicago: American Medical Association.

Manthey, D. & Harrison, B. (1998). Foreign bodies of the ear canal. In J. Roberts & J. Hedges (Eds.). *Clinical procedures in emergency medicine* (3rd ed., pp. 1132–1133). Philadelphia: W. B. Saunders.

Roberts, J. & Hedges, J., eds. (1998). Ear irrigation. In: *Clinical procedures in emergency medicine* (3rd ed., pp. 1128–1130). Philadelphia: W. B. Saunders.

chapter 24

Treatment of Epistaxis

CPT Coding:

30901 Control nasal hemorrhage, anterior, simple (limited cautery and/or packing) any method ($138–$175)

30903 Control nasal hemorrhage, anterior, complex (extensive cautery and/or packing) any method ($194–$242)

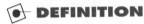 **DEFINITION**

• Epistaxis is hemorrhage in the nasal cavity.

INDICATIONS

• Treatment is required to control the bleeding that continues after direct pressure. If the source is anterior, this procedure may be the final treatment.
• For posterior bleeding, this procedure is a temporary measure.

 ALERT: Identification of the source of bleeding followed by control is crucial to the treatment of epistaxis.

PATIENT EDUCATION

• Encourage the patient to relax and reassure that bleeding will be controlled.
• Explain the procedure to the patient.

ASSESSMENT

1. Assess the patient's vital signs, mental status, skin color, orthostatic changes, and quantify blood loss.
2. Determine whether or not the patient has any underlying medical problems, such as angina, bleeding disorders, or chronic obstructive lung disease, all of which may be exacerbated due to hypovolemia or anemia.

 ALERT: If the patient is symptomatic in any of these areas, or if the blood loss is deemed significant, refer the patient to the emergency room.

3. Assess location of bleed, if possible. Most cases of anterior bleeding occur in Kisselbach's plexus.
4. Obtain history of prior epistaxis, date, location, and treatment.
5. Obtain history of prior episodes of sinusitis and allergic rhinitis.
6. Obtain history of any medication use (over-the-counter, prescription, and illicit drugs).

 ALERT: Many patients with epistaxis may be hypertensive. No direct correlation has been proven between hypertension and epistaxis. Many consider hypertension to be a stress response. Therefore, hypertension does not require treatment until the bleeding is controlled and the anxiety of the situation has been resolved.

EQUIPMENT

- Gown
- Emesis basin
- Light source (headlight is best)
- Phenylephrine (Neo-Synephrine), 0.125% to 0.5% on a cotton pledget
- Nasal speculum
- Suction equipment with an 8- to 10-French catheter
- Silver nitrate sticks
- 0.25- or 0.5-inch petroleum jelly (Vaseline) gauze and bayonet forceps

PROCEDURE	SPECIAL CONSIDERATIONS
1. Drape patient to protect clothing.	May need to administer analgesia.
2. Have patient hold emesis basin to collect any continual bleeding.	May have emesis from swallowed blood.
3. Have patient sit upright in the sniffing position, with neck flexed and head extended. The base of the nose should remain parallel with the floor.	Have patient maintain constant pressure on the nose by pinching it between the thumb and first finger.
4. Encourage patient to clear the nose of any blood clots by using forceful blowing.	
5. If bleeding is minimal, attempt to identify bleeding source.	
6. Apply topical vasoconstrictor if bleeding is too profuse to identify bleeding source.	**Continue to monitor patient for reactions to medications.**
7. Insert the nasal speculum into the naris.	
8. Use the suction catheter to evacuate blood.	

(procedure continued)

PROCEDURE	SPECIAL CONSIDERATIONS
9. Attempt to cauterize the bleeding.	May repeat vasoconstrictor if needed before attempting cautery.
10. Cauterize above the bleeding source to avoid the flow of blood.	You cannot cauterize an actively bleeding source.
11. Cauterize in a circular manner.	Cautery works well for a small circumscribed area of bleeding.
12. Wipe away excess silver nitrate.	Wiping away excess silver nitrate will prevent cauterizing other areas.
13. If bleeding persists, the next step is nasal packing.	
14. Grasp the packing 2 to 3 cm from its end with bayonet forceps.	

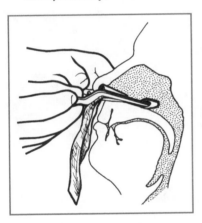

15. Place the first layer on the floor of the nose through the nasal speculum.

16. Continue to pack the nose using layers in an accordian method to fill the nose.

(procedure continued) ————————————————————————————

| PROCEDURE | SPECIAL CONSIDERATIONS |

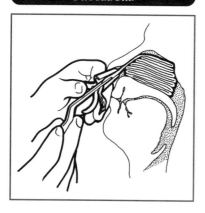

17. Secure the packing to prevent it from falling into the nasopharynx.

Illustrations from Simon, R. & Brenner, B. (1994). Emergency procedures and technique, (3rd ed). Baltimore: Williams & Wilkins.

 FOLLOW-UP

- Return to office 24 to 48 hours for packing removal, if applicable.
- May give antibiotic to prevent infection, if packing was used.
- Decongestant may be helpful.
- Advise the patient how to handle simple nosebleeds at home.
- Increase humidity in home environment.
- Keep nose lubricated.
- Avoid use of aspirin or nonsteroidal anti-inflammatory drugs (NSAIDs) for 3 to 4 days following epistaxis.
- Refer to ear, nose, and throat (ENT) specialist for recurrent epistaxis.

BIBLIOGRAPHY

Barkin, R. M. (1997). *Concepts and clinical practice: Pediatric emergency medicine* (2nd eds.). St. Louis: Mosby.

Healthcare Consultants of America. (1999). *1999 Physicians' fee and coding guide.* Augusta, GA.

Roberts, J. R. & Hedges, J. R. (1998). *Clinical procedures in emergency medicine* (3rd eds.). Philadephia: W. B. Saunders.

Stine, R. J. & Chudnofsky, C. R. (1994). *A practical approach to emergency medicine* (2nd ed.). Boston: Little Brown, 715–718.

chapter 25

Eye Irrigation: Morgan Lens

CPT Coding:

68339 Unlisted procedure, conjunctiva

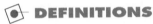 **DEFINITIONS**

- **Eye irrigation** is irrigation of the eye with copious amounts of saline.
- A **Morgan lens** is a specially designed lens that is placed on the sclera of the eye to provide continuous irrigation. It is made of hard plastic, with soft plastic tubing ending in a female adapter.

INDICATIONS

- Removal of chemical irritant, with prevention of further damage to eye

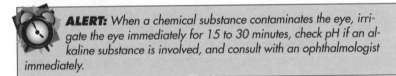

ALERT: When a chemical substance contaminates the eye, irrigate the eye immediately for 15 to 30 minutes, check pH if an alkaline substance is involved, and consult with an ophthalmologist immediately.

PATIENT EDUCATION

- Reassure the patient that the irrigation is critical to prevent damage to eye secondary to chemical or foreign body.
- Reassure the patient that a topical anesthetic will make the procedure less uncomfortable.
- Emphasize the need for ophthalmology follow-up.
- Encourage the use of safety glasses.

ASSESSMENT

1. Obtain history related to episode.
2. Assess for redness, excessive tearing, discharge, and swelling. Ask about photophobia.
3. Obtain visual acuity, if possible. (May need to wait 1 to 2 minutes after topical anesthetic instilled.)

4. Determine whether solution is acid or alkaline. Acid substances cause co-agulation of proteins, which limits the depth of injury. Alkaline substances cause liquefaction of proteins and have a tendency to penetrate through to the anterior chamber. Alkaline substances need a longer period of irrigation. A normal pH of conjunctiva (7.4 to 7.6) should be obtained before irrigation is stopped.

5. Alkali substances include lye (drain openers, oven cleaners), lime (plaster, concrete), and ammonia.

6. Acid substances include sulfuric acid (car batteries), hydrochloric acid (drain openers) and muriatic acid (swimming pool chemical).

 ALERT: Ask about contact lenses and remove if present.

7. Determine patient's ability to cooperate and hold still during procedure.

DEVELOPMENTAL CONSIDERATIONS

Child: It is very important to have the child remain still during procedure. Use of a papoose board or other means to control movement and hands is very important (see Chapter 50: Child Restraint).

EQUIPMENT

• pH strip
• Irrigating solution and IV tubing
• Topical anesthetic (tetracaine, proparacaine)
• Waterproof pad
• Basin
• Morgan lens

PROCEDURE	SPECIAL CONSIDERATIONS
Obtain pH of eye before irrigation. Retract lower lid and touch pH strip to the conjunctiva.	Retest pH during and after irrigation.
1. Assess eye throughly before proceeding.	**Choices of irrigating solution include normal saline, saline with bicarbonate (pH 7.4), Ringer's lactate, and balanced saline solution (BSS Plus, Alcon Laboratories).**
2. Instill one to two anesthetic drops to affected eye. Cleanse external eye.	
3. Position patient in side-lying position on same side as affected eye or in ENT chair.	

(procedure continued)

PROCEDURE	SPECIAL CONSIDERATIONS

4. Use towels or waterproof pad to protect clothes. Position basin below eye to catch runoff.

5. To insert lens; gently open lids.

6. Attach IV tubing to Morgan lens. Ask the patient to look up and insert the lens into the lower fornix of the eye. Ask patient to look down and insert the superior border of the lens into upper fornix of the eye using the projecting tubing.

The Morgan lens should not be used for foreign bodies in the eye because foreign bodies ca be trapped under the lens.

If patient is unsure of eye problem, fluoroscein must be instilled before the Morgan lens.

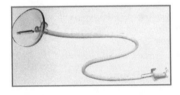

7. Open IV clamp and adjust rate to patient comfort.

At least 1 liter per eye should be used for chemical contaminant. Recheck pH before patient leaves.

8. To remove lens, ask patient to look up, retract lower lid, and pop out lower border of Morgan lens; then ask patient to look down and remove superior border of lens.

9. Dry eye with sterile gauze or cotton ball.

ALTERNATIVE PROCEDURE

- If no Morgan lens is available, irrigation of eye can be performed by directing fluid from end of IV tubing, making sure to direct stream in all directions over anterior surface of eye for at least 15 minutes.

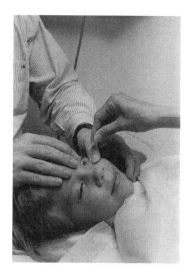

Technique for flushing for chemical irritants. (Lohr, Jacob A. [1991]. *Pediatric outpatient procedures*. Philadelphia: J.B. Lippincott Company.)

FOLLOW-UP

- The patient should be sent directly to ophthalmologist at the earliest opportunity for evaluation.
- Encourage the use of protective goggles when working around chemicals.

BIBLIOGRAPHY

American Medical Association. (1998). *Physicians' current procedural terminology: CPT.* Chicago: American Medical Association.

Kerr, R., White, G., Bernhisel, K., Mamalis, N., & Swanson, E. (1991). Clinical comparison of ocular irrigation fluids following chemical injury. *American Journal of Emergency Medicine, 9*(3), 228–231.

Lowe, S. & Saxe, J. M. (1999). *Microscopic procedures for primary care providers.* Philadelphia: Lippincott Williams & Wilkins.

McConnell, E. (1991). How to irrigate the eye. *Nursing 1991, 21*(3), 28.

Parshall, M. (1996). In P. Kidd & P. Sturt (Eds.). *Mosby's emergency nursing reference* (pp. 767–769). St. Louis: Mosby.

Sheey, S. & Lombardi, J. (1995). *Manual of emergency care* (4th ed.). St. Louis: Mosby.

chapter 26

Foreign Body: Ear

CPT Coding:

69200 Removal of foreign body from external auditory canal without general anesthesia ($98–$118)

 DEFINITION

- A foreign body is any foreign object that is found in the external auditory canal (EAC). Despite its small size, the EAC may play host to a number of types of foreign bodies. Living insects account for the majority of foreign bodies found in adults (Fritz, Kelen, & Sivertson, 1987). Items used to clean the ears may also be found (matchsticks or a cotton applicator) Children frequently place food (eg, peas and beans), organic matter (eg, grass and leaves), and inorganic objects (eg, beads and rocks) into their ear canals during play.

 INDICATIONS

- Any person complaining of symptoms of foreign body retention of the ear

 ALERT: *Patients with foreign bodies that have been pushed beyond the isthmus or are lying against the tympanic membrane (TM) should be referred to an ear, nose, and throat (ENT) specialist. Other contraindications to removal include the patient with severe hemophilia or the inability to restrain the patient adequately either physically or chemically (Dieckmann, Fiser, & Selbst, 1997).*

 ASSESSMENT

1. Obtain a thorough history about the foreign body, if known:
   – What the object is
   – How long the foreign body has been lodged
   – Attempts made by patient or family to remove the foreign body
2. Assess the patient's ear symptoms.
3. Assess the patient's hearing ability.
4. Assess the pinna for redness or tenderness.
5. Carefully examine the EAC for signs of trauma, purulent drainage, and protrusion of the foreign body.

6. Examine both the opposite ear and the nose of children to search for a possible second foreign body.

 ALERT: *Uncooperative children, or numerous unsuccessful attempts, glass or other sharp-edged objects, existent injury to the EAC or TM, or objects wedged against TM may require surgical extraction (this occurs in about a third of cases) (Ansley, & Cunningham, 1998).*

DEVELOPMENTAL CONSIDERATIONS

Adult: The patient presents with ear pain, fullness, or impaired hearing.
Child: The child may not present until an associated otitis externa with a purulent discharge has developed.

EQUIPMENT

- An adequate light source is essential
- A headlamp with a separate specula is preferred
- An otoscope with an operating head is the next best choice
- Alligator or Hartmann forceps
- Suction apparatus and catheters of different sizes (eg, 5, 8, and 10 French)
- Wire loops or blunt hooks
- Cotton-tipped applicators

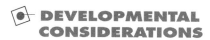

PROCEDURE	SPECIAL CONSIDERATIONS
Use the otoscope to visualize the foreign body. The technique used to remove the foreign body will vary depending on the depth of and type of foreign body. Removal of foreign bodies from the medial 2/3 of EAC is much more painful and ENT referral may be advisable. *Irrigation* is the least invasive option (see Chapter 23: Ear Irrigation). **Suction-tipped catheters** can be used, but the patient must be informed of the impending noise to prevent sudden movements from a startle reflex. Place either the blunt or soft plastic tip against the object and withdraw slowly. If using a suction instrument with a thumb-controlled release valve, cover the port to activate the suction (Manthey & Harrison, 1998).	**Never attempt to irrigate a disc battery in the EAC. It causes leakage of the alkali electrolyte solution and can cause necrosis of the EAC and TM.** Tinnitis, vertigo, significant hearing loss, or bleeding from behind the object should raise a high suspicion for an associated tympanic membrane rupture (Manthey & Harrison, 1998). **ALERT: Use of water with vegetable matter may cause the foreign body to expand.**

(procedure continued)

PROCEDURE	**SPECIAL CONSIDERATIONS**

Manual Instrumentation. This approach may be attempted with a variety of instruments. Good lighting and visualization are imperative. An assistant should hold the pinna back and out so that the otoscope can be held with one hand and the instrument can be manipulated with the other. A speculum and either a headlamp or head mirror or light source can also provide light, but magnifying loupes are usually required for adequate visualization. Use small alligator forceps to remove objects with edges that can be grasped. A small right angle hood is another choice. Place the tip past the object, rotate it 90 degrees, and then pull the object from the canal. Loops may be used in a similar fashion.

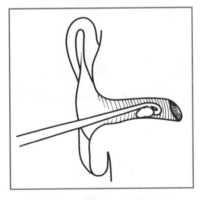

Removal of insects. Cockroaches are the most commonly found live insect in the ear. Treatment consists of instillation of various substances into the ear canal to first immobilize or kill the insect. Mineral oil or microscope oil kill the insect in approximately 45 seconds. Lidocaine has been reported to paralyze roaches and to allow easier extraction than the more viscous mineral oil. Once disabled, insects may be removed with mechanical extraction as previously described, or pieces can be suctioned out using a suction catheter.

Use of an instilled substance helps retrieval by allowing for a stationary target and also halts the disturbing and painful movement of the insect.

Substances such as benzocaine (Auralgan), water, and hydrogen peroxide are ineffective in killing insects in a reasonable amount of time.

ALTERNATIVE PROCEDURE

- If object is round (like a hair bead) and lodged in the canal, the object can be removed by hooking the hole in the bead using a right-angle hook or by putting a small drop of cyanoacrylate (Krazy glue) onto the wooden end of an applicator stick and placing the stick against the object. After several seconds, the applicator will adhere to the object.

FOLLOW-UP

- Evaluate the EAC and TM after removal of the foreign body.
- Minor lacerations or excoriations of the canal usually heal with or without antibiotic eardrops as long as the canal is kept clean and dry.
- Patients with foreign bodies that cannot be removed should be referred to a otolaryngologist.
- Also refer patients with severe ear pain, suspected TM rupture, embedded button batteries, or a concomitant canal infection.
- Instruct the patient to return if there is bleeding, a discharge, ear pain, or loss of hearing.

BIBLIOGRAPHY

American Medical Association. (1998). *Physician's current procedural terminology: CPT 1998.* Chicago: American Medical Association.

Ansley, J. F. & Cunningham, M. J. (1998) Treatment of aural foreign bodies in children. *Pediatrics, 101*(4, Part 1), 638–641.

Dieckmann, R., Fiser, D., & Selbst, S., eds. (1997). External auditory canal foreign bodies. In: *Illustrated textbook of pediatric emergency & critical care procedures* (pp. 712–713). St. Louis: Mosby–Year Book, Inc.

Fritz, S., Kelen, G., & Sivertson, K. (1987). Foreign bodies of the external auditory canal. *Emergency Medical Clinics of North America, 5,* 183.

Goldman, S. A., Ankerstjerne J. K., Welker, K. B., & Chen, D. A. (1998). Fatal meningitis and brain abscess resulting in foreign body–induced otomastoiditis. *Otolaryngology Head and Neck Surgery, 118*(1), 6–8.

Healthcare Consultants of America. (1998). *1998 Physician's fee and coding guide.* Augusta: GA.

Manthey, D. & Harrison, B. (1998). Foreign bodies of the ear canal. In J. Roberts & J. Hedges (Eds.). *Clinical procedures in emergency medicine* (3rd ed., pp. 1132–1133). Philadelphia: W. B. Saunders.

chapter 27

Foreign Body: Eye

CPT Coding:

65205 Removal of foreign body, external eye; conjunctival superficial ($70–$84)

65210 Conjunctival, embedded (includes concretionary, subconjunctival, or scleral nonperforating) ($78–$95)

65220 Removal of corneal foreign body, without slit lamp ($91–$110)

65222 Removal of corneal foreign body, with slip lamp ($110–$133)

DEFINITION

- Many foreign bodies in the eye are very painful and anxiety-provoking in the patient. Children are more prone to eye injury and foreign bodies than adults because they have not yet learned to protect their eyes or those of their playmates (ie, throwing sand)(Dieckmann, Fiser, & Selbst, 1997). Not all foreign bodies are associated with pain. Some may be difficult to detect, such as glass embedded in the cornea (Roberts & Hedges, 1998).

> **ALERT:** Immediate referral is needed for penetrating eye trauma, hyphema, or acute visual loss.

INDICATIONS

- Removal of extraocular foreign bodies
- A history of foreign body or eye being scratched
- If the patient complains of eye tearing, photophobia, redness or pain, the eye should be examined for a foreign body.

PATIENT EDUCATION

- Reassure the patient that removal of the foreign body is necessary.
- Many patients display great anxiety related to pain and fear of vision loss. Reassure these patients that it is necessary to evaluate the eye thoroughly to determine the extent of the injury. Pain can be decreased by the use of topical anethestics, anti-inflammatory medications, or cyclopegics.

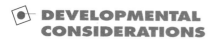 ASSESSMENT

1. Obtain a thorough history of the causative agent of the foreign body (eg, sand, glass, rust, or dust).
2. Evaluate visual acuity of both eyes (may need to instill topical anesthetic to enable the patient to open his or her eye).
3. Evaluate cardinal fields of vision.

DEVELOPMENTAL CONSIDERATIONS

Infant and Child: It is important to have the infant or child hold still during the examination and removal procedure. Use of a papoose board may be indicated to prevent injury during the procedure. Encourage parents to talk to their child in a calm manner throughout the procedure, to minimize the anxiety of both the parent and the child. When the patient is extremely uncooperative (eg, a mentally deficient individual or a young child), immediate ophthalmologic consultation is indicated.

EQUIPMENT

- Gloves
- Topical anesthetic, such as proparacaine 0.5%
- Sterile cotton-tipped applicators
- Fluorescein strips
- Wood's lamp
- Slit lamp
- Eye patch and tape (may not use)

PROCEDURE	SPECIAL CONSIDERATIONS
Wash hands thoroughly.	
Put on gloves.	
Instill 1 to 2 drops of 0.5% topical anesthetic. Wait 1 minute before beginning exam.	Topical anesthetic may have been instilled before visual acuity. **Never prescribe a topical anesthetic for home use—it retards healing.**
Examine the eye. While applying traction to the upper and lower lids, exposing as much of the eye as possible, have the patient look slowly in all directions. Examine the lower lid. Examine the intactness of the globe. The presence of erythema or microhemorrhages may be indicative of trauma or foreign bodies.	
Locate the foreign body.	Minute foreign bodies under the lid are missed with simple visual inspection. Ideally,

(procedure continued)

| PROCEDURE | SPECIAL CONSIDERATIONS |

the everted lid should be examined under magnification with loupes or a slit lamp (Roberts & Hedges, 1998).

Fluorescein is applied to the inside of the lower lid. The fluorescein is grasped by the non-orange end, and the orange end is wetted with one drop of saline. The wetted strip is then placed gently onto the inside of the patient's lower lid. The strip is withdrawn, and the patient is instructed to blink. The patient's blinking spreads the fluorescein over the eye. Use a Wood's lamp, the blue filter of a slit lamp, or a penlight with a blue filter to examine the eye in a darkened room, checking for areas of bright green fluorescence on the corneal and conjunctival surfaces.

Fluorescein is used to evaluate corneal injuries that may have been caused by the foreign body.

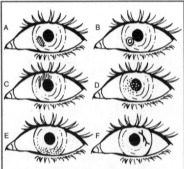

(A) Typical abrasion. (B) Abrasion around a corneal foreign body. (C) Abrasion from a conjunctival foreign body under the upper lid. (D) Abrasion from excessive wearing of a contact lens. (E) Ultraviolet exposure. (F) Herpetic dendritic keratitis.

Evert the upper eyelid. Have the patient look down as the end of an cotton-tipped applicator is pressed against the superior edge of the tarsal plate of the upper lid. The practitioner grasps the lashes and pulls down and then up to flip the lid over the applicator.

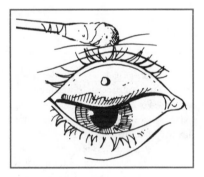

(procedure continued)

PROCEDURE	SPECIAL CONSIDERATIONS

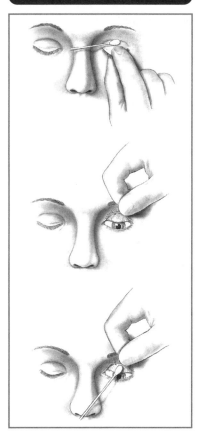

Once the foreign body is located, the technique of removal depends on whether it is embedded or not. If the foreign body is lying on the surface of the cornea, a stream of water injected from a syringe through a plastic catheter usually washes the object onto the bulbar conjunctiva. Once the foreign body is on the inner lid or bulbar conjunctiva, a wet cotton-tipped applicator can be gently touched to the conjunctiva and the object will adhere to the applicator.

Overzealous use of the applicator can lead to extensive corneal epithelial injury (Roberts & Hedges, 1998).

(procedure continued)

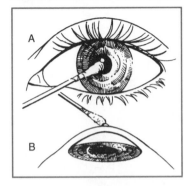

| PROCEDURE | SPECIAL CONSIDERATIONS |

Embedded foreign bodies are best removed with a commercial spud device, a short 25- or 27-gauge needle on a small diameter syringe, or a cotton-tipped applicator (Roberts & Hedges, 1998).

It is actually difficult to penetrate the sclera or cornea with a needle (Pavan-Langston, 1980). As with the removal of conjunctival foreign bodies, the eye must be well anesthetized. Position the patient where the head is well secured (preferably in a slit-lamp frame). When removing a foreign body, it is useful to have an assistant to help keep the patient's head still and to hold the eye open. The patient must be instructed to gaze or fix his or her vision on a distant object (eg, the practitioner's ear when the slit lamp is used) to stabilize the eye further. The needle or spud device is brought close to the eye *under direct vision with magnification*. While the object is in focus, the device is manipulated to pick or scoop out the foreign body.

During the removal of the foreign body, it is important for the practitioner to brace his or her hand against the patient's face. It may also be helpful to brace the elbow with a pad to provide further support of the arm as the foreign body is being removed.

Illustrations 2 and 3 from Lohr, Jacob A. (1991). Pediatric outpatient procedures. Philadelphia: J.B. Lippincott Company.

PROCEDURE	SPECIAL CONSIDERATIONS

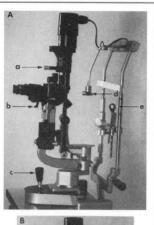

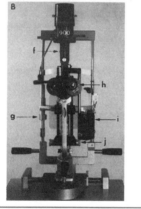

Have the patient position himself or herself upright at a 90-degree angle to the lens, with his or her chin in the chin rest and forehead against the upper strap. The room should be darkened.

The slip lamp is a magnified stereoscopic view of the eye from the lashes to the lens.

Set the light source to a narrow vertical rectangle, using the lowest possible brightness. Focus this source using the bridge of the nose to determine the intensity and shape of the beam.

Do not focus the lamp while shining the beam in the patient's eye.

(procedure continued)

PROCEDURE	SPECIAL CONSIDERATIONS
The movement of the slit-lamp beam is controlled using the joystick, both for depth of focus and lateral motion. Start the exam with the most superficial structures and then progress to deep structures. Use an arclike motion over the eye.	Do not move the lamp in a straight lateral direction.
Look at areas that might accumulate fluid due to gravity, such as the lower portion of the anterior chamber.	Blood in the anterior chamber is a hyphema.
Debris found in the anterior chamber is termed a cell-and-flare reaction, which is commonly seen in iritis.	This reaction looks like a sunbeam passing through a dusty room. It is proportional to the degree of iritis present.
Follow the plain light source with a blue filter and fluorescein stain.	The whole procedure of using a slit lamp (with experience) takes about 5 minutes.
Following the removal of the foreign body, an antibiotic ointment is applied to the interior surface of the lower lid. Good choices include gentamicin (good gram-negative coverage) or sulfacetamide 10% (few hypersensitivity reactions).	The purpose of patching is to reduce pain, decrease eye movement, and hasten healing. Recent studies indicate that patching may be more harmful due to the possibility of organism growth. **Contact lenses wearers should never wear a patch owing to the potential of _Pseudomonas_ growth.**
There is much controversy over the issue of patching the eye. Currently, the use of eye patches are not recommended.	

 FOLLOW-UP

• Instruct the patient to follow up in 24 hours. The majority of superficial abrasions heal within this time without complication. If the abrasion is healed, continue eye drops for 2 days. If healing has not taken place, refer the patient to an ophthalmologist.

 REFERRAL

• The patient should be referred in the following situations:
  – Rust ring around the foreign body
  – Herpetic lesions
  – Iritis
  – Acute vision loss

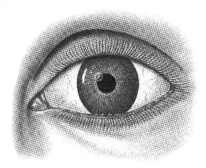

Residual rust ring following metallic corneal/conjunctival foreign body removal. (Lohr, Jacob A. [1991]. *Pediatric outpatient procedures*. Philadelphia: J.B. Lippincott Company.)

BIBLIOGRAPHY

American Medical Association. (1998). *Physicians' current procedural terminology: CPT.* Chicago: American Medical Association.

Buscemi, M., Capoferri, C., Garavaglia, A., Nassivera, C., & Nucci, P. (1991). Noncontact tonometry in children. *Optometry and Visual Sciences, 68,* 461–464.

Dieckmann, R., Fiser, D., & Selbst, S. (eds.) (1997). Eye foreign bodies. In: Su, E., *Illustrated textbook of pediatric emergency and critical care procedures* (pp. 724–726). St. Louis: Mosby–Year Book, Inc.

Hulburt, M. (1991). Efficacy of eye pad in corneal healing after corneal foreign body removal. *Lancet, 337,* 643.

Jacoby, D. (1998). A 26 year old woman with eye pain and tearing. In D. Robinson (Ed.). *Clinical decision making for nurse practitioners.* Philadelphia: J. B. Lippincott.

Jampal, H. (1995). Patching for corneal abrasion. *Journal of American Medical Association, 274*(19), 1504.

Kaiser, P. & Pineda, R. (1997). A study of topical nonsteroidal anti-inflammatory drops and no pressure patching in the treatment of corneal abrasions. *Ophthalmology, 104*(8), 1353–1359.

Kirkpatrick, J., Hoh, H., & Cook, S. (1993). No eye pad for corneal abrasion. *Eye, 7,* 468–471.

Lowe, S. & Saxe, J. M. (1999). *Microscopic procedures for primary care providers.* Philadelphia: Lippincott Williams & Wilkins.

Patterson, J., Fetzer, D., Krall, J., Wright, E., & Heller, M. (1996). Eye patch treatment for the pain of corneal abrasions. *Southern Medical Journal, 89*(2), 227–229.

Poole, S. (1996). Corneal abrasions in infants. *Pediatric Emergency Care, 11*(1), 25–26.

Roberts, J., & Hedges, J. (eds.) (1998). Foreign body of the eye & slit lamp examination. In: Manthey, D. & Harrison, B., *Clinical procedures in emergency medicine* (3rd ed., pp. 1096–1100, 1112–1115). Philadelphia: W. B. Saunders..

chapter 28
Foreign Body: Nose

CPT Coding:

30300 Removal of foreign body, intranasal; office-type procedure
($101–$119)

◉ DEFINITION

- Removal of foreign body from nose by manual extraction, manipulation with a balloon-tipped catheter or positive-pressure technique.

◉ INDICATIONS

- Caregiver observed insertion into, or suspects a foreign body in, a child's nose.
- Presence of foreign body in nose.
- Unilateral foul smell or discharge from nose.
- Persistent epistaxis.

◉ PATIENT EDUCATION

- Reassure patient (and caregiver as indicated) regarding examination.
- Provide anticipatory guidance and continually reassess for need for information.
- Advise the patient that his or her nose may feel numb or swollen from the medications used.
- Discuss the need to childproof areas where the child is playing.

◉ ASSESSMENT

1. Elicit history (Is there a known object in nose? Is it animal, vegetable, or mineral in composition?), timing, and self-care measures attempted.
2. Examine nose and throat with simple nasal speculum and light source. (Small flexible endoscope might be indicated.)

ALERT: *Otolaryngologist referral is needed in the case of a button battery, if the foreign body could not be removed, or if trauma or aspiration is likely to occur on removal.*

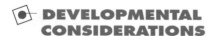

DEVELOPMENTAL CONSIDERATIONS

Child: A nasal foreign body can be difficult to remove in children. Spherical objects are especially difficult because they are hard and smooth, and difficult to grasp.

Edema and infection develops rapidly with foreign body of the nose.

Children who are unable to be calmed by environmental manipulation may benefit from restraint in a papoose board.

Be sure to check other organs for foreign bodies: it is not uncommon for children to put objects in both ears and the nose.

EQUIPMENT

• Sedation medication: midazolam or fentanyl, as appropriate
• 0.5% phenylephrine or lidocaine gel (4%)
• Alligator or bayonet forceps
• Balloon-tipped catheter
• Fine wire loop of ear curette or hooked probe

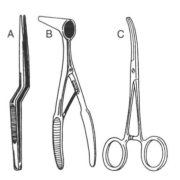

Nasal speculum (A); Bayonet forceps (B); and Curved forceps hemostat (C).

PROCEDURE	SPECIAL CONSIDERATIONS
Identification of foreign body: animal, vegetable or mineral.	Insects and other animate objects should be killed before removal. Vegetable matter tends to swell if it is hydrated and should be removed without the use of fluids.
Ensure patient's cooperation to avoid further harm.	
Anxiety can be allayed with midazolam (0.05 to 0.10 mg/kg IV or dripped into nostrils via	Fentanyl is reversible with nalaxone and also comes in lollipop form. Some patients may

(procedure continued)

PROCEDURE	SPECIAL CONSIDERATIONS

TB syringe). If necessary, conscious sedation can be achieved with fentanyl (.05 to 1.0 mg/kg, IV, repeated q 2 to 3 mins to dose of 3 to 4 mg/kg.

need to have procedure done under general anesthesia.

Use full-conscious sedation precautions. Assume the child's stomach is full. Conscious sedation means CONSCIOUS sedation, though children may doze (but are easily aroused).

Position the patient in an upright position.

This position allows visualization of more of the nasal cavity than with the head tilted back.

If object is readily visualized, consider a squirt of 0.5% phenylephrine (Neo-Synephrine) to reduce swelling or painting area with 1% lidocaine gel.

Choose a method of extraction

A. *Manual extraction*
Place the patient in the Trendelenburg position.

Use forceps (bayonet, Kelly, alligator) to snare object and remove.

Irrigation is not use because the nasopharynx is open and aspiration could occur.

Smooth objects may be removed best with suction or right-angle hooks.

Objects that may break when grasped are better removed with wire loops.

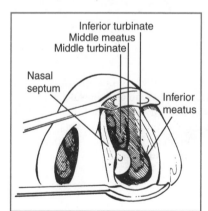

Inferior turbinate
Middle meatus
Middle turbinate
Nasal septum
Inferior meatus

B. *Balloon-tipped catheter*
Advance a 5F or 6F catheter (Fogarty balloon-tipped catheter) beyond object that is partially occluding nasal passage. Inflate balloon slightly and cautiously. Pull catheter out with balloon inflated.

The catheter is useful in removing blunt objects.

A local vasoconstrictor is helpful when mucosal edema has developed.

(procedure continued)

PROCEDURE	**SPECIAL CONSIDERATIONS**
	The balloon method is recommended in small children with a foreign body lodged posteriorly and may be less traumatic than forceps.
C. *Positive-pressure technique* Start with having patient forcefully blow his or her nose. Another method is to have caregiver or use an Ambu gag to create postive pressure.	Be prepared to cleanse the operator's face or cheeks, or both, of mucus and nasal contents.
Consider having "operator" don a protective gown. Have operator stand at patient's side (side of the unaffected nostril), lean over patient, and occlude the unaffected nostril. Instruct operator to occlude patient's mouth with operator's mouth and puff gently and quickly. Positive pressure should dislodge object. An Ambu bag can be used (if able to get an adequate mouth seal) instead of an operator.	Keep in mind the most posteriorly oriented objects might be most easily removed through the mouth. Commercial mouth covers are available. Using a positive-pressure device is probably the best choice.

ALTERNATIVE PROCEDURES

• Inspect nose for adequacy of removal and signs of infection or erosion.

FOLLOW-UP

• Instruct regarding managing nose bleeds or other complications, especially if the foreign body was a button battery (like those used in watches).
• Review treatment plan, signs and symptoms of deterioration, and actions to take. Document patient's understanding of options, treatment regimen recommended, and expected outcomes. Also document responsible party's agreement (or disagreement) with recommendation.

BIBLIOGRAPHY

Alvi, A., Bereliani, A., & Zahtz, G. D. (1997). Miniature disc battery in the nose: A dangerous foreign body. *Clinical Pediatrics, 36*(7), 427–429.

American Medical Association. (1998). *Physicians' current procedural terminology: CPT.* Chicago: American Medical Association.

Backlin, S. A. (1995). Postive-pressure techinque for nasal foreign body removal in children. *Annals of Emergency Medicine, 24*(4), 554–555.

Healthcare Consultants of America. (1998). *1998 Physicians' fee and coding guide,* Augusta, GA.

Kadish, H. A. & Corneli, H. M. (1997). Removal of nasal foreign bodies in the pediatric population. *American Journal of Emergency Medicine, 15*(1), 54–56.

Lowe, S. & Saxe, J. M. (1999). *Microscopic procedures for primary care providers.* Philadelphia: Lippincott Williams & Wilkins.

Pfaff, J. A. & Moore, G. P. (1997). Eye, ear, nose, and throat. *Emergency Medical Clnics of North America, 15*(2), 327–340.

Simon, R., & Brenner, B. (1994). *Emergency procedures and techniques.,* Baltimore: Williams & Wilkins.

chapter 29

Foreign Body: Throat

CPT Coding:

43215 Esophagoscopy with removal of foreign body ($790–$950)
74235 Removal of foreign body, radiological supervision ($545–650)
42809 Removal of foreign body from pharynx ($194–$230)

● DEFINITION

- Removal of a foreign body from the oropharynx or pharynx.

● INDICATIONS

- Sensation of something in the throat.
- History suggestive of a plausible mechanism of injury (or caregiver observed child place something in his or her mouth and the child is coughing, gagging, drooling, or otherwise exhibiting behavior suggestive of a retained foreign body).

● PATIENT EDUCATION

- Assess patient's (or caregiver's) knowledge base.
- Reassure patient regarding procedure.
- Provide anticipatory guidance and continually assess comfort and anxiety level.

● ASSESSMENT

1. Note baseline vital signs.
2. Elicit history (timing, related factors, self-care measures attempted).
3. Evaluate need for anxiolytics or local anesthetic (benzocaine [Cetacaine] or lidocaine gel).
4. Inspect oropharynx carefully to rule out abscess. (Tenderness on palpation is an unreliable sign.)

● DEVELOPMENTAL CONSIDERATIONS

Child: Toddlers are most likely to put something in their mouth. Infants and toddlers may be best treated lying on examiner's lap, tilted downward. Make sure the child is sufficiently immoblized. Use of a sheet or papoose board may be needed (see Chapter 50: Child Restraint).

EQUIPMENT

- Bayonet or alligator forceps
- Anesthetic (Cetacaine or lidocaine gel)

PROCEDURE	SPECIAL CONSIDERATIONS
Approach relaxed, cooperative adult with a calm manner.	To decrease gagging, distract adult by deflecting attention, "Open your eyes wider, wider, WIDER."
Reevaluate need for local anesthetic.	
If object is visualized, remove with grasper of choice (bayonet or alligator forceps).	
Consider direct laryngoscopy. (Pooling at indirect laryngoscopy is predictive of retained object.) Small endoscopes with grasper attachments are available for direct visualization and retrieval.	
Evaluate for need for radiographs to rule out soft tissue swelling, although x-rays studies improve management in only a few cases.	Aluminum pull-tabs from soft drink cans are not readily detectable by x-ray.

ALTERNATIVE PROCEDURE

A technique of using a 16-French Foley catheter has been used successfully. The use of a fluoroscopy table is required. Spray the oropharynx with a local anesthetic. Preinflating the catheter balloon with contrast material helps with fluoroscopic identification. The full catheter is inserted through the mouth. After the tip of the catheter is past the foreign body, the balloon is inflated. At this time, the patient is placed in the prone oblique position in a steep head-down position. The catheter is then withdrawn with moderate, steady traction, which pulls the foreign body ahead of the balloon. If steady traction does not dislodge the foreign body, then IV glucagon can be used to relax the esophagus. If this measure does not work, an endoscopy will need to be performed (Simon & Brenner, 1994).

FOLLOW-UP

- If no object is found, consider using a barium swallow to detect some other type of lesion.
- Suggest local treatment, such as cool fluids or topical anesthetics.
- Review treatment plan, signs and symptoms of deterioration (especially inability to properly handle secretions and any sign of respiratory embarrassment), and actions to take. Document patient's understanding of options,

treatment regimen recommended, and expected outcomes. Also document patient's agreement (or disagreement) with recommendation.

BIBLIOGRAPHY

American Medical Association. (1998). *Physicians' current procedural terminology: CPT.* Chicago: American Medical Association.

Jones, N. S., Lannigan, F. J., & Salama, N. Y. (1991). Foreign bodies in the throat: A prospective study of 388 cases. *Journal of Laryngology and Otology, 105*(2), 104–108.

Hilton, M. M. (1996). An unusual site to find a "swallowed" foreign body. *Journal of Accident and Emergency Medicine, 13*(4), 304.

Simon, R. & Brenner, B. (1994). *Emergency Procedures and Techniques.* Baltimore: Williams & Wilkins.

Stewart, G. D., Lakshmi, M. V., & Jackson, A. (1994). Aluminum ring pulls: An invisible foreign body. *Journal of Accident and Emergency Medicine, 11*(3), 201–203.

chapter
30
Tympanometry

CPT Coding:

92567 Tympanometry (impedance testing) ($32–$38)
92568 Tympanometry with acoustic reflex ($29–$32)

◉ DEFINITION

• Tympanometry is used to assess the movement of the tympanic membrane. The movement is translated into a graph called a tympanogram.

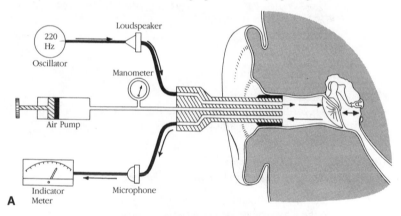

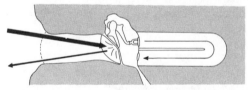

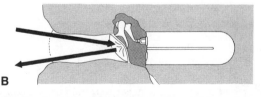

A) In tympanometry, the variable reflection of the probe tone is based on compliance. B) Schematic of a tympanometer. (Lohr, Jacob A. [1991]. *Pediatric outpatient procedures.* Philadelphia: J.B. Lippincott Company.)

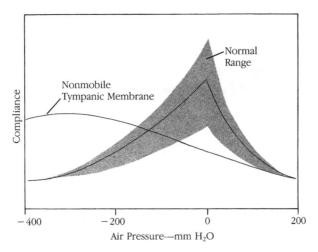

Tympanogram showing compliance as a function of pressure. (Lohr, Jacob A. [1991]. *Pediatric outpatient procedures*. Philadelphia: J.B. Lippincott Company.)

INDICATIONS

- Persistent otitis media with effusion
- Uncertainty regarding the physical examination of the tympanic membrane
- Confirmation of middle ear pathology

DEVELOPMENTAL CONSIDERATIONS

Child: Tympanometry is difficult to use in children younger than 6 months of age related to the hypercompliant condition of the ear canal (Lohr, 1991).

The child should remain still and preferably not crying. Usually, patients older than 3 years of age are more cooperative with the procedure.

 ALERT: Do not perform tympanometry if the patient had ear surgery within 4 to 6 weeks (Lohr, 1991).

PATIENT EDUCATION

- Explain the purpose of the procedure.
- The patient will feel slight pressure in the ear canal related to changes in air pressure during the procedure.
- Inform the patient that he or she needs to refrain from talking, chewing gum, crying, or yawning during the procedure.

ASSESSMENT

1. History of recurrent otitis media.
2. History of hearing loss or hearing loss detected with an audioscope.
3. Perform otoscopic examination and assess for movement of the tympanic membrane with pneumatic otoscopy.
4. Examine the middle ear for air–fluid level and retraction or perforation of tympanic membrane.

EQUIPMENT

• Tympanometer (MicroTymp 2) with tip. There are different types of tympanometers; review instructions before performing procedure.

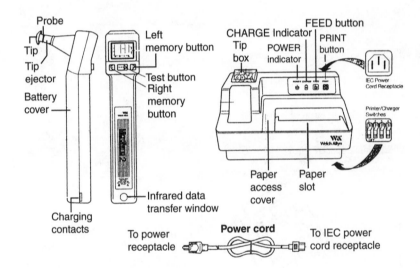

Tympanometer.

PROCEDURE	SPECIAL CONSIDERATIONS
Examine the patient's ear canal to determine the size of tip. If the patient has an increased amount of cerumen, remove it before performing test.	Select a tip that is large enough to seal the opening of the ear canal.

(procedure continued)

| PROCEDURE | SPECIAL CONSIDERATIONS |

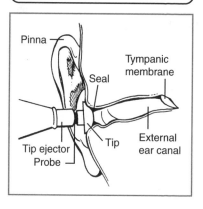

An incorrect tip size will cause a leak, making the test difficult.

Push the tip onto the probe, making sure the tip is attached correctly.

Turn on the handle by pressing the TEST button.

OPEN should appear.

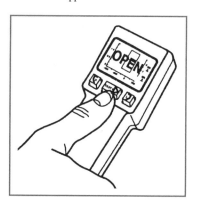

Patient should be seated. If the child is young, they may sit in parent's lap.

Grasp patient's pinna, pull up and back for adults, pull gently back to straighten child's ear canal.

(procedure continued)

| PROCEDURE | SPECIAL CONSIDERATIONS |

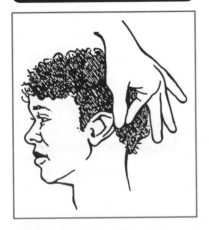

Maintain tension on the pinna while pressing the tip into the ear canal. Point the tip straight into the ear canal for adults and anteriorly for children.

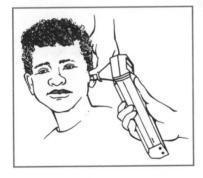

If a proper seal is obtained, look for TEST message and +200 Vea scale. Data points should be displayed from right to left as the test continues.

The test is complete when the last data point is displayed.

If LEAK, BLOCK, or OPEN message appears, reposition the tip and start again.

If the patient or instrument causes a leak, the test will be stopped but the data will be saved.

(procedure continued) ─────────────────────────────

| PROCEDURE | SPECIAL CONSIDERATIONS |

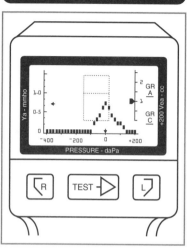 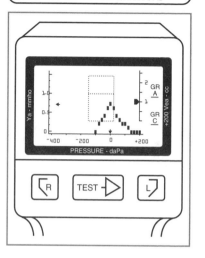

To store the results of the test, press button
related to ear that was tested.

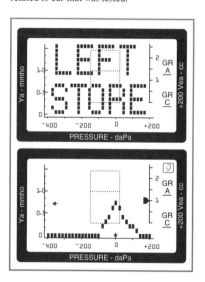

Print graph to interpret results.

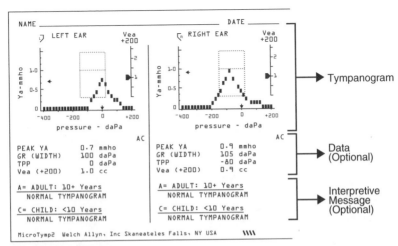

PEAK YA	0.7 mmho	PEAK YA	0.9 mmho
GR (WIDTH)	100 daPa	GR (WIDTH)	105 daPa
TPP	0 daPa	TPP	-80 daPa
Vea (+200)	1.0 cc	Vea (+200)	0.9 cc

A= ADULT: 10+ Years — NORMAL TYMPANOGRAM
C= CHILD: <10 Years — NORMAL TYMPANOGRAM

A= ADULT: 10+ Years — NORMAL TYMPANOGRAM
C= CHILD: <10 Years — NORMAL TYMPANOGRAM

→ Tympanogram

→ Data (Optional)

→ Interpretive Message (Optional)

MicroTymp2 Welch Allyn, Inc Skaneateles Falls, NY USA

Data Section of Printout

The data section displays numeric values for the four key characteristics of the tympanogram:

- **Peak Ya** – the compensated static acoustic admittance (height) of the peak, measured in acoustic millimhos (mmho).
- **Gradient (GR)** – the width of the tympanogram; the distance across the tympanogram measured at a height 50% down from the peak, measured in decapascals (daPa).
- **Tympanic Peak Pressure (TPP)** – where the tympanometric peak occurred on the pressure axis, measured in decapascals (daPa).
- **Volume of the Ear Canal (Vea)** – acoustically-determined ear canal volume, measured in cubic centimeters (cc) at +200 daPa.

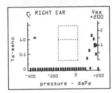

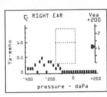

Positive Middle Ear Pressure
- Produces positive Tympanometric Peak Pressure
- Indicative of acute otitis media, if peak is extremely positive

Tympanogram with Too Much Artifact
- Caused by patient or practitioner movement
- Requires repeating measurement

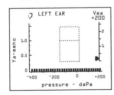

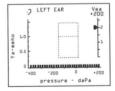

Ear Canal Occlusion
- Can produce flat tympanogram with ear canal volume lower than expected
- May also produce BLOCK message
- Requires repeating measurement

Patent Tympanostomy Tube or perforated Tympanic Membrane
- Can produce flat tympanogram with ear canal volume higher than expected
- May also produce OPEN message

Interpreting a tympanogram. (Courtesy of Welch Allyn.)

• If you are using another tympanogram, the graph will look like this:

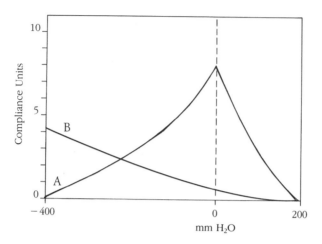

Normal tympanogram, type A; abnormal tympanogram, type B. (Lohr, Jacob A. [1991]. *Pediatric outpatient procedures.* Philadelphia: J.B. Lippincott Company.)

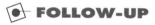

FOLLOW-UP

• Interpret results related to recurrent infections and hearing loss.
• Consider referral to an ear, nose, and throat (ENT) specialist.

BIBLIOGRAPHY

American Medical Association. (1998). *Physicians' current procedural terminology: CPT.* Chicago: American Medical Association.
Healthcare Consultants. (1998). *1998 Physicians' fee and coding guide.* Augusta, GA.
Lohr, J. A. (1991). *Pediatric outpatient procedures* Philadelphia: J. B. Lippincott.

chapter 31

Visual Evaluation

CPT Coding:

Visual acuity is not billed separately; it is considered part of the clinical examination

● DEFINITIONS

- Visual evaluation includes testing for visual acuity, cardinal fields of gaze, field defects, and color vision.
- Stabismus is misalignment of the eyes.
- Amblyopia is difference in the visual abilities of each eye. Suspected when there are more than two or more levels of difference between eyes on visual acuity test. The leading cause of nonocular vision loss in people between 20 and 70 years of age (Broderick, 1998).
- Visual fields are also known as peripheral vision.
- Cardinal fields of gaze tests the integrated function of the six extraocular eye muscles and three cranial nerves:
  - III: oculomotor
  - IV: trochlear
  - VI: abducens

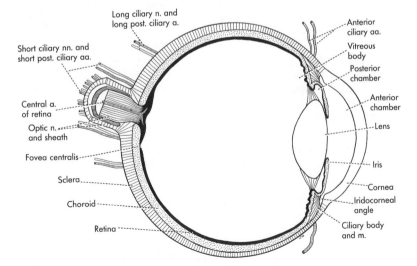

Schema of the eyeball in the horizontal section. (Rosse, C. & Gaddum-Rosse, P. (1997). *Hollinshead's textbook of anatomy.* Philadelphia: Lippincott-Raven Publishers.)

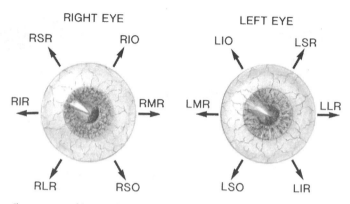

The primary actions of the extraocular muscles. Left eye: LSR, left superior rectus; LLR, left lateral rectus; LIR, left inferior rectus; LSO, left superior oblique; LMR, left medial rectus; LIO, left inferior oblique. Right eye: RIO, right inferior oblique; RMR, right medial rectus; RSO, right superior oblique; RLR, right lateral rectus; RIR, right inferior rectus; RSR, right superior rectus. (Bartley [1992]. *Essentials of ophthalmology.*)

- Color testing consists of colored dots arranged in such a way that patients with abnormal color discrimination cannot read them. Each test has very specific directions for testing.
- Visual acuity tests central vision and primarily cranial nerve II (optic nerve). Measured as a fraction in which the numerator indicates distance of the patient from the chart (usually 20 feet) and the denominator indicates the distance a normal eye can read the line. The smaller the fracture, the worse the myopia. A person whose vision is not corrected to better than 20/200 is considered legally blind.

⊙ INDICATIONS

- All patients who present with red eye or eye complaints
- Parental suspicion of visual or alignment abnormality
- Visual acuity: Perform the test as soon as children are able to cooperate and follow directions.
- Before beginning school
- History of ocular trauma
- During well-child checks
- Work or Department of Transportation (DOT) physicals
- Patients at risk for eye disorders: positive family history of eye misalignment

⊙ PATIENT EDUCATION

- Describe the importance of identifying eye problems as soon as they develop.

ASSESSMENT

1. Determine whether or not there are any eye complaints. Identify when the difficulty was first noticed
2. Discuss mechanism of injury: foreign body, trauma, occupational, and so on.
3. Determine when last eye exam was done
4. Determine if the patient normally wears corrective lenses: glasses, contacts
5. Past medical history: past surgery of eye, including refractive surgery (radial keratotomy [RK], laser, and so on)
6. Past medical history: diabetes or thyroid, preterm birth
7. Complete a thorough eye exam, including an external exam, visual testing, and ophthalmoscopic examination.

 DEVELOPMENTAL CONSIDERATIONS

Infant: Term infants have a visual acuity of about 20/200. Peripheral vision is well developed, but central vision does not develop until later. At age 2 to 3 months infants gain voluntary control of the eye muscles. Colors can be differentiated by about 8 months. A single image can be perceived by about 9 months. Infants shut their eyes tightly when an eye examination is attempted. It is difficult to separate the eyelids.

Child: Visual acuity is tested when the child is cooperative and can follow directions, usually about 3 years of age. Expected normal visual acuity for children is

- 3 years 20/50
- 4 years 20/40
- 5 years 20/30
- 6 years 20/20

Approximately 5% to 10% of children have vision problems. Up to 3% of children younger than 6 years of age have strabismus; up to 40% of these children develop amblyopia.

Pregnant women: Mild corneal edema occurs, especially in the third trimester. Changes may be seen in the visual acuity during pregnancy. However, no prescription changes should be made during pregnancy; wait at least 1 month after delivery for any changes to be made.

Elderly: A decrease in the flexibility of the lens and weakening of the ciliary muscle of the iris around the age of 45, known as presbyopia, decreases an individual's ability to see near objects. The lens continues to develop fibers, which are compressed centrally. These changes may cause loss of integrity of the lens and contribute to cataract formation. Increased intraocular pressure may also occur with aging, leading to glaucoma. Risk factors for glaucoma include age greater than 40 years, family history of glaucoma, black race, and diabetes.

◉ EQUIPMENT

- Penlight
- Snellen, Illiterate E chart, picture chart

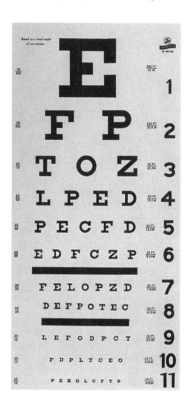 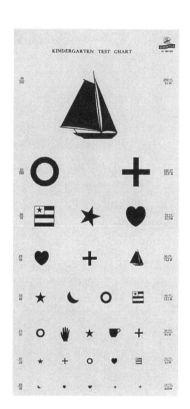

- Ishihara or Hardy-Rand-Rittler plates for color vision
- Near-vision chart for adults (Rosenbaum Pocket Visual Screener)
- Cotton wisp
- Eye cover
- Testing for visual acuity

PROCEDURE	SPECIAL CONSIDERATIONS
Position the patient 20 feet away from the Snellen, Illiterate E, or picture charts. Test each eye separately. Cover one eye with an opaque card. Ask the patient to identify all the letters beginning at any line. Determine the smallest line in which the patient can identify all the letters and record the visual	Make sure the area is well lit. Use the Allen object recognition chart for preliterate young children or older children with mental disabilities. Always test without glasses first. When testing the second line, have the patient read from right to left.

(procedure continued)

PROCEDURE	SPECIAL CONSIDERATIONS
acuity. Using the Illiterate E, have the patient point his or her fingers in the direction of the E on the chart. Demonstrate how to do it first.	Make sure not to hurry the patient when asking the letters.
	A difference of two lines between the scores for each eye should make you suspect amblyopia (for example 20/30 and 20/50). It is important to detect and treat amblyopia as early as possible to prevent blindness.
Near vision: Use a hand-held card such as the Rosenbaum Pocket Visual Screener. Have the patient read the smallest line possible.	Make sure the card is held the correct distance (approximately 14 inches) from the patient.

TESTING FOR VISUAL FIELDS (PERIPHERAL VISION)

PROCEDURE	SPECIAL CONSIDERATIONS
Sit or stand opposite the patient at eye level, approximately 30 inches apart. Have the patient cover the right eye while you cover your left eye (the open eyes are directly opposite). Extend your hand so that it is midway between the patient and yourself. Move your fingers centrally with the fingers wiggling. Have the patient tell you when he or she is able to see the fingers. Compare the patient's vision with your own.	Sophisticated instruments are available to check visual fields. Expected fields of vision (rough estimate): 60 degrees nasally 90 degrees temporally 50 degrees superiorly 70 degrees inferiorly

BINOCULAR ALIGNMENT

• Hirschberg corneal light reflex test

PROCEDURE	SPECIAL CONSIDERATIONS
Look for obvious deviation of one eye. If there is a misalignment, have the child look up, down, right, and left to determine whether the deviation is the same in all fields. Observe the corneal light reflection in each eye. If you	Esotropia is a nasal or inward deviation. It is the most common primary strabismus in children. Hold light approx. 10″ away from patient in the midline and at eye level.

(procedure continued)

PROCEDURE	SPECIAL CONSIDERATIONS
are not sure if a deviation exists, do the cover/uncover test described below.	Looking for a corneal light reflection is a way to determine whether a more subtle deviation is present.

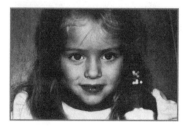

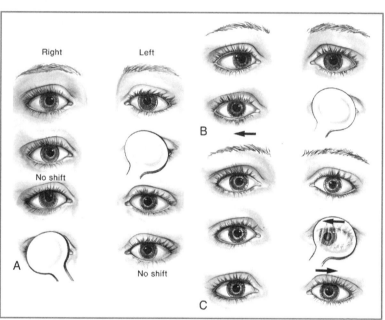

 COVER/UNCOVER TEST

PROCEDURE	SPECIAL CONSIDERATIONS
Have the child stare at a light source approximately 12 inches away. Cover the right eye. Watch for any movement in the left eye.	The cover/uncover test is a more sensitive test for strabismus.

(procedure continued)

PROCEDURE	SPECIAL CONSIDERATIONS
Now move the cover to the left eye. Watch for any movement in the right eye.	Movement of the left eye indicates an abnormal response.
Repeat the test covering and uncovering the left eye.	Any movement (especially if there was left eye movement) indicates that the right eye needs a constant visual stimulus to remain fixated.
	Refer the patient to an ophthalmologist if strabismus is identified.

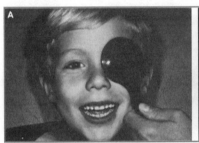
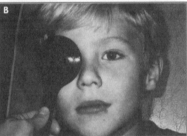

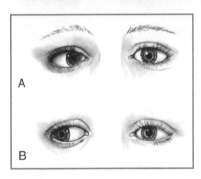

SUMMARY OF TESTING BY AGE GROUP

Age Group	Testing Procedures	Specifics of Testing	Referral Needed
Infants and newborns	Test eye fixation on an object Test ability to track object (age 6 months)	Hold the infant upright and slowly move your face in front of the infant. Normal response is to follow your face.	No synchronous eye movement by age 5 months to 6 months.

table continued

Age Group	Testing Procedures	Specifics of Testing	Referral Needed
	Cover/uncover test	Use three fingers placed in front of one eye. Look at the other eye as a face or object is moved in front of it.	If either of these tests are abnormal, refer the patient to ophthalmologist.
	PERRLA (pupils round, react to light and accommodation)	Checks third cranial nerve function.	
	Visual field testing	Shine a light at the periphery of vision. The infant should turn his or her head in that direction.	
	Funduscopy	Deferred until the child is 2–6 months old due to the difficulty of opening the eye (American Academy of Ophthalmology recommends fundus exam at age 3 to 4 years).	
	Red reflex—bilateral evaluations	These evaluations should be performed in every newborn. Observe for opacities, or dark or white spots. These spots may indicate congenital cataracts or retinoblastoma.	No red reflex seen.
Young children	Check vision in each eye and visual field defects	Use a favorite toy to attract the child's attention. Cover one eye and pass the toy from the periphery into each of the visual fields. The child will respond with facial brightening or making noises. Repeat with the other eye. The child may cry if the normal eye is covered.	
	Strabismus	Have child look at an object (toy or mother) in distance. Shine a light on the cornea. The reflection should be symmetric. Momentary eye wandering is common up to 3 to 4 months of age.	

table continued

Age Group	Testing Procedures	Specifics of Testing	Referral Needed
Older children	Test visual acuity	Use Illiterate E or picture chart. Review the names of objects prior to using the picture chart. Depending on the child's exposure he/she may not know the names of the items.	<4/6 correct on 20-foot line or two-line difference between eyes.
	Visual fields Strabismus	As described earlier (cover/uncover).	Any eye movement on cover test warrants referral.
Adults	Distance acuity: Snellen Near vision Visual fields Strabismus Color vision (if indicated)	As described earlier Color vision testing: test the patient in a well-lit room, wearing corrective lenses. Record the number of charts that cannot be read.	<4/6 correct on 20-foot line or two-line difference between eyes.

 ALTERNATIVE PROCEDURES

• None

 FOLLOW-UP

• Any abnormal findings detected on visual testing should be referred for further testing and evaluation to an ophthalmologist.

BIBLIOGRAPHY

American Medical Association. (1998). *Physicians' current procedural terminology: CPT*. Chicago: American Medical Association.

Broderick, P. (1998). Pediatric vision screening for the family physician. *American Family Physician, 58*(3), 691–704.

Healthcare Consultants of America. (1998). *1998 Physicians' fee and coding guide*. Augusta, GA.

Pfenninger, J. & Fowler, G. (1994). *Procedures for primary care physicians*. St. Louis: Mosby.

Seidel, H., Ball, J., Dains, J., & Benedict. G. (1995). *Mosby's guide to physical examination* (3rd ed.). St. Louis: Mosby.

chapter 32

Nebulizer and Metered-Dose Inhaler (MDI)

CPT Coding:

94640 Nonpressurized inhalation treatment for acute airway obstruction ($31–$36)

 DEFINITION

Nebulizers and MDIs deliver medication to the pulmonary system for the treatment of bronchospasm.

 INDICATIONS

- Nebulizers and MDIs are used to treat bronchospasm in children and adults.
- MDIs are also used to deliver steroids, mucolytics, and ergotamine tartrate for migraine headaches.
- Gentamicin and other antibiotic solutions have been used in a nebulized route for antimicrobial therapy.
- Aerosolized racemic epinephrine is employed to treat croup, and aerosolized pentamidine can be used in the treatment of *Pneumocystis carinii* pneumonia.

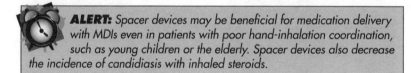

ALERT: Spacer devices may be beneficial for medication delivery with MDIs even in patients with poor hand-inhalation coordination, such as young children or the elderly. Spacer devices also decrease the incidence of candidiasis with inhaled steroids.

 ASSESSMENT

1. Ventilatory function
2. Precipitating factors
3. Duration of current episode
4. History of similar episodes
5. Need for prior hospitalization

6. Current medical regimen and compliance
7. Family history
8. History of coronary artery disease (CAD), pulmonary emboli, and smoking (pack per day [ppd]/years)
9. Physical exam: note patient's general appearance, level of distress, mental status, vital signs, skin color, character of effort, use of accessory muscles, lung sounds (such as wheezing and crackles), and vital signs.

 ALERT: Oxygen-powered nebulization may be contraindicated in the case of CO_2-retaining patients.

PATIENT EDUCATION

• Emphasize the need to perform proper technique.
• Identify completion of treatment.
• Identify complications associated with medication.

EQUIPMENT

• Nebulizer machine
• 1–3 mL of beta-agonist with normal saline
• Mouthpiece or ventilation mask

PROCEDURE	SPECIAL CONSIDERATIONS
Have patient inhale slowly and deeply.	Continue to monitor patient's mental and respiratory status.

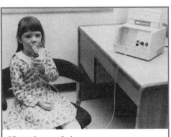

Via t-tube mouthpiece.

(procedure continued)

PROCEDURE	SPECIAL CONSIDERATIONS

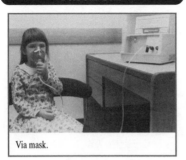

Via mask.

Patient needs to inhale slowly and deeply repeatedly until the medication delivery has been completed. An audible click will indicate that the medication is completed.

Once the treatment is completed, reassess the patient for improvement of condition.

Can repeat the nebulizer treatment, if necessary.

Common side effects of medication include nervousness, dizziness, palpitations, tachycardia, hypertension, diaphoresis, and tachypnea.

(Figures from: Lohr, Jacob A. [1991]. *Pediatric outpatient procedures.* Philadelphia: J.B. Lippincott Company.)

FOLLOW-UP

- Encourage compliance with medical regimen.
- Return for exacerbation of condition, complications with device, or prolonged side effects from medication.
- Refer to the emergency department for acute exacerbation of condition without relief from nebulizer treatments.
- Schedule return office visit after 1 to 2 weeks for reevaluation.

METERED-DOSE INHALER USE

- An MDI may be used as an alternative treatment for bronchospasm.

PATIENT EDUCATION

- Emphasize the need to follow proper technique.
- Emphasize frequency and compliance with treatments.
- Provide information regarding environmental conditions causing exacerbations.
- Provide instructions on how the device works and the use of spacers and masks to assist in the delivery of medication.

• Demonstrate how to test for quantity of medication remaining in inhaler.
• Identify complications related to delivery of medications.

⟨●⟩ EQUIPMENT

• MDI

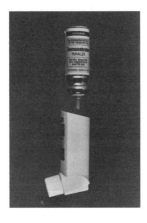

Metered dose inhaler. (Lohr, Jacob A. [1991]. *Pediatric outpatient procedures.* Philadelphia: J.B. Lippincott Company.)

• Spacer (the tube type)

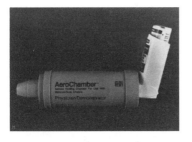

Spacer attached to metered dose inhaler. (Lohr, Jacob A. [1991]. *Pediatric outpatient procedures.* Philadelphia: J.B. Lippincott Company.)

PROCEDURE	SPECIAL CONSIDERATIONS
Shake well several times. Remove the protective cap from the MDI. Check the mouthpiece for foreign material.	With aerosol medications that are being used for the first time or have not been used for a period of time, spray into the air initially.
	The tube spacer can be constructed with a mask to fit infants, children, and elderly patients. This system maximizes drug delivery to those who can tolerate a face mask but cannot use the mouthpiece of the standard MDI device.

(procedure continued)

PROCEDURE	SPECIAL CONSIDERATIONS
Have the patient breathe out. Place the MDI at the designated soft end of the spacer (if using spacer). The patient's mouth is placed at the mouthpiece.	When using the mask, apply gentle pressure against the face, covering the nose and mouth to ensure a good seal is obtained.
Instruct the patient to breathe slowly and deeply through his or her mouth. Have the patient or parent depress the canister completely. Have the patient hold their breath as long as possible. Have patient remove the inhaler before exhaling.	Crying children can still breathe through the mask system. Maintain facial contact after MDI activation until several breaths have been taken.
If it is necessary to repeat the procedure, wait 1 minute and shake the MDI before repeating.	The inhaler device should be cleaned. Remove canister and rinse plastic case and cap in warm water. When it is dry, replace canister and replace cap.

FOLLOW-UP

- Encourage proper technique. Have patient return demonstration.
- Encourage compliance with medical regimen.
- Return for exacerbation of condition, problems with device, or prolonged side effects from medication.
- Understand when to go to the emergency department.

BIBLIOGRAPHY

American Association Respiratory Care. (1996). Clinical practice guidelines: Selection of device for delivery of aerosols. *Respiratory Care, 41*(7), 647–653.

American Association Respiratory Care. (1994). Clinical practice guidelines: Delivery of aerosols. *Respiratory Care, 39*(8), 803–807.

American Medical Association. (1998). *Physicians' current procedural terminology: CPT.* Chicago: American Medical Association.

Healthcare Consultants of America. (1998). *1998 Physicians' fee and coding guide.* Augusta, GA.

Roberts, J. R. & Hedges, J. R. (1998). *Clinical procedures in emergency medicine* (3rd ed.). Philadelphia: W. B. Saunders.

chapter 33

Peak Flowmeter

CPT Coding:

94150 Vital capacity, total ($22–$26)

 ## DEFINITION

Peak flow measurements (PFM) provide a rapid evaluation of airway passages. Peak expiratory flow rate (PEFR) is the quickest expulsion of air forced out after a maximum inspiratory effort.

 ## INDICATIONS

• Because spirometry depends on the effort of the patient, and some patients, specifically children, may not be able to cooperate adequately for valid test results to be obtained, PFMs are recommended. Peak air flow is also reduced in obstruction, and because peak flow measurements do not depend on a sustained effort, this is often a preferable test for measuring the degree of bronchospasm, particularly in children.
• The peak flowmeter is also useful in the assessment of upper airway or laryngeal obstruction.

PATIENT EDUCATION

• Assure the patient that this is a noninvasive test.
• Patient needs to perform peak flow measurement as directed.
• Emphasize the need for accurate record keeping.

ASSESSMENT

1. Ventilatory function is primary assessment
2. Precipitating factors
3. Duration of current episode
4. History of similar episodes
5. Severity of attack in relation to prior episodes
6. Need for prior hospitalizations
7. Current medications and compliance
8. Family history
9. History of coronary artery disease (CAD), pulmonary emboli, smoker(pack per day [ppd]/years)
10. Physical exam: Note general appearance, level of distress, vital signs,

mental status, skin color, character of effort, accessory muscle use, and lung sounds, such as wheezing and crackles.

ALERT: *Inadequate assessment and thus treatment of severe bronchospasm may contribute to an increased mortality rate in these patients.*

 EQUIPMENT

• Peak flowmeter with disposable mouthpiece

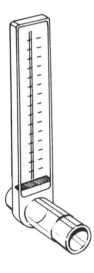

Peak flow meter. (Courtesy of HealthScan Products, Inc.)

PROCEDURE	SPECIAL CONSIDERATIONS
1. The patient should stand.	
2. Have the patient inhale maximally.	Mouth goes around mouthpiece.
3. Place mouthpiece in mouth.	Do not place the tongue in the mouthpiece.
4. Exhale forcibly into the peak flowmeter.	**It is not necessary to make a sustained effort.**
5. Repeat procedure two times.	If the patient coughs or errors occur, rest and instruct to take additional maximum inspiratory effort.
6. Record the best reading.	

Normal Predicted Average Peak Expiratory Flow (liters per minute)

The National Asthma Education and Prevention Program recommends that a patient's "personal best" be used as his/her baseline peak flow. "Personal best" is the maximum peak flow rate that the patient can obtain when his/her asthma is stable or under control. The following tables are intended as guidelines only.

NORMAL MALES*

Age (Years)	Height				
	60" (152)	65" (165)	70" (178)	75" (191)	80" (203)
20	554	575	594	611	626
25	580	603	622	640	656
30	594	617	637	655	672
35	599	622	643	661	677
40	597	620	641	659	675
45	591	613	633	651	668
50	580	602	622	640	656
55	566	588	608	625	640
60	551	572	591	607	622
65	533	554	572	588	603
70	515	535	552	568	582
75	496	515	532	547	560

NORMAL FEMALES*

Age (Years)	Height				
	55" (140)	60" (152)	65" (165)	70" (178)	75" (191)
20	444	460	474	486	497
25	455	471	485	497	509
30	458	475	489	502	513
35	458	474	488	501	512
40	453	469	483	496	507
45	446	462	476	488	499
50	437	453	466	478	489
55	427	442	455	467	477
60	415	430	443	454	464
65	403	417	430	441	451
70	390	404	416	427	436
75	377	391	402	413	422

NORMAL CHILDREN AND ADOLESCENTS[†]

Height (in)	Height (cm)	Males & Females	Height (in)	Height (cm)	Males & Females
43	109	147	55	140	307
44	112	160	56	142	320
45	114	173	57	145	334
46	117	187	58	147	347
47	119	200	59	150	360
48	122	214	60	152	373
49	124	227	61	155	387
50	127	240	62	157	400
51	130	254	63	160	413
52	132	267	64	163	427
53	135	280	65	165	440
54	137	293	66	168	454

* Nunn, AJH, Gregg I: *Brit Med J* 298:1068-1070, 1989.

† Polgar G, Promadhot V: *Pulmonary Function Testing in Children: Techniques and Standards.* Philadelphia, W.B. Saunders Company, 1971.

NOTE: All tables are averages and are based on tests with a large number of people. The peak flow rate of an individual can vary widely. Individuals at altitudes above sea level should be aware that peak flow readings may be lower than those at sea level, which are provided in the tables.

FOLLOW-UP

- The patient is encouraged to notify the health care provider of any changes in respiratory status.
- The patient is instructed on how to record peak flow rate measurements at home.
- To obtain the best PEFR reading, it is recommended to take the measurement once daily when the patient awakens in the morning.
- Bring a copy of the peak flow measurements to each office visit.
- Two ways to establish the patient's best PEFR values include the following:
  - The National Asthma Education Prevention Program (NAEPP) guidelines suggest the patient can estimate his or her best PEFR after 2 to 3 weeks of obtaining morning measurements established by recording the best out of three readings for each morning session. (Measurement is obtained without resetting the PFM indicator after each attempt).
  - The American Thoracic Society (ATS) recommends that the patient record all three readings at each morning monitoring session before establishing a best PEFR value. (Measurement is obtained subsequent to resetting the PFM indicator after each attempt.)

BIBLIOGRAPHY

American Medical Association. (1998). *Physicians' current procedural terminology: CPT.* Chicago: American Medical Association.

American Association Respiratory Care. (1995). Clinical Practice Guideline. *Respiratory Care, 40*(7), 760–768.

Roberts, J. R., Hedges, J. R., (1998). *Clinical procedures in emergency medicine* (3rd ed.). Philadelphia: W. B. Saunders.

chapter 34
Spirometry

CPT Coding:

94010 Spirometry, including graphic record, total and timed vital capacity, expiratory flow rate ($98–$118)

DEFINITION

• Spirometry is the measurement of lung volumes, capacities, and flow rates obtained through a forced expiratory maneuver to analyze the extent and severity of airway obstruction and the restriction of the amount of air that can be expired. A graphic representation (a spirogram) of the maneuver should be a part of the results. Either a volume-time or flow-volume display is acceptable.

CHART 34-1   Combinations of Symbols and Abbreviations

Blood gas symbols may be combined in the following ways:

P_{O_2} = Oxygen tension or partial pressure of oxygen

Pa_{O_2} = Arterial oxygen tension or partial pressure of oxygen in arterial blood

$P_{A_{O_2}}$ = Alveolar oxygen tension or partial pressure of oxygen in the alveoli

P_{CO_2} = Carbon dioxide tension or partial pressure of carbon dioxide

Pa_{CO_2} = Partial pressure of carbon dioxide in arterial blood

Pv_{CO_2} = Partial pressure of carbon dioxide in venous blood

S_{O_2} = Oxygen saturation

pH = Hydronium (hydrogen) ion concentration

pH_a = Hydronium (hydrogen) ion concentration in arterial blood

Sa_{O_2} = Percentage saturation of oxygen in arterial blood as measured by hemoximetry (direct method)

Sv_{O_2} = Percentage saturation of oxygen in venous blood

Sp_{O_2} = Percentage saturation of oxygen in arterial blood as determined by pulse oximetry (indirect method)

Tc_{O_2} = Total carbon dioxide content

(From: Fischbach, F. [1996] A Manual of Laboratory & Diagnostic Tests (5th ed.). Philadelphia: Lippincott-Raven.

• The objective of spirometry is to assess ventilatory function. Spirometry includes, but is not limited to, the measurement of forced vital capacity (FVC), the forced expiratory volume in the first second (FEV_1), and other forced expiratory flow measurements of maximum voluntary ventilation (MVV).

CHART 34-2   LUNG VOLUME SYMBOLS:
PULMONARY FUNCTION
TERMINOLOGY

This list indicates terms used in measuring lung volumes as well as the units used in expressing these measurements.

FVC = *Forced vital capacity:* maximal amount of air that can be exhaled forcibly and completely following a maximal inspiration (units; L)

FEV_1 = *Forced expiratory volume* in 1 second: volume of air expired during the first second of the FVC maneuver (units: L)

FEV_3 = *Forced expiratory volume* in 3 seconds: volume of air expired during the first 3 seconds of the FVC maneuver (units: L)

FEV_1/FVC = Ratio of a timed forced expiratory volume to the forced vital capacity (eg, FEV_1/FVC) (units: percent)

$FEF_{200-1200}$ = *Forced expiratory flow* between 200 mL and 1200 mL flow of expired air measured after the first 200 mL and during the next 1000 mL of the FVC maneuver (units: L/sec)

FEF_{25-75} = *Forced expiratory flow* between 25% and 75%: flow of expired air measured between 25% and 75% of the FVC maneuver (units: L/sec)

PEFR = *Peak expiratory flow rate:* maximum flow of expired air attained during an FVC maneuver (units: L/sec or L/min)

PIFR = *Peak inspiratory flow rate:* maximum flow of inspired air achieved during a forced maximal inspiration (units: L/sec or L/min)

FEF_{25} = Instantaneous flow rate at 25% of lung volume achieved during an FVC maneuver (units: L/sec or L/min)

FEF_{50} = Instantaneous flow rate at 50% of lung volume achieved during an FVC maneuver (units: L/sec or L/min)

FEF_{75} = Instantaneous flow rate at 75% of lung volume achieved during an FVC maneuver (units: L/sec or L/min)

FIVC = *Forced inspiratory vital capacity:* maximal amount of air that can be inhaled forcibly and completely following a maximal expiration (units: L)

FRC = *Functional residual capacity:* volume of air remaining in the lung at the end of a normal expiration (units: L)

IC = *Inspiratory capacity:* maximal amount of air that can be inspired from end tidal expiration (units: L)

IRV	= *Inspiratory reserve volume:* maximal amount of air that can be inspired from end tidal inspiration (units: L)
ERV	= *Expiratory reserve volume:* maximal amount of air that can be expired from end tidal expiration (units: L)
RV	= *Residual volume:* volume of gas left in the lung following a maximal expiration (units: L)
VC	= *Vital capacity:* maximal volume of air that can be expired following a maximal inspiration (units: L)
TLC	= *Total lung capacity:* volume of gas contained in the lungs following a maximal inspiration (units: L)
DL_{CO}	= Carbon monoxide diffusing capacity of the lung—rate of diffusion of carbon monoxide across the alveolar–capillary membrane (ie, rate of gas transfer across the alveolar–capillary membrane (units: $mL/mm^{-1}/torr^{-1}$)
D_L/V_A	= Carbon monoxide diffusing capacity per liter of alveolar volume (units: $mL/mm^{-1}/torr^{-1}\ L^{-1}$ of alveolar volume)
CV	= *Closing volume:* volume at which the lower lung zones cease to ventilate, presumably as a result of airway closure (units: percentage of VC)
MVV	= *Maximal voluntary ventilation:* maximal number of liters of air a patient can breathe per minute by a voluntary effort (units: L/min)
VisoV̇	= *Volume of isoflow:* volume in which flow was the same with air and with helium during an FVC maneuver (units: L/min)

(From: Fischbach, F. [1996] A Manual of Laboratory & Diagnostic Tests (5th ed.). Philadelphia: Lippincott-Raven.

 ALERT: *Spirometry is contraindicated in severe cases of bronchospasm or if the patient is uncooperative.*

 INDICATIONS

- Assessment of pulmonary function
- Quantify the severity of known lung disease
- Assess the change in lung function over time or following administration of, or change in, therapy
- Assess the potential effects or response to environmental or occupational exposure
- Assess the risk of surgical procedures known to affect lung function
- Assess impairment or disability, or both (eg, rehabilitation, legal reasons, military).

ALERT: Contraindications to performing spirometry are
- Hemoptysis of unknown origin (forced expiratory maneuvers may aggravate the underlying condition)
- Pneumothorax
- Unstable cardiovascular status (forced expiratory maneuver may worsen angina or cause changes in blood pressure) or recent myocardial infarction or pulmonary embolism
- Thoracic, abdominal, or cerebral aneurysms (danger of rupture due to increased thoracic pressure)
- Recent eye surgery (eg, cataract)
- Presence of an acute disease process that might interfere with test performance (eg, nausea, vomiting)

PATIENT EDUCATION

- Explain the purpose and the procedure of the test. Emphasize that this is a noninvasive test; however, it does require cooperation.
- Withhold bronchodilators for 4 to 6 hours before study, if tolerated.

ASSESSMENT

1. Always start with the patient's ventilatory function.
2. Precipitating factors
3. Duration of the current episode
4. History of similar episodes, if so, when was the last episode
5. Severity of attack in relation to prior episodes
6. The need for prior hospitalization
7. Current medication and compliance
8. History of coronary artery disease (CAD), smoking, pulmonary emboli
9. Any complications related to treatments
10. Family history
11. Physical exam: Note general appearance, vital signs, level of distress, mental status, skin color, character of effort, use of accessory muscles, presence of diaphoresis, lung sounds (such as local or diffuse wheezing), extent of air movement.

 ALERT: Inadequate assessment of bronchospasm may contribute to an increased rate of mortality.

 ALERT: Patients may experience some lightheadedness and shortness of breath. These symptoms are usually brief. If they are severe, testing is terminated.

DEVELOPMENTAL CONSIDERATIONS

Physical impairment and younger age may limit the patient's ability to perform spirometry.

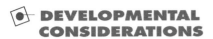 EQUIPMENT

• Disposable mouthpiece connected to spirometer
• A nose clip is encouraged so that only mouth breathing is possible.

PROCEDURE	SPECIAL CONSIDERATIONS
1. Have the patient inhale maximally, holding his or her breath momentarily.	The patient may be sitting or standing.
2. Follow with a forcible, maximal exhalation.	
3. Allow the patient to rest.	
4. Repeat the procedure twice.	A minimum of three tracings need to be obtained. The two best should compare within 5% of one another (Fischbach, 1996). Spirometry can be performed before and after adminstration of a bronchodilator. Wait 15 minutes to perform testing.
A minimum of three acceptable FVC maneuvers should be performed. If a subject is unable to perform a single acceptable maneuver after eight attempts, testing may be discontinued.	Acceptability includes no hesitation or false start; no cough, especially during the first second of the maneuver; and no early termination of exhalation (a minimum exhalation time of 6 seconds is recommended).

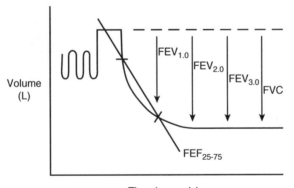

Typical volume-time spirogram illustrating the measurements of FVC, FEV_1, FEV_2, FEV_3, and FEF_{25-75}.

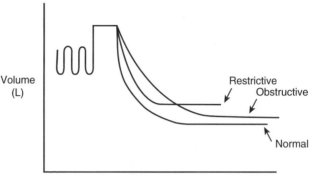

Examples of normal, obstructive, and restrictive volume-time spirograms.

⬤ FOLLOW-UP

• Evaluate complaints of fatigue, shortness of breath, or chest pain or discomfort.
• Monitor and provide rest, as necessary.
• Patient should be sent directly to the emergency department for unresolved respiratory distress.
• Referral to a pulmonary specialist is recommended for advanced or unknown pulmonary disease.

BIBLIOGRAPHY

American Association for Respiratory Care. (1991). Clinical practice guideline: Spirometry. *Respiratory Care, 136,* 1414–1417.

American Medical Association. (1998). *Physicians' current procedural terminology: CPT.* Chicago: American Medical Association.

American Thoracic Society. (1995). Standardization of spirometry: 1994 update. *American of Journal Respiratory Care Medicine, 15*(3), 1107–1136.

Fischbach, F. (1996). *A manual of laboratory diagnostic tests* (5th ed.). Philadelphia: J. B. Lippincott.

Healthcare Consultants of America (1998). *1998 Physicians' fee and coding guide.* Augusta, GA.

Morrissey, W. L., Smith, M. D., & Matthew, H. (1992). Inhalation techniques and oxygen delivery. In *Current Emergency Diagnosis and Treatment* (4th ed.), Saunders, C., Ho, M. (eds). Norwalk, CT: Appleton and Lang, 30–32.

Respiratory Care. (1996): American Association for Respiratory Care—Clinical practice guidelines. *Respiratory Care, 41*(7), 629–636.

Roberts, J. R., Hedges, J. R. (1998). *Clinical procedures in emergency medicine* (3rd ed.). Philadelphia: W. B. Saunders.

chapter
35

Anoscopy

CPT Coding:

46600 Anoscopy, diagnostic, with or without collection of specimen(s) by brushing or washing (separate procedure) ($57–$70)

◉ DEFINITION

Anoscopy is the visualization of the anus and distal rectum using a clear plastic speculum and light source.

◉ INDICATIONS

- Rectal bleeding not accounted for by an external hemorrhoid
- Painful defecation
- Suspected rectal fissure, trauma, or foreign body

◉ PATIENT EDUCATION

- Assess patient's knowledge base and ascertain fears.
- Reassure patient regarding procedure.
- Provide anticipatory guidance and continually assess comfort and anxiety level.
- No bowel preparation is needed.

◉ ASSESSMENT

1. Note baseline vital signs.
2. Elicit history (timing; related factors; amount of bleeding, discharge, or pain; associated symptoms; trauma; sexual practices; environmental (especially travel) factors; self-care measures attempted).
3. Examine the perianal and buttocks area for any lesions. Inspect for external hemorrhoids. Have patient bear down gently. Observe character of discharge or blood.

◉ EQUIPMENT

- Rectal anoscope

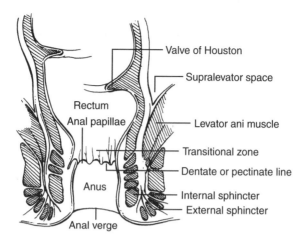

Rectal anatomy.

- Xylocaine gel
- K-Y jelly
- Gloves
- Light source: ordinary flashlight or gooseneck lamp
- Cotton swabs on forceps may be needed to clean the area

PROCEDURE	SPECIAL CONSIDERATIONS
Place patient in left lateral Sims' position.	Consider lubricating finger with xylocaine gel to increase comfort for the patient.

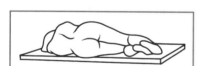

Perform digital exam.

Seat obturator into rectal speculum. Ensure that obturator fits properly without making a sharp edge.

Introduce the well-lubricated speculum and obturator into rectum, with the patient bearing down gently. Direct the anoscope gently toward the midline anteriorly, following the direction of the anal canal. Hold the obturator in place with thumb until the instrument is fully inserted.

(procedure continued)

PROCEDURE	SPECIAL CONSIDERATIONS

Remove obturator. Use a light source to illuminate the rectum, observing for source of bleeding, presence of fissure, or foreign body. Rotate the anoscope 360 degrees to inspect all of the areas of the anus circumferentially.

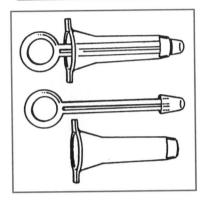

(First figure from: Simon, R. & Brenner, B. [1994]. Emergency procedures and techniques, [3rd ed.]. Baltimore: Williams & Wilkins.)

ALTERNATIVE PROCEDURES

• None

FOLLOW-UP

• If the source of bleeding is not associated with a hemorrhoid (or is continuous), consider double-contrast barium enema and sigmoidoscopy. A gastroenterology consult or referral may be indicated.
• Review the treatment plan, signs and symptoms of deterioration, and actions to take. Document patient's understanding of options, treatment regimen recommended, and expected outcomes. Also, document patient's agreement (or disagreement) with recommendation.

BIBLIOGRAPHY

American Medical Association. (1998). *Physicians' current procedural terminology: CPT.* Chicago: American Medical Association.

Healthcare Consultants of America (1998). *1998 Physicians' Fee and Coding Guide.* Augusta, GA.

Helfand, M., Marton, K. I., Zimmer-Gembeck, M. J., & Sox, H. C. (1997). History of visible rectal bleeding in a primary care population. Initial assessment and 10-year follow up. *Journal of the American Medical Association, 277*(1), 44–48.

Jones, D. J. & Irving, M. H. (1992). ABC of colorectal disease. Investigation of colorectal disorders. *British Medical Journal, 304,* 1312–1313.

Metcalf, J. V., Smith, J., Jones, R., & Record, C. O. (1996). Incidence and causes of rectal bleeding in general practice as detected by colonoscopy. *British Journal of General Practice, 46*(404), 161–164.

Simon, R., & Brenner, B. (1994). *Emergency procedures and techniques* (3rd ed.). Baltimore: Williams & Wilkins.

chapter
36
Arthrocentesis

CPT Coding:

20600 Aspiration of fingers or toes (small joint) ($65–$77)
20605 Aspiration of wrist, ankle, or elbow (intermediate joint)($69–$82)
20610 Aspiration of shoulder, knee, or hip (major joint)($78–$93)

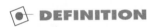 **DEFINITION**

Arthrocentesis is the insertion of a needle into a joint of the body and the withdrawal of fluid.

INDICATIONS

- Decrease a painful acute hemarthrosis or tense effusion
- In suspected joint infection, collect joint fluid for analysis
- Diagnosis of nontraumatic joint disease by analysis of synovial fluid
- Diagnosis of bony or ligamentous injury by confirmation of the presence of blood in the joint
- Intra-articular injection of long-acting corticosteroids
- Through the use of local anesthetics, differentiate the source of pain as intra-articular or extra-articular

 ALERT: Contraindications for arthrocentesis include the following:
- Local infection of the overlying skin
- Severe coagulopathy
- Bacteremia
- Patients receiving anticoagulants
- Uncooperative patients
- Presence of joint prosthesis unless the procedure is being performed to rule out infection

PATIENT EDUCATION

- Explain the procedure and the purpose for performing it.
- Discuss the complications and risks.
- Explain that an anesthetic will make the procedure more tolerable.

ASSESSMENT

1. Perform a history and physical exam on the patient.
2. Determine whether or not the patient has any contraindications for this procedure.
3. Perform an assessment of the particular joint to be injected.
4. Identify the relevant anatomic landmarks.
5. Determine the patient's ability or desire to cooperate during this procedure.

DEVELOPMENTAL CONSIDERATIONS

- Typically used to determine whether or not a child has septic arthritis.
- Perform this technique only when lab results coupled with a thorough history and physical do not produce a clear diagnosis for a child with joint swelling, limited motion, and pain.

EQUIPMENT

- Sterile gloves
- Iodine-based or similar antiseptic solution
- Local anesthetic (1% or 2% lidocaine) and 25-gauge needle with syringe
- 18- to 25-gauge needle of adequate length, 30- to 55-mL syringe, sterile basin, and hemostat
- 2 × 2 gauze pad
- Sterile bandage

PROCEDURE	SPECIAL CONSIDERATIONS
Use sterile technique throughout this procedure.	
Identify the landmarks for the particular joint to be aspirated.	
Cleanse the skin over the site with antiseptic solution.	
Infiltrate the skin with local anesthetic.	
Insert the needle and syringe combination through the same needle tract. Refer to the diagrams and descriptions for specific insertion sites of individual joints to be aspirated.	Avoid striking the periosteum of the adjacent bone ends because of the presence of nerve endings. Be careful not to cut into the articular cartilage of the joint.

(procedure continued)

PROCEDURE	SPECIAL CONSIDERATIONS

Fully aspirate the synovial fluid of this joint. If the synovial fluid stops flowing into the syringe, this may indicate that the joint is fully drained, the needle is clogged with debris, or the needle tip may have exited the joint space into soft tissue. Slight position changes of the needle, rotation of the bevel, or reinjecting some aspirate may alleviate flow problems.

Withdraw the needle and place pressure over the injection site to prevent bleeding.

Cleanse the skin and dress the injection site with a sterile bandage.

Synovial fluid may be examined as the clinical picture warrants. The hemostats may be used to hold the needle if the syringe must be changed during the procedure or if the needle breaks from the hub.

KNEE (MEDIAL APPROACH)

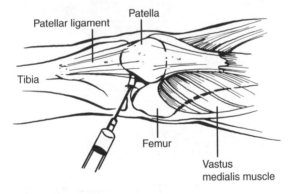

Arthocentesis of the knee joint.

- With the patient supine, extend the legs fully.
- Medial approach to the joint is located at the midpoint of the patella, approximately 1 cm medially to the medial edge.
- Insert an 18-gauge needle between the patella and medial femoral condyle into the joint.

SHOULDER (ANTERIOR APPROACH)

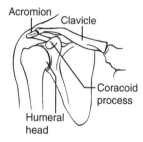

Arthocentesis of the shoulder joint.

- The patient is in a sitting position, with the extremity resting in the lap.
- Palpate the glenohumeral joint, which is 45 degrees inferior and lateral to the coracoid process.
- Insert a 20-gauge needle in an anterior posterior fashion into the joint.

ELBOW

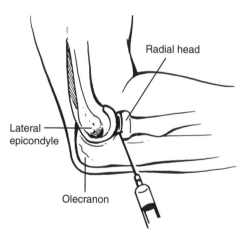

Arthocentesis of the elbow joint.

- The patient is sitting, with the arm flexed to 90 degrees.
- Palpate the tip of the olecranon process and the lateral epicondyle of the humerus.
- Insert a 22-gauge needle at a 45-degree angle and parallel to the radius and ulna at a point halfway between the olecranon process and the medial epicondyle.

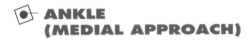

ANKLE (MEDIAL APPROACH)

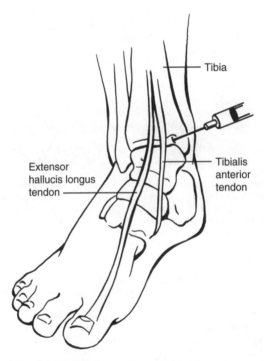

Tibia

Extensor hallucis longus tendon

Tibialis anterior tendon

Arthocentesis of the ankle joint.

- The patient is lying supine, with the ankle in the neutral position.
- Palpate the medial malleolus, the tibialis anterior tendon, extensor hallucis longus tendon, and the dorsalis pedis artery.
- Insert a 20-gauge needle slightly anterior and lateral to the medial malleolus and medial to the extensor hallucis longus tendon, avoiding the dorsalis pedis artery. The needle should be inserted toward the tibiotalar joint.

ALTERNATIVE PROCEDURES

- If the patient does not want an arthrocentesis or has contraindications the use of cold or moist heat, antiinflammatory drugs and non-weight bearing to the affected joint may be helpful in decreasing the joint inflammation.

FOLLOW-UP

- Instruct the patient to contact the health care provider if evidence of infection develops.
- Have the patient contact the health care provider if the joint develops severe pain or redevelops a large amount of joint fluid.

BIBLIOGRAPHY

American Medical Association. (1998). *Physicians' current procedural terminology: CPT.* Chicago: American Medical Association.

Benjamin, G. (1998). Arthrocentesis. In J. R. Roberts & J. R. Hedges (Eds.), *Clinical procedures in emergency medicine* (3rd ed., pp. 919–932). Philadelphia: W. B. Saunders.

Bird, H. (1994). Intra-articular and intralesional therapy. In J. Klippel & P. Dieppe (Eds.), *Rheumatology* (1st ed., pp. 3.7.1–3.7.4). London, UK: Mosby–Year Book Europe Limited.

Coumas, J., Howard, B., & Jacobson, E. (1996). Diagnostic imaging of rheumatologic disorders. In J. Noble (Ed.), *Textbook of primary care medicine* (2nd ed., pp. 962–978). St. Louis, MO: Mosby–Year Book, Inc.

Gatter, R. A. (1996). Arthrocentesis technique and intra-synovial therapy. In W. J. Koopman (Ed.), *Arthritis and allied conditions: A textbook of rheumatology* (13th ed., pp. 751–760). Baltimore, MD: Williams & Wilkins.

Healthcare Consultants of America. (1998). *1998 Physicians' fee and coding guide.* Augusta, GA.

Mosca, V. & Sherry, D. (1990). Juvenile rheumatoid arthritis and seronegative spondyloarthropathies. In R. Morrissy (Ed.), *Lovell and Winter's pediatric orthopedics* (3rd ed., pp. 297–324). Philadelphia: J. B. Lippincott.

Pousada, L. & Osborn, H. (1986). *Emergency medicine for the house officer.* Baltimore, MD: Williams & Wilkins.

Steinbrocker, O. & Neustadt, D. (1972). *Aspiration and injection therapy in arthritis and musculoskeletal disorders.* Hagerstown, MD: Harper & Row.

Snider, R. (1997). *Essentials of musculoskeletal care.* Rosemont, IL: American Academy of Orthopedic Surgeons.

chapter 37

Fracture Immobilization

CPT Coding:

29105 Application of long arm splint (shoulder to hand) ($93–$124)
29125 Application of short arm splint (forearm to hand), static ($65–$79)
29126 As above but dynamic ($85–$105)
29130 Application of finger splint, static ($42–$51)
29131 As above but dynamic ($62–$75)
29200 Strapping, thorax ($47–$56)
29260 Strapping, elbow or wrist ($46–$55)
29280 Strapping, hand or finger ($37–$45)
29505 Application of long leg splint (thigh to ankle or toes) ($96–$115)
29515 Application of short leg splint (calf to foot) ($81–$98)
29540 Strapping, ankle ($48–$58)
29550 Strapping, toes ($42–$50)

DEFINITIONS

- Immobilization is the splinting of fractures and is helpful in the recovery of soft tissue trauma such as sprains and contusions. "Splints are appliances that restrict the mobility of a body part" (Hart, Rittenberry, & Uehara, 1999, p. 92). Immobilization provides comfort (decreases pain) and protects the injured part from further trauma. It also promotes proper healing and minimizes the potential for subsequent neurovascular injury.
- Splints are used for immobilization of injuries. They have the advantage of permitting soft tissue swelling and do not interfere with circulation. These splints are used as an initial immobilization method; a definitive cast is usually applied after the swelling has decreased.
- Dynamic splints are those used for sprains (usually distal interphalangeal [DIP] or proximal interphalangeal [PIP] joints). The injured finger or toe is splinted to the adjacent normal finger or toe, which provides support yet permits motion.
- Other orthopedic definitions:

Condition	Definition
Dislocation	Total disruption of joint with loss of congruity between articulating surfaces.
Subluxation	Partial dislocation. Partial articular contact remains between bone surfaces.

(table continued)

Condition	Definition
Sprain	Tear in the ligamentous fibers that stabilize a joint.
	Grade I: small number of fibers are torn. No ligamentous instability exists, but tenderness and swelling are present.
	Grade II: moderate number of fibers are torn. Some degree of instability noted on exam.
	Grade III: complete disruption of fibers and gross instability on exam.
Strain	Injury to musculotendinous unit that results from stretching or contraction of the muscle.
	Graded from minor to severe, with severe strains involving complete disruption of the muscular unit.

From Hart, R., Rittenberry, T., & Uehara, D. (1999). Handbook of orthopaedic emergencies (p. 15). Philadelphia: Lippincott Williams & Wilkins.

INDICATIONS

- Musculoskeletal injuries that may benefit from short-term immobilization.
- Fractures to maintain alignment of the bony fragments until more definitive treatment (casting) is performed.
- Immobilization allows for more efficient reabsorption of edema and blood.
- Immobilization of fractures decreases the incidence of fat embolism.

PATIENT EDUCATION

- Warn the patient about the feeling of warmth that occurs when the splint is applied and is setting.
- Instruct patients with injuries that have the potential for development of significant swelling (eg, crush injuries, forearm and lower leg fractures) to seek follow-up evaluation in 24 to 48 hours.
- Instruct them to monitor for signs of vascular compromise.
- Discuss proper cast care, such as (give written instructions):
  - Avoiding getting the casting material wet; use a plastic bag to protect the cast when applying ice to the injury.
  - Avoid placing objects under the material to relieve itching.
  - Avoid weight bearing on ankle and foot casts.
  - Do not stress splint for 24 hours because the splint is still "curing" and will not be at its maximal strength for 24 hours.
  - Elevate the extremity as appropriate, applying ice to the affected area.
- Helpful suggestions for activities of daily living (ADLs) include placing a garbage bag over the splint and securing it with rubber bands while bathing.
- Remind the patient not to submerse the splint underwater directly.
- Commercial products are also available for placement over the splint to prevent it from becoming wet.
- If the patient experiences itching, a blow dryer held over the site for a few

seconds may provide some relief. (Warn patients about holding the dryer in one place for too long because burning may occur.)

• Begin rehabilitation exercises as soon as possible after injury to prevent contractures and loss of conditioning.

• Arrange follow-up visit.

ASSESSMENT

1. Obtain a thorough history: allergies, medications, past medical history, last meal, and events preceding the injury.
2. Obtain a history to determine the mechanism of injury.
3. Determine any treatment given before arrival.
4. Ask about prior history of musculoskeletal trauma.
5. Inquire about tetanus toxoid history.
6. Is fracture stable or unstable?
7. Assess for any associated injury to surrounding vessels, skin, nerves, or organs. Remember that hemorrhage may occur with fractures of the femur, pelvis, or multiple fractures.
8. Complete a thorough assessment: five Ps: pain (point tenderness), pallor, pulses, paresthesia, and paralysis. Compare the injured extremity with the noninjured extremity. Look for abnormal angulations, shortening of the extremity, external or internal rotation, crepitus, edema, or exposed bone, tendons, ligaments, or muscle.
9. Review commonly associated injuries of fractures and dislocations.

Fracture/Dislocation	Associated Injury
Clavicular shaft fracture	Subclavian vessels, brachial plexus, acromioclavicular joint
Shoulder dislocation	Brachial plexus, axillary nerve, subclavian vessels
First rib fracture	Subclavian vessels
Midshaft humeral fracture	Radial nerve
Supracondylar humeral fracture	Median nerve, brachial artery
Avulsion fracture of medial epicondyle	Ulnar nerve
Radial head dislocation	Posterior interosseus nerve
Distal radius or ulnar fracture	Median nerve, ulnar nerve
Proximal ulnar shaft fracture	Radial head dislocation
Posterior hip dislocation	Sciatic nerve, acetabular fracture
Knee dislocation	Popliteal artery, tibial and common peroneal nerve
Upper fibular fracture	Peroneal nerve
Ankle dislocation	Anterior and posterior tibial artery
Calcaneual fracture	Lumbar compression

From Hart, R., Rittenberry, T., & Uehara, D. (1999). Handbook of orthopaedic emergencies (p. 14). Philadelphia: Lippincott Williams & Wilkins.

10. Determine the range of motion (ROM) of the injured extremity and evaluate muscle strength.
11. Note any lacerations or hematomas.
12. Keep the extremity elevated as much as possible during the examination.

◉ DEVELOPMENTAL CONSIDERATIONS

Child: Children's bones are not completely calcified and therefore are more flexible than those of adults, so incomplete fractures may be seen (greenstick or buckle fractures).

The growth of bones occurs at the epiphyses; these areas may be mistaken for fractures on x-ray studies. These areas are weaker than other parts of the bone and are more susceptible to injury. Injury to the growth plate can interfere with subsequent bone growth. Injuries to the growth plate are classified using Salter-Harris terminology.

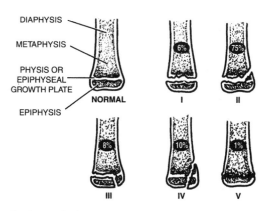

The Salter-Harris classification. (Hart, R., Rittenberry, T., Uehara. D. [1999]. *Handbook of orthopaedic emergencies.* Philadelphia: Lippincott-Raven.)

Torn ligaments are rare in children; the more likely injury to consider is a growth plate injury.

Fractures in children are able to remodel with growth. This ability is dependent on the age of the child, the degree of fracture, and the location as well as other factors.

Common fractures in children include

Clavicle: most common in children
Forearm: fall on outstretched arm
Elbow: may be difficult to recognize
Nursemaid's elbow: forced hyperextension and supination of the forearm
Femur: high-energy trauma and multisystem trauma

Elderly: Increased incidence of osteoporosis increases the risk of fracture, and fractures are frequently comminuted due to aging process of bone. Digits in particular often show arthritic changes with resulting joint stiffness after even brief immobilization.

Falls are a common cause of fractures in the elderly, with femur fracture a frequent result.

Fractures may occur spontaneously in patients with osteoporosis.

Pregnancy: Change of the center of gravity in pregnant women may predispose them to falls.

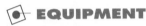 EQUIPMENT

- Plaster of paris: Modern day plaster of paris is available impregnated into strips of a crinoline-type material that keeps the plaster molded into the desired shape while drying. It is commercially available in widths of 2, 3, 4, or 6 inches.
- Webril: Dense cotton padding used over the stockinette to provide padding and protection of the skin over bony prominences. (Available in 3-, 4-, 6-inch widths.)
- Elastic bandages: Use elastic (Ace) bandages to secure the splint to the extremity.
- Orthopedic felt: Apply ½-inch thick felt to pad bony prominences such as the olecranon, radial and ulnar styloids, patella, fibular head, and medial and lateral malleoli.
- Utility knife or shears: Used to cut and shape dry plaster or to cut prefabricated splint rolls to the desired length.
- Bucket: Use a stainless steel bucket to dip the splinting material for moistening.
- Protective clothing: Wear protective gloves, gowns, and safety glasses, particularly when using plaster of paris, to protect clothing and prevent skin or eye injury from plaster dust or wet plaster.
- Metallic splints: These splints are available with sponge rubber padding on one side; they can be cut and shaped as needed.

PROCEDURE	SPECIAL CONSIDERATIONS
Stockinette and Webril are applied before the cast material is applied.	Make sure the right side of the commercial product is applied next to the skin.
	In most cases, a circumferential cast is never applied. Only a partial cast for immobilization is used.

For custom-made splints:

Position the limb before stockinette or Webril is applied.	Some people argue that stockinette is not necessary; just using Webril is sufficient and speeds application.

(procedure continued) ──────────────────────────────

PROCEDURE

Apply a single layer of stockinette so that approximately 4 inches extends beyond the splint on both ends. Use 3 inches on upper extremities and 4 inches for lower extremities.

Then apply Webril. It can stretch and tear, allowing for soft tissue swelling. Apply to all areas to be covered by the splint, extending past the splint by about 1 inch. Apply approximately two to three layers. Wrap so the Webril overlaps 50% of preceding wrap. Use 2 inches for hands/feet, 3 to 4 inches for upper extremities, and 4 to 6 inches for lower extremities.

SPECIAL CONSIDERATIONS

What is the difference between cotton and synthetic cast padding or stockinette? Cotton is less expensive. Synthetic padding is better at handling moisture. If you want to wear a fiberglass cast into water, you will need synthetic padding. Cotton is fine for most casts.

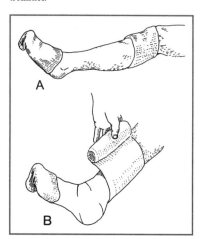

A

B

Prefabricated plaster splint rolls:

Commercial products include both stockinette and Webril with plaster or fiberglass so it can be applied in just one layer.

Then apply plaster of paris, fiberglass, or prefabricated splint roll: For whatever product that is chosen, select splint width and cut to desired length. In general, use width slightly greater than the diameter of the limb being splint:

• If fiberglass is used, immediately reseal the bag.

• If using plaster of paris rolls, assemble ap-

Plaster can clog drains, so do not prepare it directly in a sink or use a sink with a plaster trap to prevent clogging.

What is the difference between fiberglass and plaster of paris? Fiberglass is significantly more expensive. It is also waterproof, lighter, stronger, and sets and can bear weight in 30 minutes. Unlike plaster of paris, fiberglass is more difficult to remove but it makes a

(procedure continued)

PROCEDURE	SPECIAL CONSIDERATIONS

proximately six to eight layers stacked vertically.

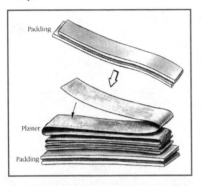

Padding

Plaster

Padding

reusable cast. Fiberglass comes in a range of colors. A lot of people prefer the thickness, the weight, and the feel of plaster of paris. It takes 24 to 48 hours for plaster to set completely.

Dip the splinting material through cool water (70°–85°) until bubbling stops.

Remember that an exothermic chemical reaction is begun when the splinting material comes in contact with water; the patient will feel heat when the cast is applied.
The reaction is accelerated by increasing the temperature of the water. The warmer the water, the quicker the plaster of paris sets. **If warm water is used, enough heat is generated to burn the patient.**

Roll or fold splint and squeeze out excess water.

Smooth out splint with a gloved flat hand on a flat surface.

Apply splint to patient and gently smooth with a flat palm to conform with extremity. (An assistant may be needed to hold the splint in place.)

Wrap the splint with elastic bandage under slight tension. Overlap preceding layer by 50%. Secure with tape or metal clips.

Choice of ACE bandage: (2 inches best for hands and feet; 3 to 4 inches best for upper extremities; and 4 to 6 inches best for lower extremities.

Mold splint to affected extremity for 2 to 4 minutes for fiberglass and 10 to 15 minutes for plaster of paris.

Have the patient hold still until the exothermic reaction subsides.

(Figures from Simon, R. & Brenner, B. [1994]. *Emergency procedures and techniques,* (3rd ed). Baltimore: Williams & Wilkins.)

SPECIFIC SPLINTING TECHNIQUES

Upper Extremities:

Type of Injury	Patient Population	Recommended Splint
Clavicle: Most fall onto ipsilateral shoulder (87%).	Usually greenstick or nondisplaced fractures in children. Older children and adults: Complete fracture is common fracture usually in middle third of bone.	None for children or sling only in those younger than 6 years of age. Patients older than 10 years: Figure-eight clavicle strap. There is controversy as to the use of clavicle strap versus sling. Studies comparing outcomes have not demonstrated any difference, and the sling is better tolerated.

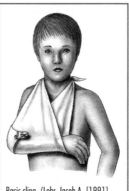

Basic sling. (Lohr, Jacob A. [1991]. *Pediatric outpatient procedures.* Philadelphia: J.B. Lippincott Company.)

| Elbow: Supracondylar fracture: Fall onto outstretched arm with elbow in extension or directly onto the elbow. Olecranon: Direct blow. | Supracondylar fracture is most common elbow fracture in children. Fracture of lateral humeral condyle is the second most common, followed by medial epicondylar fracture (direct blows to epicondyle). Radial fractures are the most common elbow injuries in adults. | Long arm posterior splint (from distal metacarpals to proximal humerus) and sling or double sugar tong splint and sling. Use 4- to 5-inch width (6 inches in larger patients). Measure from proximal humerus to the palmar crease. Splint forms a gutter along ulnar surface of the hand and forearm; and posterior surface of elbow and humerus, leaving fingers free. |

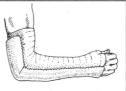

Posterior arm splint. (Simon, R. & Brenner, B. [1994]. *Emergency procedures and techniques,* (3rd ed.) Baltimore: Williams & Wilkins.)

Extremity Position	Comments
Pull shoulders back tightly as in military position. Apply spint as if applying backpack (see illustration). Sling: Hand should be higher than elbow (flex elbow slightly more than 90 degrees). The hand and wrist should be inside the sling. 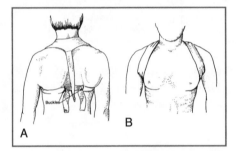	Used for 3 to 5 weeks for children. Adults will require 6 weeks or more. Adults will require closer follow-up due to possible extensive callus formation. Refer an adult to orthopedics in 1 week if fracture is not completely reduced using splint or if fracture is lateral or medial third. Have the patient remove the harness for bathing; warn the patient or parents about the bump of callus that forms during healing, which remodels and disappears over a period of 6 to 9 months.
Apply a posterior splint with elbow at 90 degrees and wrist slightly extended (10 to 20 degrees), with thumb in neutral position (thumb up).	Assessment of neurovascular status is very important. Remember to check for other commonly associated fractures: Proximal radius, radial head, coronoid process or olecranon. Splint children with localized tenderness and swelling due to the possibility of occult fractures. Follow-up should be done by orthopedic surgeon.

table continued

(table continued)

Type of Injury	Patient Population	Recommended Splint
		Double sugar tong: Same length as above, with two layers: posterior and anterior surfaces. 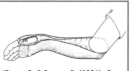 (Simon, R. & Brenner, B. [1994]. *Emergency procedures and techniques*, (3rd ed). Baltimore: Williams & Wilkins.)
Wrist and distal forearm: Fall onto outstretched hand. Wrist: Fall onto outstretched hand. Colles' fracture: Fall with wrist in dorsiflexion.	Children: Forearm fractures are among most common; usually does not result in intra-articular injury Scaphoid fractures are the most common carpal fractures; Colles' fracture occurs most frequently in patients 60 to 70 years of age.	**Volar splint** (use 3- to 4-inch widths) Apply splint from distal palmar creases to before the elbow. Cut splint from fingertips to proximal forearm. 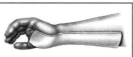 (Lohr, Jacob A. [1991]. *Pediatric outpatient procedures*. Philadelphia: J.B. Lippincott Company.) **Sugar tong** (use 3- to 4-inch widths) Apply from distal palmar creases to the elbow, around the elbow and back to the dorsum of the hand (MCP joint). Holds arm in supination or pronation without a circumferential cast. Apply arm sling after splint has set. **Thumb spica** (3- to 4-inch widths) Used for management of scaphoid fractures, gamekeeper's thumb, or nonrotated, nonangulated, nonarticular fractures of the thumb. The splint extends from the metacarpophalangeal joints, up the dorsal forearm, around the elbow, and down the volar aspect of the forearm to the palmar crease.

Extremity Position	Comments
Put elbow in 90 degrees of flexion with wrist in 10 to 20 degrees of extension, and thumb and fingers free. The distal end of the splint should be folded back onto itself, making a shelf on which the fingers can rest.	Used for simple fractures and not rotational abnormalities or significant displacement. Owing to the high number of complications, the best plan is to splint and then refer for follow-up in 2 to 4 days.
	Remember that solitary fractures of the ulna or radius are unusual due to the close relationship of the bones. Treatment should be dictated by clinical suspicion for scaphoid fractures because 10% are not seen initially on x-ray study.
	Any unstable scaphoid fractures should be examined by orthopedist.
	Colles' fractures should be followed by an orthopedist.

table continued

(table continued)

Type of Injury	Patient Population	Recommended Splint
Thumb spica position: fore-arm in neutral position, mid-way between supination and prona-tion. Keep wrist in 30 degrees of ex-tension, thumb ab-ducted and the interpha-langeal joints in slight flex-ion.		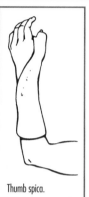Thumb spica.
Hand splints: Fractures of fourth or fifth metacarpals (boxer frac-tures) due to direct blow (as in punching a solid ob-ject).	None specific.	**Ulnar gutter splint:** Extends from the fingertips to just below elbow, permitting movement of elbow joint. Make the splint wide enough to cover both the volar and dorsal surfaces of the fourth and fifth metacarpals (use 4-inch plaster, 3- to 4-inch Ace, sling). 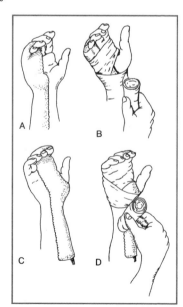

Extremity Position	Comments
Gutter: Wrist splinted at 15 degrees of extension and metacarpophalangeal joints at 50 to 90 degrees of flexion, first three digits free.	Goal is to obtain the best functional result. Because hand movement is so vital, close follow-up of hand injuries is necessary. Splinting will be in place for about 2 weeks, followed by range of motion exercises. Most patients can return to work in 2 to 4 weeks.

table continued

(table continued)

Type of Injury	Patient Population	Recommended Splint

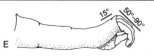

(Simon, R. & Brenner, B. [1994]. *Emergency procedures and techniques*, (3rd ed). Baltimore: Williams & Wilkins.)

Finger: Stable phalangeal fracture, avulsion fracture of the extensor tendon attachment to the distal phalanx.

Dorsal (volar) functional finger splint: Dorsal splint is the most commonly used: apply to back of hand, extending from nail to past wrist joint.

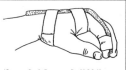

(Simon, R. & Brenner, B. [1994]. *Emergency procedures and techniques,* (3rd ed). Baltimore: Williams & Wilkins.)

Distal dorsal splint (Fingertip):
Used for extensor tendon attachment to distal phalanx (mallet finger) or distal phalanx (tuft) fractures.

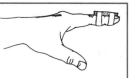

(Simon, R. & Brenner, B. [1994]. *Emergency procedures and techniques,* (3rd ed). Baltimore: Williams & Wilkins.)

Extremity Position	Comments
Dorsal functional finger splint: Fingers held at approximately 50 to 90 degrees of flexion at metacarpophalangeal and 15 to 20 degrees of flexion at the interphalangeal joints. Motion is allowed at wrist. **Fingertip splint:** Full extension to slight hyperextension of distal interphalangeal joint. Splint should be placed on distal interphalangeal joint without interfering with motion of proximal interphalangeal. **Dynamic finger splint:** Allows motion at metacarpophalangeal joint.	**Remember to remove any rings when the fingers are injured.** Distal (fingertip) splint: Position must be maintained for 6 to 8 weeks with the splint in place. The splint should not be removed or the finger flexed. Nocturnal splinting will be needed for 2 to 4 additional weeks. Dynamic finger splinting is used with first and second degree sprains of PIP and DIP joints. Tuft fractures: 2 to 4 weeks of protection in cage or splint. Pediatric injuries: Most fractures should be referred to specialist for follow-up.

table continued

(table continued)

Type of Injury	Patient Population	Recommended Splint

Hairpin splint: Protection of fingertip.

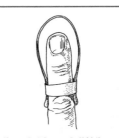

(Simon, R. & Brenner, B. [1994]. *Emergency procedures and techniques*, (3rd ed). Baltimore: Williams & Wilkins.)

Dynamic finger splinting: Used in soft tissue injuries. Splint the injured finger to the adjacent finger. Insert Webril or cotton beween fingers and tape as shown.

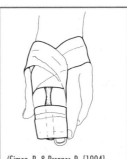

(Simon, R. & Brenner, B. [1994]. *Emergency procedures and techniques*, (3rd ed). Baltimore: Williams & Wilkins.)

Extremity Position	Comments

table continued

(table continued)

Type of Injury	Patient Population	Recommended Splint
Thumb injuries: Fracture of first metacarpophalangeal joint or proximal phalanx, or soft tissue injuries to the thumb. Usually occurs with direct blows to thumb or axial loading when hand strikes a solid object.	Patients in fist fight (Bennett's fracture).	Thumb spica: (use 4-inch plaster, Webril 3-inch, Ace one 3-inch and one 4-inch). Measure plaster from thumbnail to proximal forearm. Apply splint to the lateral half of forearm. Plaster edges should meet on the medial aspect of thumb to maintain abduction. Secure with Ace bandage. (See Distal Forearm Injury earlier.)

Extremity Position	Comments
Wrist extended to 15 degrees, thumb abducted in position of function (similar to position of hand holding a glass). Fingers 2 to 5 are free.	

Lower Extremities:

Type of Injury	Patient Population	Recommended Splint
Knee: ligamentous or soft tissue injuries to the knee. ACL and PCL: Anterior and posterior stability. MCL and LCL: Side-to-side stability.	ACL: Deceleration, flexion, and rotation (running at full speed, followed by sudden stop). PCL: Dashboard injury (rarely an isolated injury). MCL: (Most commonly injured knee ligament) trauma to lateral aspect of knee. LCL: Uncommon: Trauma to medial aspect of knee. Meniscus: Twisting of a flexed knee.	Knee immobilizers are available in a variety of sizes. The knee immobilizer has virtually replaced plaster or fiberglass splints for immobilization of mild to moderate knee sprains and soft tissue injury. The advantages of the knee immobilizer is that they are lightweight, easy to apply and remove, and can be placed over the patients clothing. To determine the proper size and fit, place the immobilizer next to the injured leg, aligning the patellar cutout area with the knee. The immobilizer should extend from just a few inches above the malleoli to just beneath the crease of the buttocks. Place the immobilizer around the knee, with the metal supports along the medial and lateral aspects of the knee and hold in place by securing the Velcro fasteners.

(Simon, R. & Brenner, B. [1994]. *Emergency procedures and techniques*, (3rd ed). Baltimore: Williams & Wilkins.)

Extremity Position	Comments
Full extension of knee.	Crutches should be given to prevent weight bearing. Follow-up knee injuries with orthopedic referral.

table continued

(table continued)

Type of Injury	Patient Population	Recommended Splint
Ankle: Inversion or eversion injuries, including second- or third-degree ankle sprains, fractures of distal tibia and fibula.	The majority of ankle injuries involve the lateral ligaments. Lateral malleolar fracture is the most common fracture of the ankle. Usually an inversion injury.	**Short leg posterior gutter splint:** (4-inch plaster, Webril 3- to 4-inch rolls; Ace 3- to 4-inch rolls) extend from toes to below the knee. Measure from the metatarsophaleangeal joint to the level of the fibular head. Place Webril between toes and make sure prominences (especially malleoli) are well padded. Apply splint, carefully molding around malleoli and instep for a secure fit. Use 12 layers if making custom splint.

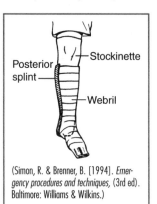

(Simon, R. & Brenner, B. [1994]. *Emergency procedures and techniques,* (3rd ed). Baltimore: Williams & Wilkins.)

Sugar tong splint: May be added to posterior splint for additional ankle stability. A U-shaped lateral splint extending around the medial and lateral sides of the leg to just below the fibular head.

Extremity Position	Comments
Ankle is held at 90 degrees so that knee flexion is maintained. The easiest way to apply splint is to have the patient lie prone, with knee and ankle flexed at 90 degrees.	Grade I ankle injuries can be managed by conservative (RICE) means. Follow-up 1 wk with PCP. Grade II to III ankle injuries RICE, follow-up with orthopedics in 1 week. Lateral malleolar fracture: Short leg splint, RICE, non-weight bearing, follow-up orthopedics in 1 week.

table continued

(table continued)

Type of Injury	Patient Population	Recommended Splint
		(Simon, R. & Brenner, B. [1994]. *Emergency procedures and techniques*, (3rd ed). Baltimore: Williams & Wilkins.)
		Semi-rigid orthotics: May be used for minor ligamentous and soft tissue injuries of the foot and ankle not requiring complete immobilization. Commercial products are available that resemble sugar tong splints (Aircast Inc.). The splints are applied over the patient's socks. Additional air can be added when the initial swelling has resolved. The oval plate is placed under the heel, and the sides extend up the lateral and medial calf.
Foot: Fractures or soft tissue injuries of the foot. Usually due to direct trauma, indirect trauma or overuse injury.	Calcaneus is the most commonly fractured tarsal bone, associated with falls from heights. Forefoot fractures of the metatarsals occur when a heavy object falls on the foot. Frequently, there is more than one fracture. March fractures: second and third metatarsals: stress fractures.	Postoperative shoe: slip shoe over foot. It fastens with Velcro straps or ties.

Extremity Position	Comments
Ankle free, sole of foot supported.	Patient may bear weight.

table continued

(table continued)

Type of Injury	Patient Population	Recommended Splint
Toes: Soft tissue injuries or fractures of the toes.	Toe injuries occur with direct trauma or forced hyperextension.	Toes 2 to 5 can be splinted using dynamic splinting. Dynamic splint: buddy taping. Injured toe is splinted by an adjacent toe. Place a small piece of Webril between two toes to be taped. Apply tape circumferentially around toes. Do not pull the tape too tight. See p. 250 for example of dynamic splint cap.

🔘 REFERRAL AND CONSULTATION

- Immediate orthopedic intervention is required for the following fractures:
  - Long bone fractures
  - Displaced fractures
  - All fractures with neurovascular compromise
  - Significant instability or mortise widening of joints
- Surgical intervention is required for the following fractures:
  - Displaced intra-articular fractures
  - Arterial injury with fracture

🔘 FOLLOW-UP

- Patients with fractures should be referred for follow-up in 2 to 3 days once the initial edema has subsided sufficiently for placement of a circumferential cast.
- Patients with moderate to severe sprains may be followed in the office and referred if complications arise. Follow-up for most injuries should occur in 3 to 5 days, depending on the type and location of the injury:
  - Simple nondisplaced fractures
  - Grade II to III sprains
- Any minor sprains that do not respond to conservative management should have orthopedic follow-up.
- Follow-up any patients who complain of increased pain, burning, or irritation under the splints.

BIBLIOGRAPHY

American Medical Association. (1998). *Physicians' current procedural terminology: CPT.* Chicago: American Medical Association.

Durbin, D. (1997). Splinting. In R. Dieckmann, D. Fiser, & S. Selbst (Eds). *Illustrated textbook of pediatric emergency & critical care procedures* (pp. 613–624). St. Louis: Mosby–Year Book.

Chudnofsky, C. (1998) Splinting. In J. Roberts, & J. Hedges (Eds). Splinting techniques.

Extremity Position	Comments
	Tape second toe to third toe instead of great toe.

Clinical procedures in emergency medicine (3rd ed., pp. 852–872). Philadelphia: W.B. Saunders.

Hart, R., Rittenberry, T., & Uehara, D. (1999). *Handbook of orthopaedic emergencies.* Philadelphia: Lippincott Williams & Wilkins.

Healthcare Consultants of America. (1998). *1998 Physicians' fee and coding guide.* Augusta, GA.

Simon, R. & Brenner, B. (1994). *Emergency procedures and techniques* (3rd ed.). Baltimore: Williams & Wilkins.

chapter
38

Corticosteroid Joint Injection

CPT Coding:

20600 Injection of fingers or toes (small joint) ($65–$77)
20605 Injection of wrist, ankle, or elbow (intermediate joint) ($69–$82)
20610 Injection of shoulder, knee, or hip (major joint) ($78–$93)

DEFINITION

Corticosteroid joint injection involves insertion of a needle into a joint of the body and injecting corticosteroid medication into that joint.

INDICATIONS

- To control pain quickly at a joint that has sterile inflammation
- When systemic antiinflammatory agents have not been effective or are contraindicated
- Patients with active rheumatoid arthritis, osteoarthritis, or crystal-induced arthritis (gout or pseudogout)
- Through the use of local anesthetics, differentiate the source of pain as intra-articular or extra-articular.

 ALERT: Contraindications for joint injections include the following:

- Acute trauma
  - Instability of the joint
- Septic arthritis
- Nerve or tendon injection
- Osteonecrosis
- Local infection of the overlying skin
- Severe coagulopathy
- Bacteremia
- Avascular necrosis
- Patients receiving anticoagulants
- Uncooperative patients

PATIENT EDUCATION

- Explain the procedure and purpose for performing it.
- Discuss the complications and risks (ie, infection, bleeding, skin discoloration, and fat atrophy).

- Explain that an anesthetic will make the procedure more tolerable.
- Discuss the possibility of a postinjection pain flare-up for approximately 24 to 48 hours. Approximately 10% of patients may experience this problem.
- Inform the patient that he or she can take antiinflammatory medications and apply ice over the injection site, or both, if a postinjection flare-up of pain occurs.

ASSESSMENT

1. Perform a history and physical exam on the patient.
2. Ask the patient if this joint has been injected with corticosteroids in the past, when this occurred, was there a positive effect, and how long did the results last? A joint should not be injected again for 3 to 4 months.
3. Diabetics may experience transient hyperglycemia.
4. Alternative therapies should be explored if a joint has been regularly injected with corticosteroids for 1 year.
5. Determine whether or not the patient has any contraindications for this procedure.
6. Perform a thorough assessment of the particular joint to be injected.
7. Identify the relevant anatomic landmarks.
8. Determine the patient's ability or desire to cooperate during this procedure.
9. Determine the appropriate steroid to inject and the appropriate dosage.

Corticosteroids and Dosage for Intra-articular Injection Listed According to Decreasing Length of Action

Steroid for Injection	Dose for a Large Joint	Dose for a Small Joint
Triamcinolone hexacetonide	20 mg	2 to 6 mg
Triamcinolone acetonide	20 mg	2 to 6 mg
Prednisolone tebutate	25 mg	2.5 to 7.5 mg
Betamethasone sodium phosphate	1 mL	0.25 to 0.5 mL
Betamethasone sodium acetate	1 mL	0.25 to 0.5 mL
Methylprednisolone acetate	40 mg	3.5 to 10.5 mg
Triamcinolone diacetate	20 mg	2 to 6 mg
Prednisolone acetate	30 mg	3 to 9 mg
Dexamethasone acetate	5 mg	0.5 to 1.5 mg

DEVELOPMENTAL CONSIDERATIONS

- Steroid injection may be useful for patients in whom medical therapy has failed and surgery is not indicated for their treatment of arthritis.
- When a child has only a few joints that are affected by arthritis, intra-articular steroid injection may prove to be of benefit.

EQUIPMENT

- Iodine-based or similar antiseptic solution and sterile gloves
- Local anesthetic (1% or 2% lidocaine), 25-gauge needle with syringe
- 18- to 25-gauge needle of adequate length, syringe, hemostat, and solution to be injected
- 2 × 2 gauze pad
- Sterile bandage

PROCEDURE	SPECIAL CONSIDERATIONS
Assess the joint to be injected thoroughly.	
Position the patient as appropriate for the particular joint to be injected. Refer to the diagrams and descriptions for specific insertion sites of individual joints to be injected.	
Identify the landmarks for the particular joint to be injected.	
Use sterile technique throughout this procedure.	
Cleanse the skin over the site with antiseptic solution.	
Infiltrate the skin with local anesthetic.	
If a significant effusion is present, this should be aspirated fully before injection. (See Chapter 36: Arthrocentesis.)	
Insert the needle and syringe combination through the same needle tract. Refer to the diagrams and descriptions for specific insertion sites of individual joints to be aspirated.	Avoid striking the periosteum of the adjacent bone ends because of the presence of nerve endings. Be careful not to cut into the articular cartilage of the joint.
Inject the corticosteroid and anesthetic solution into the joint.	Insert the needle slightly deeper if the fluid does not flow well. The needle may not be in the joint space.

(procedure continued)

PROCEDURE	SPECIAL CONSIDERATIONS

Withdraw the needle and place pressure over the injection site to prevent bleeding.

Cleanse the skin and dress the injection site with a sterile bandage.

KNEE (MEDIAL APPROACH)

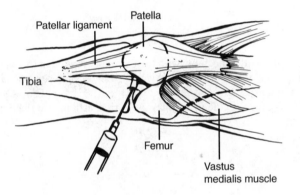

Injection of the knee joint.

- With the patient supine, extend the legs fully.
- The medial approach to the joint is at the midpoint of the patella, approximately 1 cm medially to the medial edge.
- Insert an 18-gauge needle between the patella and medial femoral condyle into the joint.

SHOULDER (ANTERIOR APPROACH)

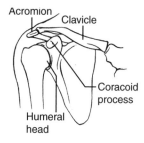

Injection of the shoulder joint.

- Patient is in a sitting position, with the extremity resting in the lap.
- Palpate the glenohumeral joint, which is 45 degrees inferior and lateral to the coracoid process.
- Insert a 20-gauge needle in an anteroposterior fashion into the joint.

ELBOW

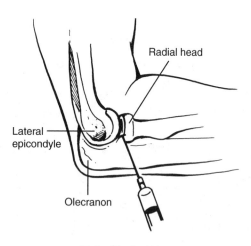

Injection of the elbow joint.

- The patient is sitting, with the arm flexed to 90 degrees.
- Palpate the tip of the olecranon process and the lateral epicondyle of the humerus.

• Insert a 22-gauge needle at a 45-degree angle and parallel to the radius and ulna at a point halfway between the olecranon process and the medial epicondyle.

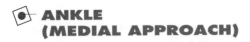

ANKLE (MEDIAL APPROACH)

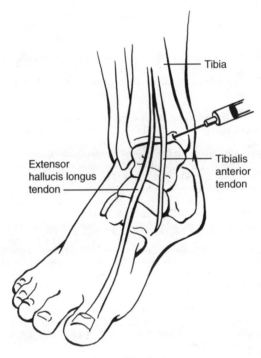

Tibia

Tibialis anterior tendon

Extensor hallucis longus tendon

Injection of the ankle joint.

• The patient is lying supine, with the ankle in the neutral position.
• Palpate the medial malleolus, the tibialis anterior tendon, the extensor hallucis longus tendon, and the dorsalis pedis artery.
• Insert a 20-gauge needle slightly anterior and lateral to the medial malleolus and medial to the extensor hallucis longus tendon, avoiding the dorsalis pedis artery. The needle should be inserted toward the tibiotalar joint.

ALTERNATIVE PROCEDURES

• Continue with appropriate oral medications (antiinflammatory medications, arthritic agents, and so on).

• Recommend possible surgical management as warranted for the patient's condition.

FOLLOW-UP

• Instruct the patient to follow up if he develops evidence of infection.
• Have the patient follow up if the joint develops severe pain or redevelops a large amount of joint fluid.

BIBLIOGRAPHY

American Medical Association. (1998). *Physicians' current procedural terminology: CPT*. Chicago: American Medical Association.

Benjamin, G. (1998). Arthrocentesis. In J. R. Roberts & J. R. Hedges (Eds.), *Clinical procedures in emergency medicine* (3rd ed., pp. 919–932). Philadelphia: W. B. Saunders.

Bird, H. (1994). Intra-articular and intralesional therapy. In J. Klippel & P. Dieppe (Eds.), *Rheumatology* (1st ed., pp. 3.7.1–3.7.4). London, UK: Mosby–Year Book Europe Limited.

Coumas, J., Howard, B., & Jacobson, E. (1996). Diagnostic imaging of rheumatologic disorders. In J. Noble (Ed.), *Textbook of primary care medicine* (2nd ed., pp. 962–978). St. Louis, MO: Mosby–Year Book, Inc.

Gatter, R. A. (1996). Arthrocentesis technique and intra-synovial therapy. In W. J. Koopman (Ed.), *Arthritis and allied conditions: A textbook of rheumatology* (13th ed., pp. 751–760). Baltimore, MD: Williams & Wilkins.

Healthcare Consultants of America (1998). *1998 Physicians' fee and coding guide*. Augusta, GA.

Mosca, V. & Sherry, D. (1990). Juvenile rheumatoid arthritis and seronegative spondyloarthropathies. In R. Morrissy (Ed.), *Lovell and Winter's pediatric orthopedics* (3rd ed., pp. 297–324). Philadelphia: J. B. Lippincott.

Pousada, L. & Osborn, H. (1986). *Emergency medicine for the house officer*. Baltimore, MD: Williams & Wilkins.

Steinbrocker, O. & Neustadt, D. (1972). *Aspiration and injection therapy in arthritis and musculoskeletal disorders*. Hagerstown, MD: Harper & Row.

Snider, R. (1997). *Essentials of musculoskeletal care*. Rosemont, IL: American Academy of Orthopedic Surgeons.

chapter 39

Ring Removal

CPT Coding:

(N/A)

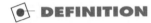 DEFINITION

This procedure involves removal of a ring that is interfering with circulation of the finger.

INDICATIONS

- To relieve constriction by a ring caused by swelling
- To prevent vascular compromise by a ring when there has been an injury to the ringed extremity

PATIENT EDUCATION

- Explain the procedure to the client. Explain risks of constriction and answer questions. Rings made of precious metals can often be repaired by a jeweler if they are damaged by cutting. If cutting, explain that small abrasion and cuts may occur when the ring is pulled from the finger.
- If one is cutting off the ring, obtain written consent per institutional policy before the procedure.

ASSESSMENT

1. Obtain the medical history from client and assess the client as indicated by report or injury. Injury anywhere on the ringed extremity indicates ring removal.
2. Assess ringed digit for swelling, warmth, color, and capillary refill.
3. Assess tightness of ring and determine whether or not ring can be removed manually.
4. If one is unable to remove the ring manually, determine whether to use the string method of removal or the cutting method of removal. The string method is the method of choice for prophylactic ring removal. If it is unsuccessful, the ring should be cut. If there is any evidence of vascular compromise on assessment of the ringed digit, the ring should be cut immediately.

DEVELOPMENTAL CONSIDERATIONS

Child: Instruct the client using age-appropriate language. Allow the child to inspect the equipment as appropriate. Involve the parent or guardian in procedure.

Adult and Elderly Patients: Wedding bands, engagement rings, and other pieces of jewelry can hold great meaning for these individuals. Explaining that a ring might be repaired, treating it with care, cleaning away blood, and keeping it within sight of the client will decrease anxiety.

STRING METHOD

Equipment
• Gloves (if blood or body fluids are present)
• 3-foot string (No. 1 silk Mersilene)
• Umbilical tape
• Optional: small bar of soap

PROCEDURE	SPECIAL CONSIDERATIONS
Anchor one end of the string close to the patient's ring.	Anchor with your nondominant hand.
Wrap the string firmly around the finger, starting at the distal side of the ring and wrapping toward the tip of the toe or finger until it passes the point of maximal swelling or diameter. Leave a few inches of string unwrapped for grasping.	Lay the string close together but not overlapping. Some patients may need a digital block if the pain increases from the compression of the string.

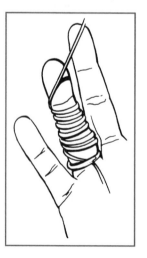

(procedure continued)

PROCEDURE	**SPECIAL CONSIDERATIONS**
Pass the proximal end of the string underneath the ring, from distal side to proximal side. Hemostats may be needed to pass the string under the ring to the proximal side.	The string should pass smoothly underneath the ring. It should not be wrapped around the ring.

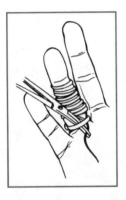

Gradually unwrap the string starting from the proximal side. Apply tension and work the ring outward as you unwrap.	If it is wrapped smoothly and firmly, the string will have compressed the tissue just enough for the ring to gradually pass over. The patient may be uncomfortable during this step.

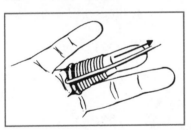

If the ring has not been removed, repeat this step as necessary to pass the ring over bony or tight area.	Some advocate "waxing" the string with bar soap as an aid to removal. If repeated attempts are unsuccessful, consider cutting the ring.

CUTTING METHOD

Equipment
- Gloves (if blood or body fluids are present)
- Ring cutter
- Hemostats
- Cotton or loosened 2 × 2 gauze

PROCEDURE	SPECIAL CONSIDERATIONS
Insert the smooth curved blade of the ring cutter underneath the ring.	The circular "saw" portion of the ring cutter should be superior to the ring.

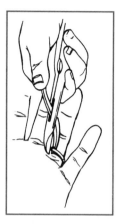

Clamp the ring tightly between the blade and the saw by squeezing the handles with your left hand. With your right hand, turn the small handle on the saw to cut into the ring. Turn the saw's handle until the ring has been severed.	If the saw is spinning or not cutting effectively, grasp the ring more tightly with the ring cutter.
Insert a small amount of cotton under the severed ends of the ring as protection for the client. Bend the severed ends away from the client and carefully remove the ring (hemostats may be needed to do this).	The severed ends of the ring may be quite sharp.
Reassess circulation of the ringed finger or toe. Assess skin for abrasions caused by ring removal and treat as necessary.	

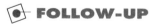 **FOLLOW-UP**

• As indicated by client's injury or report.

BIBLIOGRAPHY

American Medical Association. (1998). *Physicians' current procedural terminology: CPT.* Chicago: American Medical Association.
Haynes, J. Ring Removal from an edematous finger.

Healthcare Consultants of America. (1998). *1998 Physicians' fee and coding guide.* Augusta, GA.

Pfenninger, J. & Fowler, G. (1994). *Procedures for primary care physicians.* St. Louis: Mosby.

Proehl, J. (1993). Ring removal. In J. Proehl (Ed.), *Adult emergency nursing procedures* (pp. 378–380). Boston, MA: Jones and Bartlett Publishers.

Rosen, P. & Sternbach, G. (1983). *Atlas of emergency medicine* (2nd Ed). Baltimore: Williams & Wilkins.

Trott, A. (1991). *Wounds and lacerations: emergency care and closure* (p. 179). St. Louis: Mosby.

chapter 40

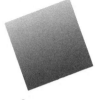

Trigger Point Injection

CPT Coding:

20550 Injection of a trigger point ($72–$85)

DEFINITION

A trigger point is any site on the body that, when stimulated, brings about in a specific area abrupt pain similar to, or reproducing, pain felt without stimulus at the same site.

INDICATIONS

• To deliver pain relief from a painful trigger point

 ALERT: Contraindications for trigger point injections include the following:
  • Local infection of the overlying skin
  • Severe coagulopathy
  • Bacteremia
  • Patients who are receiving anticoagulants
  • Uncooperative, agitated, or confused patients

PATIENT EDUCATION

• Explain the procedure and the purpose for performing it.
• Discuss the complications and risks.

ASSESSMENT

1. Perform a thorough history and physical on the patient to eliminate other causes of myofascial pain.
2. In a methodical fashion, find the trigger points for this patient. This may be accomplished by using the tips of the examiner's fingers over the areas with pain to find these trigger points.
3. When a trigger point is located, the patient may find that pressure on this site will cause an increase in the pain. The trigger point may feel tight, bandlike, or ropelike.
4. Address the trigger points through treatment of the most painful one first.

EQUIPMENT

- Iodine-based or similar antiseptic solution, latex gloves
- 25- or 27-gauge needle, 5-mL syringe, and local anesthetic or saline for injection
- Moist heat

PROCEDURE	SPECIAL CONSIDERATIONS
Position the patient on the treatment table. The supine position is preferable to abate a syncopal episode after injection.	
Assess the patient and determine where the trigger points are located.	
Cleanse the skin over the site with antiseptic solution.	
While stabilizing the trigger point between two fingers, insert the needle into the trigger point at the area of maximum pain intensity. The needle should be inserted through the skin at an acute angle and parallel to the bandlike trigger point.	Blood in the syringe on aspiration (vascular insertion) or paresthesia or severe pain (nerve insertion) indicates improper needle placement. Reposition the needle as needed.

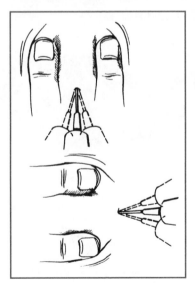

(procedure continued)

PROCEDURE	SPECIAL CONSIDERATIONS
Inject 0.5 to 2.0 mL of the fluid into the trigger point using a fanlike method.	When treating multiple trigger points, no more than 20 mL per day should be injected.

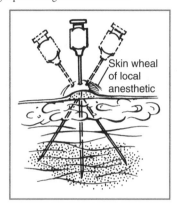

Skin wheal of local anesthetic

Stretching of the muscle groups after injection is key to adequate treatment of patients with trigger points.

Apply moist heat to the site over the trigger point injection.	May decrease postinjection discomfort.

ALTERNATIVE PROCEDURES

- Stretch and spray
- Stretch without spray
- Ischemic compression
- Massage
- Ultrasound
- Myofascial release

FOLLOW-UP

- Physical therapy
- Repeat injection
- Relaxation therapy
- Therapeutic exercise
- Massage

BIBLIOGRAPHY

Healthcare Consultants of America. (1998). *1998 Physicians' fee and coding guide.* Augusta, GA

Sola, A. (1998). Trigger point therapy. In J. R. Roberts & J. R. Hedges (Eds.), *Clinical procedures in emergency medicine* (3rd ed., pp. 890–901). Philadelphia: W. B. Saunders.

Travell, J.& Simons, D. (1992). *Myofascial pain and dysfunction: The trigger point manual.* Baltimore: Williams & Wilkins.

chapter
41 | Cervical Cap Fitting

CPT Coding:

57170 Diaphragm or cervical cap fitting with instructions ($59–$73). (This does not include the cost of the cervical cap.)

DEFINITIONS

• The cervical cap is a rubber, thimble-shaped, barrier birth control device that fits tightly against the cervix and remains in place through suction.
• Fitting is the art of measuring and procuring a cervical cap to cover the cervix completely with an adequately tight fit and adequate suction.

INDICATIONS

• Woman desires barrier contraceptive method.

ASSESSMENT

Elements That Must be in Place for Cervical Cap to be Successful

1. Desire or need of individual woman for barrier contraceptive method (including comfort in touching genitals)
2. Anatomic configuration of the cervix that allows adequate fit of the cervical cap (length of at least 1.5 cm and width of 1.0 to 2.5 cm, and uterus not acutely anteflexed)
3. No allergy to latex or spermicidal agents
4. Negative history of constipation, which may dislodge the cap (Secor, 1995)
5. Normal recent Pap smear results
6. At least 6 weeks postpartum, or after spontaneous or induced abortion
7. Absence of active genitourinary infection
8. Negative history of toxic shock syndrome
9. No cervical biopsy or cryosurgery within the past 6 to 12 weeks

PATIENT EDUCATION

- Assure the patient that most women can be fitted with and use a cervical cap successfully.
- Inserting and removing the cap takes practice. The patient may try different positions until she determines the best position for insertion and removal. Figure 43-1.8 shows suggested positions. Figure below shows appropriate cap fit.

Cap fit

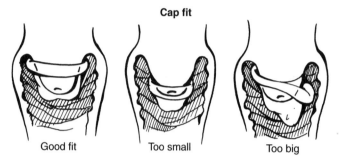

Good fit   Too small   Too big

Cap fit. (Chalker, R. [1987]. *The complete cervical cap guide.* [p. 45] New York: Harper and Rowe.)

- The cervical cap works through suction, so proper fitting is necessary.
- 1/4 teaspoon of contraceptive agent of choice (cream, jelly or foam that is compatible with latex) is inserted into the dome of the cervical cap ONLY. Care should be taken so that the agent does not come in contact with the rim of the cap or the outside of the cap, because this situation will interfere with the suction required for adequate contraceptive effect of the cap.

 ALERT: *Because of the danger of toxic shock syndrome, the cap should never be left in place during menstruation.*

DEVELOPMENTAL CONSIDERATIONS

Adolescents. The cervical cap is relatively difficult to use and may not be the best choice for unmarried or young adolescents.

Postpartum. Patients should be refitted after every delivery.

EQUIPMENT

- Glove and speculum
- Fitting set of cervical caps
- Private exam room and correct size cervical cap
- Cervical cap fitting set, soap, water, and disinfectant

PROCEDURE	SPECIAL CONSIDERATIONS

View cervix and vagina. Perform gonorrhea and chlamydia cultures. Inspect for signs of asymptomatic infections or nabothian cysts.

Infections should be resolved before cap fitting. Nabothian cysts may alter the symmetry of the cervix.

Perform a bimanual exam for location and position of cervix, and to estimate the size of the base of cervix as well as its configuration and angle of uterus. The middle and index fingers are inserted into the vagina, and the middle finger is used to measure the diameter of the base of the cervix (where it meets the vaginal fornix).

A cervix that is too short, asymmetric, significantly scarred, or flush with the vaginal vault may preclude adequate fitting of cervical cap (Hatcher et al, 1998). An extremely ante-flexed uterus may predispose to cap dislodgement during intercourse.

Select a cervical cap size to begin fitting session. Sizes include 22 mm, 25 mm, 28 mm and 31 mm.

Cap should be deep enough that the cap does not rest on the os. Cap size should almost be identical to the diameter of the base of the cervix.

Insert cap into vagina by folding the rim and compressing the dome. Place the cap over the cervix and then release the compression on the cap. Check fit all around the rim (there should be no gap).

The patient may feel a tugging sensation when the suction occurs during cap insertion. Attempts at fitting with more than one cap is not unusual and, in fact, is expected. The patient should feel the cap with her finger when it is properly in place.

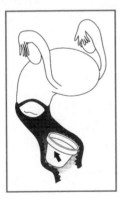

Attempt to dislodge the cap with one finger. After a moment, grasp the dome and gently tug. The cap should remain in place.

(procedure continued)

| PROCEDURE | SPECIAL CONSIDERATIONS |

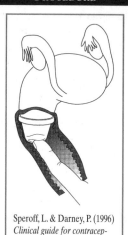

Speroff, L. & Darney, P. (1996)
Clinical guide for contraception, Baltimore: Williams &
Wilkins.

Remove the cap by grasping dome with finger and thumb, easing cap forward, and reaching posterior rim of cap. Break suction with finger. Remove the cap.

Never attempt to remove cap without breaking the suction first.

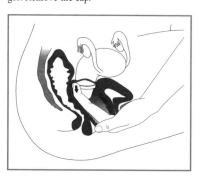

The patient should be allowed to practice as long as necessary to feel comfortable and confident in her ability to insert and remove the cap for effective use. Check for fit when patient is ready.

The patient should be patiently instructed and encouraged as much as necessary. This may take as long as 45 minutes.

The sample cervical caps should be thoroughly cleaned, disinfected, and dried before storage. Caps should be stored in a clean, covered container, away from temperature extremes.

ALTERNATIVE PROCEDURE

• If the patient cannot be fitted or is unable to insert and remove the cap, an alternate method of birth control should be discussed.

 FOLLOW-UP

• If there are any doubts about the patient's skill in using the cap, the patient should return in 1 week with the cap in place to be checked for placement.
• Recommend replacement of cervical cap every 3 years.

BIBLIOGRAPHY

Chalker, R. (1987). *The complete cervical cap guide.* New York: Harper & Row.

Fogel, C. I. & Woods, N. F. (1995) *Women's health care.* Thousand Oaks: Sage.

Hatcher, R. A., Trussell, J., Stewart, F., Kowal, D., Guest, F., Stewart, G. K., Cates, W., & Policar, M. S. (1994). *Contraceptive technology* (16th ed). New York: Irvington.

Healthcare Consultants of America (1998). *1998 Physicians' fee and coding guide,* Augusta, GA.

Secor, M. C. (1995). Cervical cap. In Hawkins, J. W., Roberto-Nichols, D. M., & Stanley-Haney, J. L. (eds) *Protocols for nurse practitioners in gynecologic settings* (5th ed.). New York: Tiresias.

Speroff, L. & Darney, P. (1996). *Clinical guide for contraception.* Baltimore: Williams & Wilkins.

chapter
42
Treatment of Condyloma Acuminatum

CPT Coding:

57061 Destruction of vaginal lesions, simple; any method ($152–$189)
57065 Extensive, any method ($523–$640)
46900-46917 Anal lesions ($104–$365)
56501-56515 Vulvar lesions ($135–780)

DEFINITION

The human papillomavirus (HPV) causes condyloma acuminatum (genital warts). Treatment is indicated for visible genital warts, particularly those that are symptomatic.

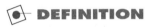 INDICATIONS

- The primary goal of treating visible genital warts is the removal of symptomatic warts, (eg, blocking the vaginal orifice, itching or burning).
- Improve cosmetic appearance.
- Reduce the amount of HPV.

 ALERT: There is a high level of anxiety associated with the diagnosis of HPV, educate over time.

PATIENT EDUCATION

- Genital warts are caused by HPV infection.
- Warts may regress spontaneously, remain the same, or progress.
- Treatment of genital warts does not guarantee elimination of the HPV infection.
- Transmission of HPV to sexual partners and to infants during the birth process remains a risk.
- Need for follow-up continues even after treatment eradicates the lesions.
- There is a potential risk for malignancy.
- The patient will need regular cytologic screening throughout life.

ASSESSMENT

1. Obtain a medical history related to condyloma acuminata. Chief reasons for seeking care are painless papules, pruritus or discharge. The usual history is of multiple lesions.
2. Obtain sexual history, including sex with men, women, or both. Obtain information about the patient's sexual practices: Oral-genital contact has a potential for oral, laryngeal, or tracheal muscosal lesions. Anal intercourse in both males and females has the potential for internal anal lesions.
3. Eruptions can be pearly, filiform, fungating, cauliflower, or plaquelike in appearance.
4. Multiple sites are usually involved—search systematically. Eruptions may be anywhere in the genital area where skin-to-skin contact occurs.
5. Presence of external condyloma acuminata in women warrants a vaginal speculum examination to search for vaginal and cervical lesions.
6. Presence of external condyloma acuminata in men warrants a search for urethral lesions.
7. If the patient practices anal intercourse, search for internal anal lesions. Note: Lesions may be around anus even if the patient does not practice anal intercourse.
8. Assess for evidence of other sexually transmitted diseases (STDs), such as ulcerations, adenopathy, vesicles, or discharge.
9. Assess for immunosuppression in clients with treatment failure and frequent recurrence of condyloma acuminatum.

DEVELOPMENTAL CONSIDERATION

• Children with HPV infection must be assessed for sexual abuse.

> **ALERT:** None of the available treatments is superior to other treatments. No evidence indicates that the available treatments eradicate or affect the natural course of HPV. Treatment must be guided by the preference of the client, the cost, and experience of the health provider.

OFFICE TREATMENT

Equipment
• Podophyllum in a compound of tincture of benzoin
• Cotton applicators
• Petroleum jelly

PROCEDURE	SPECIAL CONSIDERATIONS
Apply petroleum jelly with cotton applicator around wart to protect normal skin.	**Contraindicated in pregnancy.**

Apply petroleum jelly with cotton applicator around wart to protect normal skin.

With cotton applicator (may use the stick end of the applicator), apply podophyllum directly to warts.

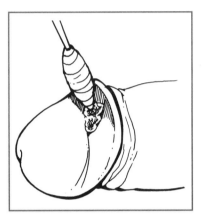

Allow to air dry before allowing surfaces to touch.

Instruct patient to wash off in 1 to 2 hours after the first application and 1 to 4 hours after subsequent treatments.

Repeat weekly for 4 weeks.

May apply to urethral meatal warts if it can be visualized in entirety. Mucosal attachment must be clearly visible.

Contraindicated in pregnancy.

Check the date on the podophyllum, because it has a short half-life.

Limit the application to ≤0.5 mL of podophyllum or ≤10 cm of warts per session to avoid toxicity.

Avoid contacting normal mucosa with podophyllum.

Not recommended for cervical or vaginal warts.

Podophyllum is systemically absorbed. Symptoms of toxicity: seizures, painful urination, breathing difficulty, dizziness, heartbeat irregularities, numbness, and tingling of hands and feet.

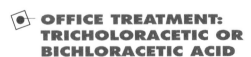

OFFICE TREATMENT: TRICHOLORACETIC OR BICHLORACETIC ACID

Equipment
• Trichloroacetic (TCA) or dichloroacetic (Bichloracetic [BCA]) acid
• Petroleum jelly
• Cotton applicators
•Sodium bicarbonate (household baking soda)

PROCEDURE	SPECIAL CONSIDERATIONS
Apply petroleum jelly around area to be treated.	Safe during pregnancy.
Apply a small amount of TCA or BCA only to warts and allow to air dry.	
Apply sodium bicarbonate to remove unreacted acid if application is in excess.	
Repeat weekly.	

 ## OFFICE TREATMENT: CRYOTHERAPY

Equipment
- Cryotherapy liquid nitrogen
- Cotton-tipped applicators (fluff cotton to hold more liquid)
- Styrofoam cup containing approximately ½ inch of liquid nitrogen

PROCEDURE	SPECIAL CONSIDERATIONS
Place several swabs in cup to allow time to cool and soak up liquid nitrogen.	Always use a separate container for soaking the cotton swabs to avoid contaminating the stock liquid.
Rotate the swabs to maintain the freezing temperature.	Vent to the outside.
Freeze each wart twice for 10 to 15 seconds. Allow time for area to thaw between applications.	(See Chap. 8: Skin Lesions, p. 58, for illustrations of freezing.)
Press on the wart until an ice coat forms and extends to 1 to 3 mm beyond the base.	
Requires three to four weekly or biweekly treatments.	Avoid applying too much pressure because it increases the rate and depth of freezing.
Patient education: Blistering and pain may occur. If open areas result, an antibiotic ointment may be applied.	

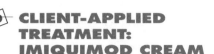

CLIENT-APPLIED TREATMENT: IMIQUIMOD CREAM

Equipment
• Imiquimod 5% cream

PROCEDURE	SPECIAL CONSIDERATIONS
Patient should apply with finger at bedtime, three times per week for up to 16 weeks.	**Contraindicated in pregnancy.**
Teach patient to apply Monday, Wednesday, and Friday.	Medication works at the cellular level, so if days are skipped, it does not deactivate in the cells.
Wash area with mild soap and water 6 to 10 hours after application.	

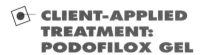

CLIENT-APPLIED TREATMENT: PODOFILOX GEL

Equipment
• Podofilox 0.5% gel (Condylox)
• Cotton-tipped applicators

PROCEDURE	SPECIAL CONSIDERATIONS
Apply directly to warts twice a day (morning and night).	**Contraindicated in pregnancy.**
Repeat the treatment twice a day for 3 days and then do not treat for 4 days. Three days of medication, then 4 days off medication.	Patient has to be able to see the wart. Medication is systemically absorbed.
Treat for up to 4 weeks.	
Stop the treatment as soon as the warts disappear.	
Return to the health care provider when 4 weeks of treatment have been completed.	

ALERT: In the case of extensive genital warts, cervical condyloma, and warts not responding to the above-mentioned measures in 3 to 4 weeks, refer the patient to an appropriate specialist for possible surgical excision, laser therapy, or other treatment.

Biopsy is indicated for genital warts that are pigmented, indurated, fixed, or ulcerated.

In the case of mucosal and meatal warts, refer the patient to an appropriate specialist. If meatal warts are present, a urologic evaluation to assess for lesions in the urethra may be indicated.

FOLLOW-UP

- Assess all clients 3 months after treatment, because this is the most frequent timeframe for recurrence.
- An annual Pap smear is recommended for all women who have been diagnosed with HPV.

BIBLIOGRAPHY

Celum, L., Wilch, E., Fennell, C., & Stamm, W. E. (1994). *The practitioner's handbook for the management of sexually transmitted diseases* (2nd ed., pp. 55–59). University of Washington: Health Science Center for Educational Resources.

Centers for Disease Control and Prevention. (1998). 1998 guidelines for treatment of sexually transmitted diseases. *MMWR, 47*(RR-1), 88–94.

Healthcare Consultants of America. (1998). *1998 Physicians' fee and coding guide*. Augusta, GA.

Neill, E. H. & Waldrop, J. B. (1998). Changes in body image, depression, and anxiety levels among women with human papillomavirus infection. *Journal of American Academy of Nurse Practitioners, 10*(5), 197–200.

Yu, J. N. (1994). Treatment and removal of warts. *Journal of American Academy of Physician Assistants, 7*(1), 33–39.

chapter
43
Diaphragm Fitting

CPT Coding:

> 57170 Diaphragm or cervical cap fitting with instructions ($59–$73). (This does not include the cost of the diaphragm.)

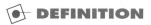 DEFINITION

A diaphragm is a barrier, dome-shaped, flexible rim, latex birth control device that is placed in the vagina to cover the cervix.

INDICATION

• Woman is interested in barrier method of birth control.

ASSESSMENT

Elements That Must be in Place for the Diaphragm to be Successful

1. Desire of the woman for a diaphragm as birth control method
2. No allergy to spermicidal agents or latex
3. Ability and willingness of woman to learn insertion and removal techniques
4. Woman has gained or lost 10 pounds or more since last diaphragm fitting
5. Woman is 6 weeks postpartum or it has been 6 weeks since a spontaneous or induced abortion
6. Woman is due for annual exam (diaphragm fit should be checked annually)
7. No history of toxic shock syndrome
8. No cervical biopsy or cryosurgery within the last 6 to 12 weeks

PATIENT EDUCATION

• Diaphragm must be fitted to the individual woman; sizes range from 50 to 105 mm in diameter.
• Urinary tract infections are more common in diaphragm users, so voiding after intercourse and using good urinary hygiene is important (Speroff & Darney, 1996).

- The patient will need to practice diaphragm removal and insertion in the exam room after the proper size is inserted. Remind the patient to wash her hands before insertion and removal.
- In actual use, the diaphragm must be used with contraceptive cream, gel, film, or foam instead of the lubricant used for practice. Two teaspoons of the contraceptive agent should be placed inside of the diaphragm, and a small amount should be spread around the rim before actual use. Oil-based products and vaginal medications should not be used with diaphragms because these products tend to damage latex.
- After intercourse, the diaphragm must be left in place for at least 6 hours but should be removed within 24 hours owing to the possibility of toxic shock syndrome. Additional spermicide should be placed in the vagina, without removing diaphragm, before each additional episode of sexual intercourse.
- The diaphragm should be washed with warm water and mild soap, rinsed, and dried after each use; store dry. A small amount of cornstarch may be applied to the dry diaphragm to prevent the latex from becoming "sticky."
- Fragranced powders or talcum should never be used because they tend to damage latex.
- The diaphragm should be held up to the light before each use to check for cracks or holes. If a crack or hole is identified, a new diaphragm should be purchased. Most diaphragms last several years with proper care.
- Note: Most diaphragms in fitting sets are manufactured with holes in the center.
- The woman should be aware of the signs and symptoms of toxic shock syndrome.

 ALERT: Because of the danger of toxic shock syndrome, the diaphragm should not be left in place during menstruation.

ASSESSMENT

1. Obtain obstetric, medical, surgical, and contraceptive history.
2. Determine the woman's ability to understand and practice correct insertion and removal of diaphragm.
3. Identify patterns of compliance. Regular use of the diaphragm is critical to its success.

DEVELOPMENTAL CONSIDERATIONS

Adolescent: Diaphragms are most appropriate and effective as birth control for older, married women. Thus, the diaphragm may not be the ideal choice for unmarried adolescents.

◉ EQUIPMENT

- Gloves, water-soluble lubricant
- Diaphragm fitting ring; a set of fitting diaphragms
- Fitted diaphragm, lubricant, private room
- Soap, water, disinfectant (what do you recommend?), storage area away from extreme temperatures

PROCEDURE	SPECIAL CONSIDERATIONS

Perform a vaginal exam with the middle and index fingers. With the tip of the middle finger placed against the vaginal wall at the cul-de-sac, lift the hand anteriorly so that the symphysis pubis touches the hand between the index finger and the thumb. Mark that point exteriorly with the thumb as you withdraw the fingers from the vagina. The distance from the tip of the middle finger to the placement of the thumb marks the approximate diaphragm size.

Although this maneuver provides an estimate of size, more than one diaphragm should be tried for fit. A diaphragm that is too large may cause discomfort, whereas a diaphragm that is too small will be ineffective.

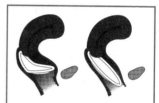

Incorrect diaphragm—too large. (Speroff, L. & Darney, P. (1996). *Clinical guide for contraception.* Baltimore: Williams & Wilkins.)

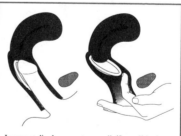

Incorrect diaphragm—too small. (Speroff, L. & Darney, P. [1996]. *Clinical guide for contraception.* Baltimore: Williams & Wilkins.)

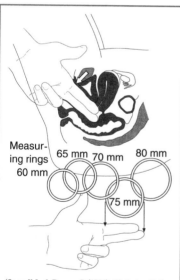

Measuring rings 60 mm 65 mm 70 mm 75 mm 80 mm

(Speroff, L. & Darney, P. (1996). *Clinical guide for contraception.* Baltimore: Williams & Wilkins.)

(procedure continued)

PROCEDURE

Select the size and type of diaphragm to fit. Sizes range from 50 to 105 mm, in increments of 3.5 to 5 mm. Most women are fitted with 65 to 80 mm (Speroff & Darney, 1996). The fit should be snug between the vaginal walls, fornix, and pubic arch but should not be uncomfortable.

Grasp the diaphragm rim edge between thumb and fingers and compress the rim edges together. This action folds the diaphragm in half so that the dome (filled with contraceptive agent) forms a hanging pouch and the rim forms two pointed ends. While spreading the lips of the labia with your other hand, insert the pointed end of the folded diaphragm into the vagina, pushing it inward and downward with the index finger as far as it will go. Then with the index finger, press the anterior edge of the diaphragm up and snugly behind the pelvic bone.

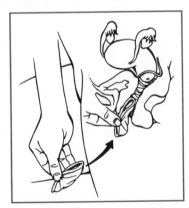

SPECIAL CONSIDERATIONS

Several types of diaphragms are available:

Flat spring: best for women with firm vaginal muscle tone or a shallow notch behind the pubic bone.

Arching spring: most women can use the arching spring; it can also be used with rectocele, cystocele, poor vaginal tone, a long cervix, or an anterior cervix of a retroverted uterus.

Coil spring: intended for women with average muscle tone and pubic arch. Many women find it difficult to place the posterior edge of the diaphragm into the posterior cul-de-sac and over the cervix.

Wide seal: this diaphragm has a cuff around the inside rim, which is intended to create a better seal between diaphragm and vaginal wall. It is available with an arcing spring or coil spring rim.

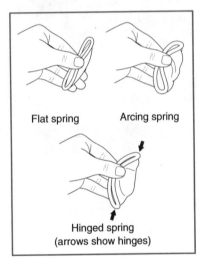

Flat spring   Arcing spring

Hinged spring
(arrows show hinges)

(procedure continued)

| PROCEDURE | SPECIAL CONSIDERATIONS |

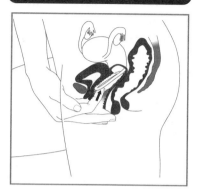

Remove the diaphragm by inserting a fingertip between the pubic bone and the front rim of the diaphragm. Pull downward on the diaphragm. When the front rim drops into the vagina, remove the diaphragm.

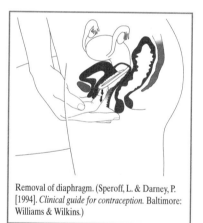

Removal of diaphragm. (Speroff, L. & Darney, P. [1994]. *Clinical guide for contraception.* Baltimore: Williams & Wilkins.)

The patient should be give the opportunity to practice insertion and removal of the diaphragm.

The patient may try to insert the diaphragm lying down, in a seated position, or standing with one foot on a stool.

(procedure continued)

PROCEDURE | SPECIAL CONSIDERATIONS

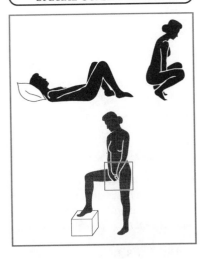

After practicing, the placement of the diaphragm should be checked.

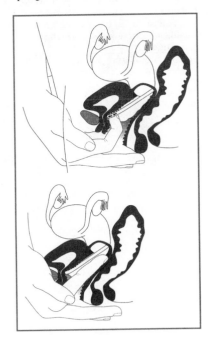

(procedure continued)

PROCEDURE	**SPECIAL CONSIDERATIONS**

At least 45 minutes should be allowed for practice. The woman should insert the fitting diaphragm rather than the fitting ring because it is more realistic.

Sample diaphragms should be washed, disinfected, and dried carefully before storing.

 FOLLOW-UP

- The patient should return 1 week after fitting with the diaphragm in place so that the practitioner can check the fit and use of the diaphragm.
- It is recommended that the woman replace the diaphragm every 3 years unless other circumstances dictate a change in diaphragm size.

BIBLIOGRAPHY

American Medical Association. (1998). *Physicians' current procedural terminology: CPT.* Chicago: American Medical Association.

Hatcher, R. A., Stewart, F. H., Trussell, J., Kowal, D., Guest, F., Stewart, G. K., Cates, W., & Policar, M. S. (1994). *Contraceptive technology* (16th ed.). New York: Irvington.

Healthcare Consultants of America. (1998). *1998 Physicians' fee and coding guide.* Augusta, GA.

Speroff, L. & Darney, P. D. (1996). *A clinical guide for contraception* (2nd ed.). Baltimore: Williams & Wilkins.

chapter 44

Depo-Provera (Depot Medroxyprogesterone Acetate [DMPA]): Injectable Contraceptive Administration

CPT Coding:

90782 Therapeutic intramuscular injection ($21–$27). The total cost is approximately $35–$37 per injection, excluding office visit charge

DEFINITION

Depo-Provera is an injectable contraceptive consisting of microcrystals of DMPA suspended in aqueous solution; it has a molecular structure similar to naturally occurring progesterone. DMPA is designed to offer sustained release of progesterone. Levels of progesterone are maintained for up to 4 months after injection, resulting in a 2- to 4-week "grace period," during which protection is provided.

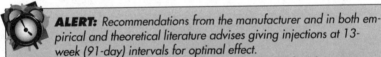

ALERT: Recommendations from the manufacturer and in both empirical and theoretical literature advises giving injections at 13-week (91-day) intervals for optimal effect.

DMPA's primary mechanism of action is suppression of ovulation secondary to suppression of follicle-stimulating hormone (FSH) and luteininzing hormone (LH) and prevention of the LH surge. Secondary mechanisms of action include (1) thickened cervical mucus and (2) altered endometrium, which serve as barriers to sperm penetration and implantation, respectively.

INDICATIONS

- Women of childbearing age who are seeking to prevent pregnancy or to space pregnancies with the aid of a contraceptive measure that offers the following advantages:
  - Not coitus-related
  - Provides for private use. Only the woman and her care provider know the drug is being used
  - Long acting (13 weeks for each dose)

- High contraceptive efficacy (Expected failure rate = <1%; typical failure rate = <1% reversible)
- Does not contain estrogen. Can be used in women with contraindications to estrogen (eg, younger than 35 years of age, smokers)
- Cost effective
- Need for advantages of drug, such as decreasing risk of pelvic inflammatory disease (PID); ectopic pregnancy; endometrial and ovarian cancer; decreased menstrual complications, such as dysmenorrhea and anemia; inhibition of intravascular sickling and increased red blood cell (RBC) survival in women with sickle cell anemia
- Efficacy not reduced by anticonvulsants, so good choice for women with seizure disorders
- Can be used safely in lactating women after 6 weeks of consistent breast-feeding; may increase protein quantity and quality in breast milk
- No increase in risk for breast cancer
• Inappropriate candidates are women who desire pregnancy within 1 to 2 years, and women who are unwilling or unable to comply with treatment schedule and/or menstrual pattern changes or any weight gain.

◉ PATIENT EDUCATION

• Review other contraceptive options.
• Provide information specific to DMPA. Provide copy of Food and Drug Administration (FDA)—approved, detailed patient labeling pamphlet or other written hand-out for reinforcement of information: mechanism of action; mode of administration; effectiveness; adverse effects; advantages and disadvantages; and charges. **Explain dosing schedule for optimal effectiveness, stressing need for return for reinjections on schedule.**
• Side effects of DMPA include menstrual changes, weight gain, headache, breast tenderness, fluid retention, decreased libido, depression, acne, hair loss, and decreased bone density.
• Discuss the delayed return to fertility associated with use of DMPA.

> **ALERT:** DMPA cannot be immediately reversed or neutralized; therefore, when DMPA is discontinued, effects continue until the drug is completely metabolized. The mean interval before return of ovulation is 4.5 months; the delay to conception is about 9 months. In a small number of women, fertility is not re-established until 18 months. The duration of use of DMPA does not appear to be related to return of ovulation.

• Review the menstrual cycle as a context for understanding DMPA's action and the changes in the menstrual pattern associated with DMPA. The most widely noted short-term side effect is menstrual changes—unpredictable, irregular bleeding and spotting in first few months—accounting for most discontinuation of drug. Frequency and length of bleeding episodes decrease, and there is a 50% incidence of amenorrhea after 9 to 12 months.

- Inform that DMPA does not protect against sexually transmitted (STDs); discuss safe sexual practices to be used in addition to the drug.
- Teach the following warning signs to report while using DMPA:
  A. Sharp chest pain, coughing up blood, or sudden shortness of breath
  B. Sudden severe headache, vomiting, dizziness, fainting, or problems with speech or vision
  C. Severe pain or swelling in the lower extremities
  D. Unusually heavy vaginal bleeding
  E. Persistent pain or infection at injection site
  F. Severe pain or persistent tenderness in lower abdomen
- Discuss the common side effect of weight gain (4 pounds per year is the average for the first 3 years). Advise about use of healthy diet and exercise to minimize drug-associated weight gain.
- Advise that decreased bone density may occur during use, but that it is reversible. Any risk continues to be investigated. Advise patient to take calcium citrate 500 mg/day PO to minimize any drug-associated bone demineralization. Teach about high-calcium foods.

◉ ASSESSMENT

1. Question about following contraindications to DMPA: allergy; hepatic disease; history of cerebrovascular accident (CVA), myocardial infarction (MI), breast cancer, or phlebitis; possible pregnancy; and vaginal bleeding of undetermined origin.
2. Ask whether the patient has a history of epilepsy, migraine, asthma, cardiac or renal dysfunction, or depression, which would involve caution and necessitate (until special protocols approved) consultation with physician before administration.
3. Ask about how common changes in the menstrual patterns will affect lifestyle and sexual relationship, appreciating that lack of support by male partner is a common reason for dissatisfaction with and discontinuation of DMPA. Does the patient believe in the myth that failure to bleed monthly is somehow harmful?
4. Conduct a brief sexual assessment to identify possible decreased libido.
5. Determine planned timing for future pregnancy.
6. List other medications that the patient is currently taking.

 ALERT: DMPA should not be given to women taking aminoglutethimide (Cytraden) (used in Cushing's disease).

7. Determine that the woman meets the following criteria for optimal administration of DMPA:
   a. Schedule the appointment within 5 days of the onset of menses to ensure that the patient is not pregnant and to prevent ovulation in first month of use

b. No later than 1 week after voluntary interruption of pregnancy or miscarriage

c. Within the first 5 days postpartum, unless the patient is breastfeeding

d. At 6 weeks postpartum, if the patient is consistently breastfeeding (use back-up during the first week)

e. With oral contraceptive pills (OCPs) or an intrauterine (IUD) in use during preceding cycle, give DMPA during first 5 days of onset of menses. No back-up is needed. If no alternative exists for starting DMPA "off-cycle," advise abstinence for 2 weeks, then perform a pregnancy test. If the results of the test are negative, give drug.

f. Back-up method for 7 days

ALERT: *Reinjections are administered at 13-week (91-day) intervals. If the patient is less than 1 week late for injection (<14 weeks since last dose, do a pregnancy test, and assure consistency of protective intercourse. Give dose if pregnancy is ruled out. If pregnancy cannot be ruled out at this time, advise no intercourse (or persistent condom use) for 2 weeks, with return visit for pregnancy test. If the results of the test are negative, give DMPA.*

8. Ensure recent physical examination, including Pap smear, and current weight, blood pressure, and hematocrit measurements. **Do not administer DMPA if the patient's hematocrit is less than 30 without consultation. With history of bleeding/spotting, repeat hematocrit before reinjection.**

◉⊢ DEVELOPMENTAL CONSIDERATIONS

Child: DMPA is not a first choice contraceptive for girls younger than 15 years of age. Concern exists about the bone demineralization that may occur in the short term, especially in puberty, when maximal bone mineralization is occurring. If the benefits of reliable contraception outweigh the risk of reversible, decreased bone density, calcium intake should be supplemented with calcium citrate 500 mg/day.

Teens: With teens, praise their responsibility for seeking contraception, making sure that they are fully informed, including knowledge of safe sexual practices. Linking contraceptive choice with their life goals increases compliance.

Lactating Women: DMPA should be given to lactating women only after lactation has been fully established at 6 weeks postpartum.

ALERT: *Before the injection, ensure that the woman has received adequate information on which to base her decision about taking the drug and that she has signed an informed consent.*

 ## EQUIPMENT

- Sterile 1- to 2-mL syringe with a 21- to 23-gauge needle: Needle gauge depends on size and muscle mass in woman and whether drug will be given in deltoid or gluteal muscle
- Vial of Depo-Provera 150 mg/mL
- Alcohol swab
- Adhesive bandage

PROCEDURE	SPECIAL CONSIDERATIONS
Shake vial vigorously to ensure that suspension of the microcrystals of drug are suspended.	
Draw the solution into the sterile syringe using aseptic technique.	
Inject a 150-mg/mL dose 1 mL IM **slowly** in either deltoid muscle or in the upper outer quadrant of the gluteal muscle using proper injection technique to minimize trauma to nerves, risk of infection, bruising, and pain.	**Do not use Depo-Provera 400 mg/mL. That dose is used to treat neoplasia.** The manufacturer prefers the gluteal injection site. Deltoid site should be reserved for women with a large muscle mass. Deltoid injections tend to be more painful.
Hold pressure over injection site after administration of medication. **Do not massage.**	
Apply to injection site if needed.	

 ## ALTERNATIVE PROCEDURE

- Discuss other options for family planning if woman does not want to continue to use DMPA.

 ## FOLLOW-UP

- Give appointment card for the next injection before leaving clinic. Help the woman associate appointment with a familiar date to optimize remembering the return visit. If clinic sends "reminder cards," be certain to ask if sending one is appropriate to ensure that concerns about privacy and confidentiality are met.

⦿ MANAGEMENT OF BREAKTHROUGH BLEEDING

- Provide reassurance that breakthrough bleeding is a common side effect during the first few months, that it does not represent a medical problem, and that it will likely decrease with length of use.
- Administer one to two cycles of monophasic OCPs; a short course (3 weeks) of estrogen (2 mg daily of estradiol or 1.25 mg daily of conjugated estrogen to stabilize endometrium); or ibuprofen 800 mg daily for 5 to 14 days. Using the Climara estrogen patch for 1 week; repeat for two cycles also may be helpful.
- **Investigate persistent heavy bleeding; refer the patient to a gynecologic specialist, if necessary.**

BIBLIOGRAPHY

American Medical Association. (1998). *Physicians' current procedural terminology: CPT.* Chicago: American Medical Association.

Darney, P. D. & Kaisle, C. M. (1998). Contraception-associated menstrual problems. *Dialogues in Contraception, 3*(5), 1–11.

Grimes, D. A. & Wallach, M. (1998). *Modern contraception.* Totowa, NJ: Emron.

Hatcher, R. A., Trussell, J., Stewart, F., Stewart, G. K., Kowal, D., Guest, F., Cates, W. & Policar, M. S. (1994). *Contraceptive Technology.* New York: Irvington Publishers.

Healthcare Consultants of America. (1998). *1998 Physicians' fee and coding guide.* Augusta, GA.

Kaunitz, A. M. (1993). DMPA: A new contraceptive option. *Contemporary OB/GYN-NP,* 5–12.

Kaunitz, A. M. & Rosenfield, D. (1994). Injectable contraception (pp. 183–188). In Corson, S. L., Derman, R. J., & Tyner, L. B. *Fertility Control.* London, Canada: Goldwin.

Kaunitz, A. M. & Jordan, C. W. (1997). Two long-acting hormonal contraceptive options. *Contemporary Nurse Practitioner, 42*(2), 27–28, 31, 35–36.

Moore, R.(1994). *Contraception issues & options for young women.* Fair Lawn, N.J.: MPE Communications. Medroxyprogesterone acetate for contraceptive use. *AWHONN Clinical Commentary.*

Overview of DMPA: Drug interactions with OCPs. *The Contraceptive Report, 3*(5), 2–8.

Peters, S. (1996). After baby—choosing a contraceptive method. *ADVANCE for Nurse Practitioners, 6,* 31–34.

Speroff, L. & Darney, P. D. (1992). *A clinical guide for contraception.* Baltimore: Williams & Wilkins.

Speroff, L., Glass, R. H. & Kase, N. G. (1994). *Clinical gynecologic endocrinology and infertility.* Baltimore: Williams & Wilkins.

chapter
45

| Female Condom

CPT Coding:

N/A

 DEFINITION

The female condom is a soft, thin polyurethane sheath with a flexible ring on each end. It is a disposable vaginal barrier that is designed to prevent pregnancy and provide protection from sexually transmitted diseases and acquired immunodeficiency syndrome (AIDS).

 INDICATIONS

• Prevent pregnancy
• Prevent transmission of sexually transmitted disease and AIDS.

 ALERT: The female condom has a 5% pregnancy rate with perfect use and a 21% pregnancy rate with typical use. Typical use is defined as incorrect or nonuse.

 PATIENT EDUCATION

• Advise the patient that the female condom can be inserted minutes to hours before intercourse. Maximum wear time is 8 hours.
• Advise patient that the female condom should remain in place after coitus for 6 hours.
• Advise the patient that the female condom comes in one size and is designed to fit most women.
• Advise the patient that the female condom has a shelf life of 3 years.
• The female condom is available over the counter at most pharmacies: The patient cost of the female condom ranges from $2.75 to $3.00 per each condom. They can be purchased in boxes of three or six.
• Instruct the patient that a spermicide is not indicated for use with the female condom.
• Advise the patient that the female condom can be worn during the menstrual cycle, but it should be removed immediately after coitus.

• The female condom is not designed for use with the male condom. This will cause displacement of one or both of the devices.

 ALERT: *The female condom is designed for a single use only.*

ASSESSMENT

1. Assess barriers to learning.
2. Assess readiness to learn proper technique used for insertion of female condom.
3. Provide indications for use and document.

EQUIPMENT

• Female condom

PROCEDURE	SPECIAL CONSIDERATIONS
In upright position, place a leg on a stool. Pinch the inner ring with the index finger of the dominant hand and insert condom into the posterior vagina and release ring.	The condom is prelubricated, and no spermicide is indicated.
	The sheath covers the cervix, lines the vaginal wall, and extends over the labia.
	If the inner ring dislodges during intercourse, the sheath will continue to move with the penis.
	Fitting is not required by a health professional.

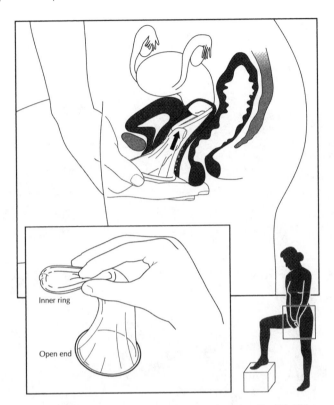

Position of woman for insertion of female condom and positioning after insertion. (Speroff, L. & Darney, P. [1996]. *Clinical guide for contraception.* Baltimore: Williams & Wilkins.)

 ## TROUBLESHOOTING GUIDELINES REGARDING INSERTION AND PLACEMENT

- If the client states that the female condom is noisy, suggest applying a water-based lubricant to the condom or the penis.
- If the client complains that the device adheres to the penis and does not stay in the vagina, suggest applying a lubricant to the device or the penis.
- If the partner can feel the inner ring of the condom at the distal aspect of the vagina, suggest that the device be reinserted and the inner ring pushed as far up inside the vagina as it will go, or check to be sure that the sheath is not twisted.
- If the client states that the outer ring (covering the labia) was pushed into the vagina, suggest using more lubricant.
- If either partner complains of minor irritation or discomfort, suggest reinsertion to ensure proper placement or suggest using more lubricant.

◉ FOLLOW-UP

• None needed, although it may be helpful to have the patient return to have her questions answered.

BIBLIOGRAPHY

American Medical Association. (1998). *Physicians' current procedural terminology: CPT.* Chicago: American Medical Association.

Grimes, D. A., & Wallach, M. (1997). *Modern contraception/updates from the contraception report.* Totowa, NJ: Emron.

Hatcher, R. A., Trussell, J., Stewart, F., et al. (1998). *Contraceptive technology,* 17. New York: Ardent Media, Inc.

Healthcare Consultants of America. (1998). *1998 Physicians' fee and coding guide.* Augusta, GA.

Speroff, L., & Darney, P. (1996). *A clinical guide for contraception.* Baltimore, MD: Williams & Wilkins.

chapter
46

Gonorrhea and Chlamydia Specimen Collection for Culture

CPT Coding:

87110 Chlamydia culture ($50–$64)
87270 *Chlamydia trachomatis* antigen detection by direct fluorescent antibody ($40–$53)
87320 *Chlamydia trachomatis* by enzyme immunoassay technique #87320 ($40–$53)
87490 *Chlamydia trachomatis,* direct probe technique ($63–$81)
87491 *Chlamydia trachomatis,* amplified probe technique ($101–$130)
87590 *Neisseria gonorrhoeae,* direct probe technique ($63–$81)
87591 *Neisseria gonorrhoeae,* amplified probe technique ($101–$130)

◉ DEFINITIONS

- Gonorrhea is a common sexually transmitted infection (STI) caused by the gram-negative diplococcus *Neisseria gonorrhoeae.* It may be asymptomatic and is often seen in conjunction with chlamydia.
- Chlamydia is the most common bacterial STI in the United States (Hatcher, Trussell, Stewart, Cates, Stewart, Guest, & Kowal, 1998); the condition is caused by *Chlamydia trachomatis.* Chlamydia are intracellular parasites; therefore, definitive laboratory diagnosis can be made only by cell culture (Hatcher et al., 1998).
- Culture is the laboratory propagation of cells for identification of specific infectious disease-causing organisms.

◉ INDICATIONS

- Mucopurulent cervicitis (even in otherwise asymptomatic women).
- Nongonococcal urethritis (NGU) is caused by chlamydia 50% of the time (Hatcher et al., 1998).
- In women, there is pelvic pain such as that seen with pelvic inflammatory disease (PID), unusual vaginal discharge, abnormal menses, dysuria, frequent urinary tract infections (UTIs), low abdominal pain or vaginal bleeding with intercourse, bleeding between menses, cervical motion tenderness or friable cervix. In men, the symptoms are urinary frequency, dysuria, and

purulent urethral discharge. In both men and women, pharyngitis or anal itching, pain, or discharge may be present.

> **ALERT:** Any woman with a fever higher than 101.4°F, a leukocyte count greater than 10,000, or an abdominal mass should be referred to an emergency room or physician immediately.

• The Centers for Disease Control and Prevention (CDC, 1998) recommends annual gonorrhea and chlamydia cultures for all women younger than 26 years of age who are unmarried or who are not involved in a monogamous relationship.

> **ALERT:** In most states, gonorrhea or chlamydia, or both, are reportable diseases.

PATIENT EDUCATION

• Reassure the patient that both gonorrhea and chlamydia cultures are completed quickly and simply with minimal discomfort.
• If either or both culture results are positive, all of the patient's sexual contacts or partners are likely to be infected with the organism and will need to be treated as well. Coitus should be avoided until the patient and his or her partner or partners complete the course of treatment.
• Both gonorrhea and chlamydia are treatable diseases.

ASSESSMENT

1. Obtain an obstetric, gynecologic, STI, and sexual history for women, and a genitourinary, STI, and sexual history for men.
2. Ask about any present signs and symptoms.
3. Perform a speculum exam on women, including palpation of Bartholin glands for enlargement.

> **ALERT:** The order of collection for separate specimens is (1) Pap smear, (2) gonorrhea, and (3) chlamydia. Simultaneous collection of both specimens with one swab must be completed before the Pap smear owing to the test's sensitivity to blood.

4. Examine the genitalia on men and ask if any discharge can be produced at the time of exam.
5. Determine the patient's ability to cooperate and hold still during specimen attainment.

DEVELOPMENTAL CONSIDERATIONS

Child: Vulvovaginitis is severe with gonorrhea in prepubertal girls (Ramin, Wendel, & Hemsell, 1994); therefore, examination may be difficult and will require patience, as well as assistance and support for the child. Consider sexual abuse as a primary cause.

Adolescent: Sexually active women 19-years-old and younger have a chlamydia rate 2 to 3 times higher than that of older women (Ramin et al., 1994) and thus should be screened yearly for gonorrhea and chlamydia.

Newborns: Newborns can develop ophthalmia neonatorum as they pass through the birth canals of mothers with gonorrhea or chlamydia. Thus, all pregnant women should be cultured and all newborns receive prophylactic ophthalmic ointment within 1 hour of birth.

 ## FOR SEPARATE GONORRHEA AND CHLAMYDIA SPECIMENS FOR WOMEN

Equipment
- Gloves and speculum
- Sterile cotton-tipped swab for gonorrhea specimen
- Label for plate lid
- Culture medium plate

PROCEDURE	SPECIAL CONSIDERATIONS
Insert the speculum into the vagina at a 45-degree posterior angle until clear visualization of the cervix is achieved. Lock the speculum in the open position. Use a large cotton swab to remove vaginal secretions and exudate from the exocervix.	In asymptomatic women, the appearance of mucopurulent cervicitis or a friable cervix is an indication for performing cultures.
Insert the cotton tip of the swab into the cervical os and hold it in place for 10 to 30 seconds (Seidel, Ball, Dains, & Benedict, 1999).	For a urethral culture in women, wait 1 to 2 hours after urination to obtain specimen since voiding may reduce urethral discharge.
	If an anal culture is needed, the cotton-tipped swab may be inserted into the anal canal about 2.5 cm and rotated 360 degrees. The rest of the procedure remains the same.

(procedure continued) ─────────────────────────────────────

| **PROCEDURE** | **SPECIAL CONSIDERATIONS** |

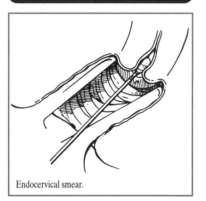

Endocervical smear.

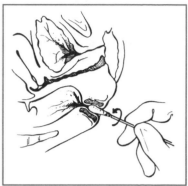

Do not touch the vaginal walls when removing the swab. Inoculate the specimen in a Z pattern over the entire culture medium (Figures A and B show this action).

Do not refrigerate the gonorrhea specimen.

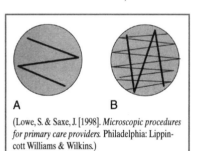

A   B

(Lowe, S. & Saxe, J. [1998]. *Microscopic procedures for primary care providers.* Philadelphia: Lippincott Williams & Wilkins.)

Place the patient's name on the label and place the label on the outside of the lid of the culture medium plate. This specimen needs to be stored in a anaerobic environment: CO_2 incubator or candle jar.

FOR SEPARATE GONORRHEA AND CHLAMYDIA SPECIMENS FOR MEN

Equipment
- Gloves
- Small cotton-tipped metal swab (Calgi) designed for urethral specimen obtainment
- Culture medium plate

PROCEDURE	SPECIAL CONSIDERATIONS

Have the patient "milk" the penis for several seconds.

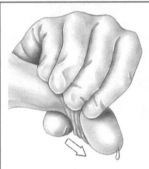

(Lohr, Jacob A. [1991]. *Pediatric outpatient procedures.* Philadelphia: J.B. Lippincott Company.)

Collect any visible exudate at the urethral meatus.

If there is no obvious discharge, insert a urogenital swab into the urethra: Grasp the glans of the penis with the nondominant hand and press gently to open the urinary meatus.

This is an uncomfortable procedure. Warn the patient beforehand.

(procedure continued)

| **PROCEDURE** | **SPECIAL CONSIDERATIONS** |

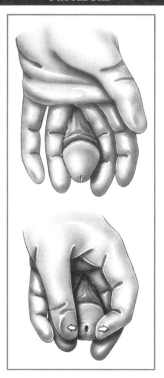

Insert the swab into the meatus about 1 to 2 cm and rotate it 360 degrees. Withdraw the swab. The remainder of the procedure is the same as the female specimen.

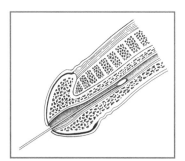

FOR COLLECTION OF CHLAMYDIA SPECIMEN OR SIMULTANEOUS DNA PROBE COLLECTION OF CHLAMYDIA AND GONORRHEA CULTURES

Equipment
- Gloves and Dacron swab with plastic or wire shaft from the test kit
- Tube containing specific specimen reagent from the test kit
- Label and pen

PROCEDURE	SPECIAL CONSIDERATIONS
Following insertion of the speculum and visualization of the cervix, insert the swab into the cervical os and rotate 360 degrees repeatedly for 30 seconds. Remove the swab without touching the sides of the vagina.	For specimen collection for men, using the wire-shaft Dacron swab, follow the directions for the actual obtainment of the urethral specimen.
Uncap the tube; insert the swab, cotton-tipped end first, into the liquid reagent in the tube. Break the plastic swab shaft at the serration (the wire shaft should fit into the length of the tube) and replace the cap.	Do not place the specimen on a medium plate.
Label the specimen tube with the patient's name.	

 ALTERNATIVE PROCEDURES

- Gonorrhea may be detected through Gram's stain. Chlamydia may be suspected when profuse white blood cells (WBCs) are found in the smear of discharge on a saline wet mount. For oropharyngeal culture, a specimen of secretion is obtained on a sterile swab from the oropharynx. (See Chapter 49: Wet Mount and Gram Stain.)

 FOLLOW-UP

- Because treatment failure is rare with good patient compliance, the most cost-effective approach is re-examination within 1 to 2 months to check for reinfection or treatment failure.

BIBLIOGRAPHY

American Medical Association. (1998). *Physicians' current procedural terminology: CPT*. Chicago: American Medical Association.

Centers for Disease Control and Prevention. (1998). Guidelines for treatment of sexually transmitted diseases. *Morbidity and Mortality Weekly Report, 47*(No. RR-1), 96.

Fogel, N. & Woods, N. F. (1995). *Women's health care: A comprehensive handbook*. Thousand Oaks, CA: Sage.

Hatcher, R. A., Stewart, F., Trussell, J., Kowal, D. Guest, F., Stewart, G. K, Cates, W., & Policar, M. (1998). *Contraceptive technology* (17th ed.). New York: Ardent Media.

Healthcare Consultants of America. (1998). *1998 Physicians' fee and coding guide*. Augusta, GA.

Ramin, S. M., Wendel, G. D., & Hemsell, D. L. (1994). Sexually transmitted diseases & pelvic infections. In A. H. DeCherney & M. L. Pernoll (Eds.), *Current obstetric & gynecologic diagnosis & treatment* (pp. 754–784). Norwalk, CT: Appleton & Lange.

Seidel, H. M., Ball, J. W., Dains, J. E., & Benedict, G. W. (1999). *Mosby's guide to physical examination* (4th ed.). St Louis: Mosby.

chapter 47

Norplant Insertion and Removal

CPT Coding:

11975 Norplant insertion ($215–$275)
11976 Norplant removal ($195–$255)
11977 Norplant removal with reinsertion ($380–$525)

DEFINITION

Norplant is a long-acting contraceptive implant inserted subdermally, usually in the medial aspect of the upper arm. It consists of six flexible closed capsules made of Silastic, each containing 36 mg of the progestin levonorgestrel. Diffusion of the levonorgestrol through the wall of each capsule provides a continuous low dose of the progestin. It provides up to 5 years of effective contraceptive protection. Two mechanisms of action are active in preventing pregnancy: inhibition of ovulation and thickening of the cervical mucus, preventing sperm penetration.

INDICATIONS

- For the prevention of pregnancy in women
- Long-term (up to 5 years) reversible contraceptive product
- Can be used by women who cannot use estrogen-containing contraceptives

> **ALERT:** Norplant is contraindicated in women with active or thromboembolic disease, undiagnosed abnormal genital bleeding, known or suspected pregnancy, acute liver disease, benign or malignant liver tumors, known or suspected carcinoma of the breast, or history of idiopathic intracranial hypertension.

PATIENT EDUCATION

Efficacy
- Norplant is one of the most effective contraceptive methods available, with an annual failure rate of less than 1%.
- Contraceptive action is fully and rapidly reversible.

Drug Interactions
- Reduced efficacy and unintended pregnancy has been reported for Norplant users taking phenytoin and/or carbamazepine.

Bleeding Irregularities
- Most women (60%) can expect some variation in menstrual bleeding patterns. Irregular bleeding, intermenstrual spotting, prolonged episodes of bleeding and spotting, and amenorrhea occur in some women. These irregularities diminish with continued use, usually after 6 to 12 months.

Delayed Follicular Atresia
- If follicular development occurs with Norplant, atresia of the follicle may be delayed and the follicle may continue to grow beyond the size it would normally attain. These lesions cannot be distinguished from ovarian cysts. Most often, these follicles spontaneously disappear and should not require surgery.

Ectopic Pregnancies
- Ectopic pregnancies have occurred among Norplant users at similar rates as with users of no method or users of intrauterine devices (IUDs). The risk may increase with duration of use or possibly with increased weight of the user.

Thromboembolic Disease
- Patients who develop active thrombophlebitis or thromboembolic disease should have Norplant removed.

Sexually Transmitted Diseases
- Norplant does not protect against sexually transmitted diseases (STDs), including human immunodeficiency virus (HIV) or acquired immunodeficiency syndrome (AIDS). For protection against STDs, it is advisable to use latex condoms with spermicide along with Norplant.

Other Disadvantages
- Weight gain, headache, nausea, dizziness, nervousness, rash, acne, change in appetite, mastalgia, scalp hair loss, hirsutism, and hypertrichosis may occur.
- Difficulty with removal can occur.

Availability of Norplant
- Norplant will be provided by the Norplant Foundation at no cost to women who meet the eligibility requirements. To qualify, women must have
  - No insurance coverage for reversible contraception
  - An annual income less than 185% of the poverty income guidelines (less than $12,247 for a single woman with no dependents, or $24,790 for a head of household with dependents); and
  - Sponsorship of a clinician for insertion and removal at no additional cost to the woman.
- An application or further information about the program is available at Norplant Foundation

P.O. Box 25223
Alexandria, VA 22314
703-706-5933, M-F, 9-5 EST

The Insertion Procedure

- Infection at the insertion site has been uncommon (0.7%). Attention to aseptic technique and proper insertion and removal reduce the possibility of infection.
- Expulsion of implants is uncommon. It is occurs more frequently when placement of the implants is extremely shallow, too close to the incision, or when infection is present. Contraceptive efficacy may be inadequate with fewer than six implants. Replacement of the expelled implant using a new sterile implant is recommended.
- Women should be counseled that they can request removal of the implants at any time for medical or personal reasons. Removal should be performed on request or at the end of the 5 years of use by personnel instructed in the removal technique.
- Norplant may be inserted at anytime in the woman's cycle provided that pregnancy has been excluded and the patient is told that a nonhormonal contraceptive should be used for at least 7 days after insertion.
- Swelling, tenderness and bruising may occur.
- A pressure dressing should be kept in place for 24 hours after insertion. The skin closures should be left on for 3 days or until they fall off. During that time, the incision site should be kept clean and dry.
- Do not bump the area or lift heavy objects until the incision heals.

Complications or Serious Side Effects That Need To Be Reported to the Clinician

- Sharp chest pain, hemoptysis, dyspnea, indicating a possible pulmonary embolism
- Pain in the calf or arm, indicating a possible thrombus
- Sudden or severe headache, vomiting, dizziness, syncope, vision loss, weakness or numbness in arm or leg, indicating a possible cerebrovascular accident (CVA) or an embolus
- Persistent headaches in an obese patient or recent weight gain, indicating possible idiopathic intracranial hypertension
- Severe pain in the abdomen, indicating a possible liver tumor, an ectopic pregnancy, or a ruptured cyst
- Signs and symptoms of depression
- Jaundice, indicating a possible liver problem

The Removal Procedure

- Patients should be counseled about the removal procedure before insertion.
- Removal is available at any time and for any reason.
- An additional charge for removal is required.
- May require an additional incision or additional visits, or both, if all implants cannot be removed at once.

ASSESSMENT

1. A complete medical history should be obtained and a physical exam should be performed before the implantation or reimplantation and at least annually during its use. The physical examination should include checking the implant site, blood pressure, breasts, liver, abdomen, extremities and pelvic organs, including cervical cytology and relevant laboratory tests.
2. If jaundice develops in any woman using Norplant, removal should be considered. Steroid hormones may be poorly metabolized in patients with impaired liver function.
3. Consideration should be given to removing Norplant in women who become significantly depressed after Norplant insertion. The symptom may be drug related.
4. An altered glucose tolerance characterized by decreased insulin sensitivity following glucose loading has been found in users of progestin contraceptives. Diabetic and prediabetic patients should be carefully monitored while using Norplant.
5. Certain endocrine tests may be affected by Norplant use:
   • Sex hormone–binding globulin concentrations may be decreased.
   • Thyroxine concentrations may be slightly decreased, and triiodothyronine uptake may be increased.

ALERT: To be sure that a woman is not pregnant at the time of insertion and to ensure complete effectiveness during the first cycle of use, it is advisable that Norplant insertion be done during the first 7 days of the menstrual cycle. Use of Norplant is not recommended before 6 weeks postpartum in breast-feeding women.

INSERTION PROCEDURE

Equipment
• The Norplant system kit contains the following items needed for insertion:
   – Six Norplant system capsules
   – #10 trocar
   – Scalpel
   – Straight and curved forceps
   – Syringe and needles for infusing local anesthetic
   – Skin closures
   – Gauze sponges
   – Stretch bandage
   – Surgical drapes
• You will need to supply the following in addition to the above:
   – Sterile gloves
   – Antiseptic solution
   – Local anesthetic

– Sterile water
– Surgical tape
– Roller gauge dressing
– Norplant insertion template
– Sterile skin marker

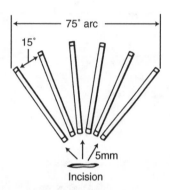

Placement of Norplant capsules. (Courtesy of Wyeth Ayerst)

| PROCEDURE | SPECIAL CONSIDERATIONS |

1. Position the patient, with arm flexed and externally rotated with her hand by her head.

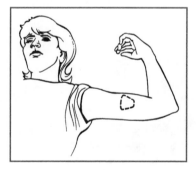

2. Identify and mark an incision site on the inner aspect of the arm, about 8 to 10 cm above the elbow fold. The distal tips should be clear of the axillary hairline.

3. Prep the arm with antiseptic.

4. Put on sterile gloves and place sterile surgical drapes under and over the arm.

5. Open the Norplant system package.

(procedure continued)

| **PROCEDURE** | **SPECIAL CONSIDERATIONS** |

6. Anesthetize the incision site in six superficial channels 4- to 5-cm long under the skin in a fan-like pattern.

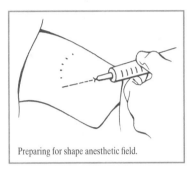

Preparing for shape anesthetic field.

7. Make a small, shallow incision about 2 mm long through the dermis with the scalpel.

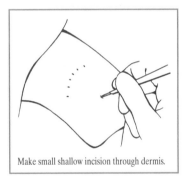

Make small shallow incision through dermis.

8. Insert the trocar with the #10 on the trocar hub and the bevel facing up, and with the obturator in place. Note that there are two marks on the trocar.

   If dimpling is seen, the trocar is not placed sufficiently under the skin.

(procedure continued)

| **PROCEDURE** | **SPECIAL CONSIDERATIONS** |

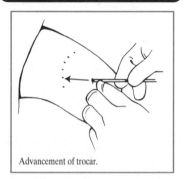

Advancement of trocar.

The mark nearer the hub is the point to which the trocar should be introduced before loading each capsule. The mark nearer the tip indicates how much of the trocar should remain under the skin following the insertion of each capsule. The trocar should never be withdrawn beyond the mark close to its tip.

9. Advance the trocar at a shallow angle until the mark nearer the tip is just outside the incision.

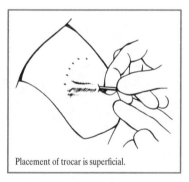

Placement of trocar is superficial.

10. Pivot the trocar and gently advance it to the mark nearer the hub, visibly tenting the skin to ensure that the channel remains superficial. Never force the trocar.

(procedure continued) ───

PROCEDURE ──┤ SPECIAL CONSIDERATIONS ├──

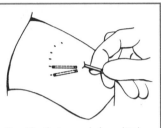

Reposition the trocar and advance it to insert each remaining capsule in a fan-like pattern.

11. Remove the obturator and introduce the capsule into the system.

12. Use the obturator to advance the capsule until you feel resistance and the tip of the implant is seen under the skin at the tip of the trocar. Never force the obturator.

13. Hold the obturator firmly with one hand and slide the barrel of the trocar back until the mark nearer the tip clears the incision. Do not remove the trocar from the incision until all six capsules have been inserted.

14. Reposition the trocar 15 degrees and advance it again to insert each remaining capsule in a fan like pattern. Stabilize the capsule inserted immediately before with the fingers, to protect it from the advancing trocar, while inserting the next capsule.

15. After the sixth capsule has been inserted, remove the trocar.

16. Apply pressure to the incision for a minute or two, or until hemostasis has been achieved.

17. Cleanse the incision area and place Steri-Strips or other skin closures over the incision.

18. Cover the insertion area with a dry gauze compress, and then wrap the area with roller gauze.

ALERT: *One of the most important factors in Norplant removal is proper insertion: use a single, subdermal plane for insertion; position and space the capsules correctly; refer to the positioning notches on the trocar during insertion; withdraw the barrel of the trocar around the obturator—never force the obturator; palpate and stabilize the previously placed capsule during insertion of the next capsule.*

◉ PATIENT COUNSELING ON REMOVAL

- Removals take longer than insertions.
- An additional incision or visit may be required if all of the capsules cannot be removed at once through a single incision.
- The adhesive bandage placed over the incision should remain in place for 3 days.
- Transient tenderness, discoloration, bruising, and swelling are to be expected for a few days postoperatively.
- Bumping the removal site should be avoided during this 3-day period.
- More serious complications are possible after removal. These complications include scarring, numbness, tingling at the removal site, and severe or persistent pain.
- Women can become pregnant after removal of the Norplant system device.

◉ REMOVAL PROCEDURE

Equipment
- Sterile gloves
- One regular and one fenestrated sterile surgical drape
- Antiseptic solution
- Local anesthetic
- 10-mL syringe
- Needles for drawing up and infusing the local anesthetic
- #11 scalpel
- 5-inch straight mosquito-clamp forceps
- 5-inch curved mosquito-clamp forceps
- Skin closures
- Sterile 4-inch square gauze bandage
- Surgical tape
- Roller gauze dressing
- Sterile water
- Sterile skin marker

PROCEDURE	SPECIAL CONSIDERATIONS

Position the patient with arm containing the capsules flexed and externally rotated, with the patient's hand by her head.

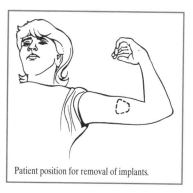

Patient position for removal of implants.

Locate the capsules by palpation and choose an incision site equidistant from the proximal capsule tips—preferably just above the original insertion site to avoid having to incise scar tissue.

Cleanse and drape the operative field.

Administer a small amount of local anesthetic under the proximal tip of each capsule.

It may be helpful to mark the location of the capsules with a sterile skin marker.

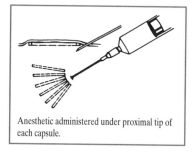

Anesthetic administered under proximal tip of each capsule.

Limit total anesthesia to 3 to 5 mL to avoid obscuring the capsules to palpation.

Make a small incision—4 mm is generally sufficient for removal and minimizes bleeding, swelling, and scarring.

(procedure continued)

| PROCEDURE | SPECIAL CONSIDERATIONS |

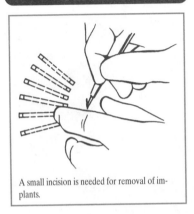

A small incision is needed for removal of implants.

Open a plane of dissection in the subdermal tissue above and beneath each capsule using the straight forceps; then guide the distal end of the nearest capsule toward the incision using gentle external finger pressure.

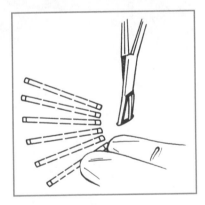

Introduce the curved forceps into the incision and beneath the capsule, with the forceps jaw closed and its tips pointing upward, then open the jaws.

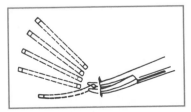

(procedure continued)

PROCEDURE	SPECIAL CONSIDERATIONS

Guide the capsule into the forceps jaws using gentle external pressure; then grasp the capsule as close as possible to its tip by gently closing the forceps around it.

Switching the curved forceps to your non-dominant hand, use the scalpel or straight forceps to expose the capsule tip by dissecting the surrounding fibrous sheath.

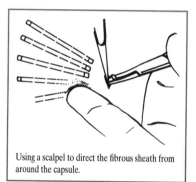

Using a scalpel to direct the fibrous sheath from around the capsule.

Once the capsule tip is exposed, grasp it with the straight forceps, release and remove the curved forceps, and gently withdraw the capsule through the incision.

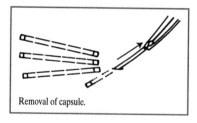

Removal of capsule.

Repeat the process for the remaining capsules. Then show the patient all six removed capsules.

Cleanse any remaining antiseptic from the patient's arm, close the incision with Steri-Strips, and complete the procedure by applying gauze bandage and roller gauze to the wound.

If the patient wishes to continue using the Norplant system, a new set of capsules may be inserted at this time in the original or contralateral arm.

◉ COMPLICATED REMOVALS

Capsules Too Far From Incision
- Capsules too distant to be retrieved through an incision close to the original insertion site generally result from errors of technique during insertion.
- These capsules require a careful choice of incision site or sites during removal.

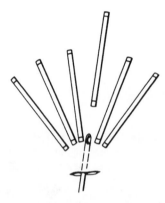

Capsule too far from incision. (Courtesy of Wyeth Ayerst)

- You may need to make an angled incision or, in some cases, a second incision near the distal tips of the capsules.

U-Shaped Capsules
- U-shaped capsules occur when the tip of a previously placed capsule is displaced by the trocar as it is advanced to insert subsequent capsules.

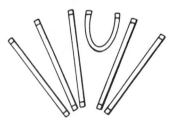

U-shaped capsule. (Courtesy of Wyeth Ayerst)

- Removal of a U-shaped capsule will usually require a second incision near one of its axillary tips.

Crimped or Corkscrew Capsules
- Crimped or corkscrew are generally caused by using the obturator to push a capsule, rather than withdrawing the trocar while holding the obturator steady.

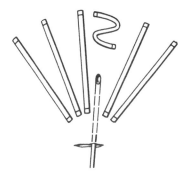

Corkscrew capsule. (Courtesy of Wyeth Ayerst)

- Crimped capsules can sometimes be removed the usual way by grasping them near the tip and removing them through the incision.
- If the proximal tip is too far to be grasped through the main removal incision, a second incision near the axillary tip may be needed.

Capsules at Different Depths

- Capsules inserted at different subdermal planes can be difficult to grasp and may require one or more additional planes of dissection to remove them.

Fractured or Nicked Capsules

- Capsule damage typically occurs intraoperatively from torsion during externalization or from overvigorous dissection of the fibrous sheath, especially over the capsule shaft.
- Incisions to open the fibrous sheath should be made on the rubbery tip of the implant, which is thicker and more resistant to incision than the capsule walls.

Impalpable Capsules

- The ability to palpate capsules clearly before removal is critical to a rapid, uneventful removal procedure.
- Palpation can often be assisted by moistening the arm with antiseptic, then drawing the shaft of a sterile applicator across the skin surface to outline the capsules.

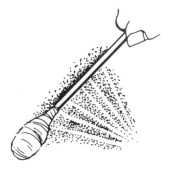

Better visualization of capsules prior to removal.

- If one or more capsules are impalpable, imaging studies may be required.
- Specifying foreign body localization can facilitate radiographic localization.
- Real-time ultrasound can also be used with a high-frequency (7–10 MHz), short focal length transducer or a stepoff pad to reduce penetration because the capsules are superficial.

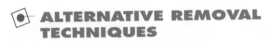

ALERT: Key elements of a standard removal are injecting a small amount of anesthetic; making an incision near the capsule tips; opening planes of dissection above and below the capsules; grasping the implant with curved forceps; externalizing the capsule tip and its fibrous sheath through the incision; dissecting the fibrous sheath to expose the capsule tip; regrasping the exposed capsule with the straight forceps; and removing the implant.

ALTERNATIVE REMOVAL TECHNIQUES

Pop-out Digital Technique

- The pop-out digital technique uses digital extrusion rather than instruments to remove the implants and a smaller 2-mm incision.
- Less anesthetic is typically required because only external manipulation is used.
- This technique can be used only with well-placed implants that are directly under the skin and are palpable.

PROCEDURE	SPECIAL CONSIDERATIONS
Position the patient with arm containing the capsules flexed and externally rotated so that her hand is by her head.	
Locate the capsules by palpation. All six capsules must be distinctly palpable for this method to be used.	
Choose an incision site equidistant from the proximal tips of all six capsules.	
Cleanse the area with antiseptic solution and drape the operative field.	Drawing the applicator shaft over the implant area after applying the antiseptic solution often reveals the location of the capsules for later reference during the removal. (See Figure 47-5).

(procedure continued)

PROCEDURE

SPECIAL CONSIDERATIONS

Administer a total of 2 to 3 mL of anesthetic intradermally at the capsule.

Using a #11 scalpel, make a small incision (approximately 2 mm) immediately below the capsule tips.

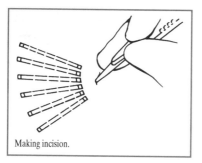

Making incision.

Placing the fingers of your nondominant hand at the axillary capsule tips, direct the proximal tip of the capsule into the incision. Remove the most palpable and accessible implants first.

With your dominant hand, use the #11 scalpel to clear the fibrous sheath from the capsule tip, using short strokes of the blade point in several directions across the tip.

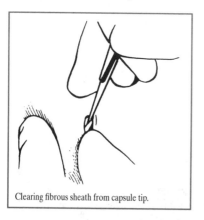

Clearing fibrous sheath from capsule tip.

When it is freed, the capsule tip will emerge from the incision, where it can be grasped with the fingers and pulled out.

(procedure continued)

| PROCEDURE | SPECIAL CONSIDERATIONS |

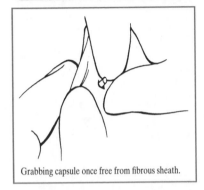

Grabbing capsule once free from fibrous sheath.

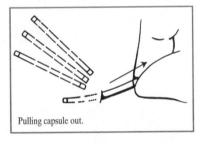

Pulling capsule out.

Repeat this procedure for the remaining capsules.

Close and bandage the incision. A pressure dressing is not necessary.

Modified U Technique

• This is a modified instrument technique that allows the capsules to be grasped anywhere along their shafts, not just at the tips, while facilitating externalization and removal of the fibrous sheath.

Equipment: Two special instruments are used: a ring-tipped forceps with an inside ring diameter of 2.2 mm and a curved vasectomy dissecting forceps.

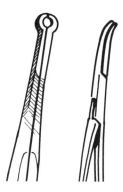

Ring-tipped forceps and vasectomy dissective forceps.

PROCEDURE | SPECIAL CONSIDERATIONS

Position the patient with arm containing the capsules flexed and externally rotated so that her hand is by her head.

Locate all six capsules by palpation; mark the location of the outermost implants and the planned incision site with a sterile marker.

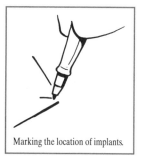

Marking the location of implants.

Prep and drape the patient.

Administer 3 to 5 mL of local anesthetic interdermally and superfically to the capsules.

Make a shallow vertical stab incision about 3 to 4 mm long between capsules 3 and 4 and close to the convergence of their tips, using the #11 scalpel.

Using straight forceps, bluntly dissect tissue planes 4 to 5 mm in width above and below the capsules.

(procedure continued)

| PROCEDURE | SPECIAL CONSIDERATIONS |

Stabilize the first capsule with external finger pressure against its long dimension distal from the incision, then introduce the closed ring tipped forceps into the incision. When you feel the forceps contact the capsule shaft, open its jaws. Direct the implant into them and close them again.

Pull the capsule toward the incision. When its ring tips are visible, reflect the forceps with its handles toward the patient's shoulder, and hold it there with your nondominant hand.

If the capsule shaft is extended and neither of its tips emerges, open a small tear in the fibrous sheath using the sharp downward facing tips of the scalpel vasectomy dissecting forceps. Then enlarge the tear by opening the forceps jaws.

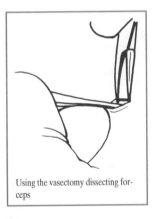

Using the vasectomy dissecting forceps

With the jaws of the dissecting forceps still open, impale the capsule shaft with one of the pointed forceps tips.

(procedure continued)

| **PROCEDURE** | **SPECIAL CONSIDERATIONS** |

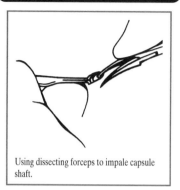

Using dissecting forceps to impale capsule shaft.

Rotate the hand holding the dissecting forceps palm upward, so the forceps tips are facing upward with the implant still impaled.

Close the dissecting forceps gently—just enough to hold the implant without cutting it—then release the ring forceps, allowing the implant to emerge from the incision.

If a capsule tip is externalized, use the point of one dissecting force to puncture the fibrous sheath at the capsule tip, then both jaws, to expand this opening. Finally, turn the dissecting forceps jaw upward and gently grasp and withdraw the capsule by its exposed tip.

Close and bandage the incision.

FOLLOW-UP

- A medical history should be obtained and a physical exam should be performed at least annually while the patient is using Norplant. The physical examination should include checking the implant site, blood pressure, breasts, liver, abdomen, extremities, and pelvic organs, including cervical cytology and relevant laboratory tests.
- Swelling, tenderness, and bruising may occur.
- A pressure dressing should be kept in place for 24 hours after insertion. The skin closures should be left on for 3 days or until they fall off. During that time, the incision site should be kept clean and dry.
- Do not bump the area or lift heavy objects until the incision heals.
- Complications or serious side effects should be reported to the clinician in a timely manner.

BIBLIOGRAPHY

American Medical Association. (1998). *Physicians' current procedural terminology: CPT.* Chicago: American Medical Association.

Hatcher, R. (1998). *Contraceptive technology* (17th ed.). New York: Irvington.

Healthcare Consultants of America (1998). *1998 Physicians' fee and coding guide.* Augusta: GA.

Klaisle, C., & Darney, P. (1995). A guide to removing contraceptive implants. *Contemporary Nurse Practitioner, 2,* 32–43.

Pfenninger, J., & Fowler, G. (1994). *Procedures for primary care physicians.* St Louis: Mosby.

Wehrle, K. (1994). The Norplant System: Easy to insert, easy to remove. *Nurse Practitioner Journal, 19*(4), 47–54.

Wyeth Ayerst. (1995). *Video library for the health care professional. Counseling guidelines & insertion techniques* (Vol. 1). Philadelphia: Wyeth Laboratories.

Wyeth Ayerst. (1995). *Video library for the health care professional. Standard removal techniques* (Vol. 2). Philadelphia: Wyeth Laboratories.

Wyeth Ayerst. (1995). *Video library for the health care professional. Alternative removal techniques* (Vol. 3). Philadelphia: Wyeth Laboratories.

chapter 48

Pap Smear

CPT Coding:

88150 Cytopathology, smears, cervical or vaginal, the Bethesda System, up to three smears, screening by a technician under physician supervision ($28–$35)

88142 Cytopathology, cervical or vaginal collected in preservative fluid, automated thin layer prep, manual screening under physician supervision ($32–$39)

88144 Cytopathology smear, cervical or vaginal with manual screening and computer-assisted rescreening under physician screening ($68–$82)

DEFINITION

A Pap (Papanicolaou) smear is a cytologic screening test for carcinoma of the cervix. Cells for cytology are obtained by scraping the endocervix.

INDICATION

• Every woman who is 18 years of age or older or is sexually active should receive a Pap smear annually or as indicated for follow-up

> **ALERT:** Some health care providers and insurance carriers are recommending Pap smear intervals of 1 to 3 years for some women. The American Cancer Society (1997) recommends annual Pap smears; however, after three or more normal smear exams, Pap smears may be done less frequently.

PATIENT EDUCATION

• Instruct patient not to douche, use vaginal preparations (such as creams, lubricants, and so on), or have intercourse for at least 24 hours before the Pap smear.
• For accuracy of results, schedule Pap smear for a time when the patient is not menstruating.
• Explain that the Pap smear is a screening test only, and any results other than normal will require follow-up (Kawada, 1994).

ASSESSMENT

1. Obtain an obstetric, gynecologic, and sexual history.
2. Assess for any signs or symptoms of vaginal infection (the Pap test may need to be deferred after treatment of infection).
3. Determine the patient's understanding of the procedure and ability to cooperate.
4. Determine the appropriate size of speculum: Pediatric for virgins, small for the majority of women, or large for larger size women.

DEVELOPMENTAL CONSIDERATIONS

Adolescents: The squamocolumnar junction (also called transformation zone) is the place on the cervix where the endocervical glands meet the squamous epithelium. The location of this area becomes higher in the cervical canal as the women becomes older. This area may be visible on the cervix of an adolescent. Adolescents may have columnar epithelium in the area around the external cervical os (Hatcher, Stewart, Trussell, Kowal, Guest, Stewart, Cates, & Policar, 1994). Preinvasive lesions, if present, usually form at the squamocolumnar junction.

Older Women: The location of the squamocolumnar junction becomes higher in the cervical canal as a women becomes older, and therefore, the feature is less visible during an exam.

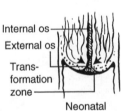
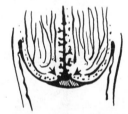

Internal os
External os
Transformation zone

Neonatal   Nulliparous reproductive age

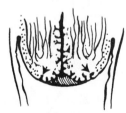
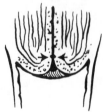

Multiparous age   Postmenopausal

Different locations of the transformation zone and the squamocolumnar junction during a woman's lifetime. The arrows mark the active transformation zone.

◉ EQUIPMENT

- Gloves
- Speculum
- Large cotton swab
- Wooden spatula
- Cytobrush
- Glass Pap smear slide
- Preservative or fixative
- Waste receptacle

PROCEDURE	SPECIAL CONSIDERATIONS
Glove both hands.	May want to double glove nondominant hand and remove the outer glove for the abdominal palpation during bimanual exam.
Placing the index finger of nondominant hand at the introitus, press down gently. While holding the speculum in the dominant hand with the blades closed, insert the speculum by sliding it along the index finger at the introitus. Tip the speculum somewhat downward toward the posterior vaginal wall. At insertion, the speculum should be held at an oblique angle. As it is guided into the vagina, the speculum will follow the natural anatomic contour and assume a "handle-down" position.	**Be sure the patient is in Sims' position, with her buttocks at the end of the exam table and her feet in the foot rests. Metal speculums may be warmed in water.** Do not use any lubricant other than plain, warm water.
The entire cervix should be visible once the speculum is opened and locked in place. Remove excess discharge before the Pap smear. A Pap smear may be performed in the presence of a small amount of blood (Hawkins, Roberto-Nichols, & Stanley-Haney, 1995).	**A cotton-tipped applicator moistened with saline should be used in lieu of the cytobrush when performing a Pap on a pregnant woman. The two specimens (from spatula and cytobrush) can be placed on the same slide, either mixing the specimens or placing them in two different spots on the same slide.**
Place the longer tip of the double tipped end of the wooden spatula into the cervical os. Scrape the entire squamocolumnar junction by rotating the spatula 360 degrees. Gently slide the spatula on the slide.	You may remove the speculum and palpate the cervix if you have difficulty visualizing it. After palpating, reinsert the speculum and visualize the cervix. **If using a DNA probe for GC and chlamydia, do BEFORE Pap smear since this test is very sensitive to blood.**

(procedure continued)

PROCEDURE	SPECIAL CONSIDERATIONS

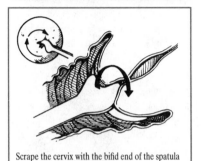

Scrape the cervix with the bifid end of the spatula for obtaining Papanicolaou smear.

Insert the cytobrush into the cervical os and twirl it 180 to 360 degrees to obtain a specimen from the endocervix.

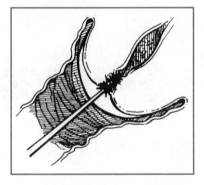

Gently roll the cytobrush onto the slide.

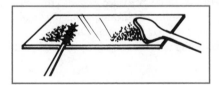

After placing both smears on the slide, immediately spray or drop cytology fixative solution onto the slide.

GC and chlamydia culture (if done) is usually obtained immediately after the Pap smear.

A smear may be used to obtain a specimen from the vaginal wall for evaluation of estrogen stimulation or for DES vaginal changes (Kawada, 1994).

This smear should be placed on a separate slide to be sent to the lab.

(procedure continued)

| PROCEDURE | SPECIAL CONSIDERATIONS |

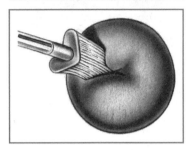

A wet mount of vaginal secretions can be performed if a vaginal infection is suspected. GC or chlamydia cultures should be completed after the Pap smear is obtained (unless DNA probe—see earlier).

A Cervexbrush can obtain both an ectodermal and endocervical sample at the same time.

Remove the speculum and continue with the rest of the pelvic exam. Place the speculum in the receptacle for soiled or contaminated items.

ALTERNATIVE PROCEDURE

- A system using a vial instead of a Pap smear slide is available (Judge, 1997). However, it is more expensive than traditional Pap smears. Called the Thinprep (CYTYC, 1998), the system uses a plastic spatula and a cytobrush or a broomlike collection device that are rinsed in the preservative solution in the vial.
- Research has been done evaluating the effectiveness of women conducting their own Pap smears using special tampons that they insert into the vagina.

FOLLOW-UP

- Patient notification systems for abnormal results vary according to the particular setting. However, notification of results, both normal and abnormal, must be accomplished in a timely manner and clearly documented.
- Follow-up for pap smears varies according to results (using Bethesda System of classification):

Result	Follow-up
Unsatisfactory for evaluation	Repeat Pap in 6 weeks (Committee on Gynecologic Practice, 1995).
Within normal limits	Repeat Pap in 1 year, or less often if 3 or more normal exams have been performed.
Infection (organism identified)	Treat infection. Repeat Pap in 2 weeks.

(table continued)

Result	Follow-up
Reactive and reparative changes	**Inflammation:** Identify infection and treat. Repeat Pap in 3 months. **Atrophy with inflammation:** Offer hormone replacement therapy (HRT). Repeat Pap in 6 months. **Hyperkeratosis:** Refer for colposcopy.
Squamous cell abnormalities	**Atypical squamous cells of undetermined significance** (ASCUS): Repeat pap in 3 months. If repeat Pap shows ASCUS, refer for colposcopy. **Low-grade squamous intra epithelial lesion (LSIL):** Refer for colposcopy and biopsy (CDC, 1998). **High-grade squamous intraepithelial lesion (HSIL):** Refer for colposcopy and biopsy (CDC, 1998). **Squamous cell carcinoma:** Refer for colposcopy and treatment.

BIBLIOGRAPHY

American Cancer Society. (1997). *Cancer facts for women* (Number 2007), New York: Author.

American Medical Association. (1998). *Physicians' current procedural terminology: CPT.* Chicago: American Medical Association.

Centers for Disease Control and Prevention. (1998). 1998 guidelines for treatment of sexually transmitted diseases. *Morbidity and Mortality Weekly Report, 47*(No RR-1), 96.

Committee on Gynecologic Practice. (1995). Absence of endocervical cells on a Pap test (Number 153). *International Journal of Obstetrics & Gynecology, 49*(2), 212.

CYTYC (1998). *PreservCyt solution sample collection and transport medium for use with the ThinPrep Pap Test* (No. 85177-00, Rev C). Boxborough, MA: CYTYC Corporation.

Hatcher, R. A., Stewart, F., Trussell, J., Kowal, D., Guest, F., Stewart, G. K., Cates, W., & Policar, M. (1998). *Contraceptive technology* (17th ed.). New York: Ardent Media.

Hawkins, J. W., Roberto-Nichols, D. M., & Stanley-Haney, J. L. (1995). *Protocols for nurse practitioners in gynecologic settings* (5th ed). New York: Tiresias.

Healthcare Consultants of America. (1998). *1998 Physicians' fee and coding guide.* Augusta, GA.

Judge, D. E. (1997). Will new technology improve Pap smears? *Journal Watch Women's Health, 2*(1), 7–8.

Kawadas, C. Y. (1994) Gynecologic history, examination, & diagnostic procedures. In DeCherney, A. H. & Pernoll, M. L. (Eds.), *Current obstetrics & gyneolcolgic diagnosis & treatment.* Norwalk: Appleton & Lange.

chapter 49

Wet Mount and Gram Stain

CPT Coding:

87210 Wet mount with simple stains, for bacteria, fungi, ova, or parasites ($15–$20)

 DEFINITION

Microscopic examination of vaginal discharge using normal saline, potassium hydroxide (10%), or gram staining as mediums for examination.

 INDICATION

• Used to differentiate complaints of vaginal discharge, including bacteria, fungus, or protozoan causes.

 PATIENT EDUCATION

• Advise the client that the procedure requires a speculum examination.
• Advise the client of minor discomfort associated with speculum examination.
• This procedure will identify causative organisms and will assist the practitioner in diagnosis and treatment.
• The collection process takes less than 5 minutes.

 ASSESSMENT

1. Conduct a thorough assessment to rule out other possibilities for vaginal discharge or itching, such as cervicitis.
2. Determine the presence of other associated symptoms, such as odor, itching, abdominal pain, or fever.
3. Determine whether or not the patient's sexual partner also is exhibiting any signs or symptoms or has recently been diagnosed with sexually transmitted infection.

 NORMAL SALINE (NS) WET MOUNT PREPARATION

Equipment
• Microscope
• Speculum, water for lubrication

- Cotton-tipped applicators
- Glass slide
- Coverslip
- Normal saline solution (NSS)

PROCEDURE	SPECIAL CONSIDERATIONS

Have all equipment ready before procedure.

Explain procedure to patient.

Introduce speculum into vagina and lock into place using water as lubricant. Place 7 to 10 drops (1 mL) of saline in a small test tube. Obtain specimen for both NSS and KOH with two cotton-tipped applicators by swabbing the mucosa along the middle third of the vaginal walls.

Immerse the one applicator quickly into the saline filled test tube (and the other into KOH: see later).

Any lubricant other than water can interfere with slide analysis.

Avoid touching the sides of the test tube with applicator.

Look at specimen within 15 minutes of collection for best results.

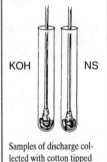

Samples of discharge collected with cotton tipped applicators, which are then placed in small test tubes prepared with a few drops of NaCL and KOH solution. Beckman (1998). *Obstetrics and Gynecology* (3rd ed.). Baltimore: Williams & Wilkins.

First use pH paper to identify the vaginal pH

Prepare the wet mount slide by gently mixing the swab in the saline.

Normal vaginal pH 3.0 to 5.5

You can use the same slide for both NSS and KOH.

(procedure continued)

| PROCEDURE | SPECIAL CONSIDERATIONS |

Place a drop of the mixture on a clean glass slide by touching the dripping swab to the slide surface.

Place a coverslip over the mixture on the slide.

Be careful that the KOH does not leach into the NSS preparation.

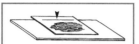

The slide preparation is covered with a coverslip for viewing. (Beckman (1998). *Obstetrics and Gynecology* (3rd ed.). Baltimore: Williams & Wilkins.)

Place on microscope stage.

Use subdued light and low condenser for wet mount preparations.

Use 10× to focus specimen initially, and then switch to 40× to identify organisms.

Examine at least 10 fields in both powers.

Interpret slide for number and type of cells, bacteria, trichomonas, hyphae, and clue cells.

Adjust the eye piece of the microscope to the examiner.

Look through the microscope with both eyes. Remove your glasses if you are near or far sighted. Bifocals should not be worn during microscopy.

A good rule of thumb is the more power, the brighter the light needed.

It may appear that the specimen is moving constantly. This is known as brownian motion and is due to the constant and unequal pressure of water against the bacteria or cells. Movement of all cells in one direction is not true motility. A motile organism, such as trichomonads, will move against the flow or spin around in one place (Lowe & Saxe, 1999).

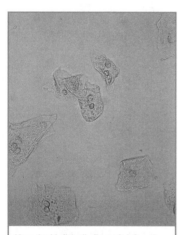

Normal epithelial cells. (Lowe, S. & Saxe, J. [1998]. *Microscopic procedures for primary care providers.* Philadelphia: Lippincott Williams and Wilkins.)

(procedure continued)

PROCEDURE	SPECIAL CONSIDERATIONS

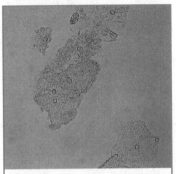

Clue cells. (Lowe, S. & Saxe, J. [1998]. *Microscopic procedures for primary care providers.* Philadelphia: Lippincott Williams and Wilkins.)

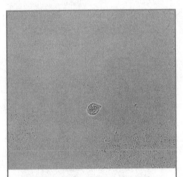

Trichomonads (Lowe, S. & Saxe, J. [1998]. *Microscopic procedures for primary care providers.* Philadelphia: Lippincott Williams and Wilkins.)

ALTERNATIVE METHOD

• Dip cotton-tipped applicator into NSS and transfer a drop to the glass slide. Roll the same applicator along the posterior and lateral vaginal walls. Remove the applicator and mix with the prepared NSS slide. Place a coverslip over the specimen. (This method tends to dry out the specimen quickly and is not recommended.)

FOLLOW-UP

• Treat based on findings of NSS wet mount.
• See summary table later.

POTASSIUM HYDROXIDE WET MOUNT PREPARATION (KOH/10%)

Equipment
- Speculum
- Microscope
- Cotton-tipped applicator
- Glass slide
- Coverslip
- Potassium hydroxide (KOH) 10%
- Exam gloves

PROCEDURE	SPECIAL CONSIDERATIONS
Introduce speculum into vagina and lock into place.	
Obtain specimen on cotton-tipped applicator by swabbing with two applicators (one for NSS) along the middle third of vaginal walls. Place the specimen on a clean glass slide. Add 1 drop of KOH.	Both the NSS and KOH can be placed on the same slide for examination. Be sure that the KOH does not leach into the NSS sample.
Smell the mixture before covering with the coverslip.	KOH causes lysis of epithelial cells, WBCs, RBCs, mucus, and other cell structures. Fungal components will remain clearly visible. "Whiff" test is when the KOH/specimen mixture is smelled. A fishy or amine odor is suggestive of bacterial vaginosis.
Examine under microscope. Examine with low and high power. Interpret slide for budding yeast and pseudohyphae.	**Examine the NSS slide first to allow KOH preparation to lyse cells and allow identification of yeast (approximately 2 to 5 minutes).**
	Adjust eye piece. Focus on 10× power and proceed to high power (40×).

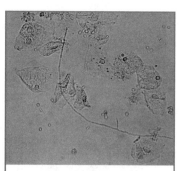

Budding yeast & pseudohyphae. (Lowe, S. & Saxe, J. [1998]. *Microscopic procedures for primary care providers.* Philadelphia: Lippincott Williams and Wilkins.)

Alternative Procedure

- Using a dropper, place a tiny dropper of KOH on slide.
- A cotton-tipped applicator is then rolled along the posterior and lateral vaginal walls.
- The applicator is then mixed with the KOH slide.
- A coverslip is placed over the specimen and then examined as above.
- Place 7 to 10 drops of KOH into the test tube.
- Obtain the specimen using the cotton-tipped applicator.
- Immerse the applicator in the KOH mixture in the test tube.
- Follow above-mentioned steps for examination.

Follow-up

- As needed based on diagnosis.
- Summary of vaginal discharge: clinical and laboratory findings

Etiology	Discharge	WBCs	pH	Wet Mount
Normal	Scant heterogeneous viscous to watery	Not increased (<5/HPF)	<4.5	Normal epithelial cells and lactobacilli
Candidiasis	Thick, white, cheesy	Increased (>5/HPF)	<4.5	Budding yeast with pseudohyphae
Trichomoniasis	Thin, frothy, and odorous	Increased (>5/HPF)	>4.5	Motile trichomonads
Bacterial vaginosis (BV)	Thin, milky, "fishy" odor (+whiff test)	Not increased (<5/HPF)	>4.5	Clue cells, lack of lactobacilli
Cytolytic vaginosis	Thick, white, cheesy	Not increased (<5/HPF)	<4.5	Lysed epithelial cells with overgrowth of lactobacilli
Atrophic vaginitis	Variable in amount, appearance and odor	Often increased (>5/HPF)	>4.5	Immature epithelial cells, lack of lactobacilli, but presence of other bacterial species
Gonorrhea, chlamydia	Most common causes of purulent discharge			Cannot be identified on wet mount or KOH

With permission from Lowe, S. & Saxe, J. (1999). Microscopic procedures for primary care providers (p. 108). Philadelphia: Lippincott Williams & Wilkins.

GRAM'S STAIN

- Gram's stain separates bacteria into two groups: gram-positive bacteria (stain purple) and gram-negative (stain pink to red). It is also helpful to identify the shape and arrangement of bacteria with Gram's stain.

Equipment
- Speculum
- Microscope
- Cotton-tipped applicator
- Heat source
- Gentian violet
- Gram's iodine
- Acetone and alcohol (decolorizer)
- Safranin
- Coverslip
- Tap water

PROCEDURE	SPECIAL CONSIDERATIONS

Insert speculum and obtain specimen using a cotton-tipped applicator.
Get two specimens if one is to be Gram stained and one is to be sent for culture.
Place thin smear of secretions on glass slide.
Allow specimen to air dry completely.

Heat fixing is done when the slide is quickly passed through a flame (specimen side up and away from the flame).
Heat fixing should be done when the slide is completely dry.
The slide should be warm but not hot.
Repeat three to four times.

An alternate way to fix the slide is to use a methanol fixation.

Flood the slide with 95% methanol for 1 minute. The methanol is drained off and then the slide is allowed to dry.
Flood slide with gentian violet (or crystal violet) preparation. Wait 5 to 10 seconds and rinse with tap water. Next, flood stain with Gram's iodine. Wait 5 to 10 seconds and rinse with water. Hold slide at a 45 degree angle.
Wash slide thoroughly with decolorizer until the drippings turn from blue to colorless. Immediately rinse slide with tap water.

Next flood the slide with safranin. Wait 5 to 10 seconds. Rinse the slide with tap water.
Air dry or blot the slide.

See procedure described in NSS wet mount. Swabs that have been rolled on a slide should not be sent for culture.
Thick smears are hard to stain properly.

To speed the drying process, a slide warmer or a 37°C incubator can be used. Using a flame to hasten drying is not recommended. Heat fixing is done so that the material remains on the slide during the staining procedure.

If the specimen is not cooled completely, the reagents will precipitate on the slide.
DO NOT OVERHEAT.
If you burn your hand from the slide, you have also burned the specimen.
Methanol is the preferred method for fixing because it preserves the cell morphology and eliminates the potential for overheating the slide.
Make sure the slide is cool before staining procedure.

Crystal violet is the primary stain. It stains all material purple.
The timing is not critical with violet stain. Gram's iodine fixes the violet to gram-positive bacteria.
Crucial step to ensure decolorizing of the primary stain from bacterial cell walls that do not have the composition of a gram-positive organism.

(procedure continued) —————————————————————————

PROCEDURE	SPECIAL CONSIDERATIONS
Place the slide on microscope stage. Focus the specimen using the 10× objective. Place a small drop of immersion oil on stained specimen and rotate lens so the 100× is in place (do not rotate 40× through the oil). Only slight adjustment of the fine focus should be needed to keep the image in sharp focus.	The decolorizing agent is acetone and alcohol. The timing in this step is not critical. Use oil immersion (100× power). The oil provides a connection between the slide and the objective (lens). This lens is sealed, so the oil will not seep into it. DO NOT USE MINERAL OIL. **Do not use 40× because the oil will get into the objective.** Condenser should be in the up position. **Be sure to remove oil with oil lens paper after using.**
Interpret the slide for clue cells, candida spores and yeast, and lactobacillus over-growth.	Endocervical discharge has many organisms that can be mistaken for gram-negative diplococci. Be cautious if you attempt to use this method to diagnose an STI. Culture or antigen detection methods are the recommended method to identify GC or chlamydia.
Quality control should be done with every specimen if Gram's stains are done infrequently.	Gram's stain may not kill all organisms on the slide, so universal precautions should be followed.

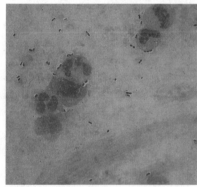

Properly done Gram's stain. (Lowe, S. & Saxe, J. [1998]. *Microscopic Procedures for Primary Care Providers.* Philadelphia: Lippincott Williams & Wilkins.)

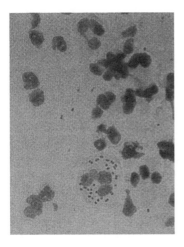

Urethral discharge with intracellular diplococci. (Lowe, S. & Saxe, J. [1998]. *Microscopic procedures for primary care providers.* Philadelphia: Lippincott Williams & Wilkins.)

Alternative Procedure
• None

Summary of Organisms Seen on Gram's Stain

Organism	Shape/Description
Gram-positive bacteria	Stained purple.
Gram-negative bacteria	Stained pink to red.
Cocci	Round or slightly oval.
Rods or bacilli	Rod-shaped organisms: may be long, fat, thin.
Spirochetes	Spiral-shaped bacteria. Does not stain with Gram's stain and will not be visible.
Epithelial cells	Large cell with small nucleus.
WBC	Polymorphonuclear cells. Smaller than epithelial cells and have multiple segments to nucleus. May be broken apart when doing Gram's stain and, therefore, are hard to identify.
Mononuclear cells	Macrophages or histiocytes: larger than polymorphonuclear cells and do not have segmented nuclei.
All cellular material	Should stain gram negative, ie, pink to red.

Follow-Up
• As needed based on diagnosis

BIBLIOGRAPHY

American Medical Association. (1998). *Physicians' current procedural terminology: CPT guide.* Chicago.

Association of Professors of Gynecology and Obstetrics (1996). *APGO educational series in women's health-diagnosis of vaginitis.* St. Paul, MN: 3M Pharmaceuticals.

Healthcare Consultants of America. (1998). *1998 Physicians' fee and coding guide.* Augusta, GA.

Lichtman, R., & Papera, S. (1990). *Gynecology: Well-woman care.* Norwalk, CT: Appleton & Lange.

Lowe, S., & Saxe, J. (1999). *Microscopic procedures for primary care providers.* Philadelphia: Lippincott Williams & Wilkins.

Monif, G. R. G. (1995). *Interpretation of wet mount preparations.* Omaha, NE: IDI Publications.

chapter
50
Child Restraints

CPT Coding: N/A

 ## DEFINITION

Restraints are physical devices used in order to perform a procedure safely. Restraints may not be necessary if the patient is positioned or restrained correctly to perform the procedure without causing harm.

 ## INDICATION

• Procedure being performed warrants no movement to prevent injury to the patient or the health care provider

 ## ASSESSMENT

1. Determine whether or not parent can assist in restraint of child or if additional personnel will be necessary.

 ## EDUCATION

• Explain to the parent and child that proper restraining is necessary to perform procedure accurately and safely.
• If a physical restraint is used, explain the rationale to the child and the parent.

 ## EQUIPMENT

• Dependent on what type of procedure is being performed. May need a blanket or papoose board.

PROCEDURE	SPECIAL CONSIDERATIONS
Examination of HEENT With Child on the Exam Table	
	These techniques can be used to perform any procedure involving the head, eyes, ears, nose, and mouth or throat (HEENT).
Place child's arms at side.	

(procedure continued)

PROCEDURE	SPECIAL CONSIDERATIONS

Parent stands at child's feet and leans over them to immobilize knees while simultaneously restraining arms down on table.

Examiner needs to restrain child's head while performing procedure.

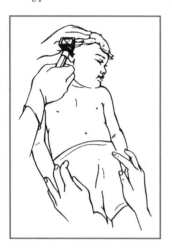

An alternative procedure to examine the pharynx of the child would be to have the parent restrain the child's arms above the head.

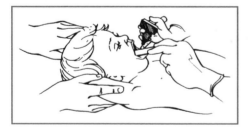

Examination of HEENT With Child on the Parent's Lap

Have the child sit on the parent's lap facing examiner.

Sit directly across from the parent.

Have the parent restrain the child's legs between their knees.

(procedure continued)

PROCEDURE	**SPECIAL CONSIDERATIONS**

Wrap one arm around and across the child's arms and chest tightly.

Have the parent use the free hand to turn child's head to one side and restrain it against his or her chest.

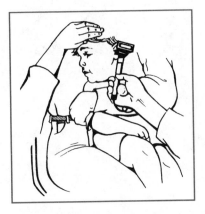

Although not shown in illustration, examiner also needs to brace hand against the child's head.

To examine the pharynx, have the parent place the hand over the child's forehead.

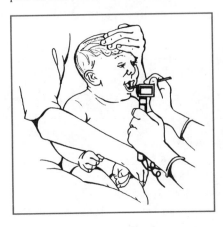

To Examine HEENT of an Uncooperative Child, Physical Restraints May Be Necessary

Restraints should not interfere with the respiratory, circulatory, and musculoskeletal systems.

For the infant, a blanket may be used to wrap the child for immobilization purposes.

(procedure continued)

PROCEDURE	SPECIAL CONSIDERATIONS

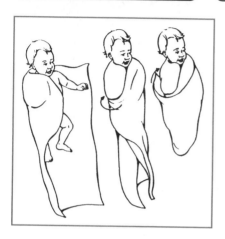

For the older child, a papoose board may be necessary.

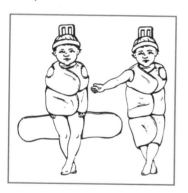

Examination of Genitals With Child on the Exam Table

This may be necessary to evaluate for possible sexual abuse or to perform catheterization in children.

Position the female patient in frog-leg position.

May need assistance with restraint depending on the procedure.

(procedure continued)

PROCEDURE	SPECIAL CONSIDERATIONS

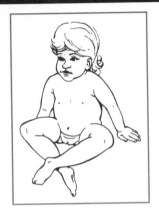

Position male patient in supine position or tailor position.

Use the position appropriate for the procedure.

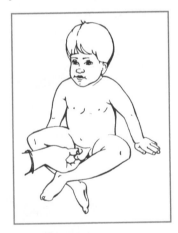

◉ FOLLOW-UP

• Allow child to be comforted by parent after restraints are used for a procedure

BIBLIOGRAPHY

Dieckmann, R. A., Fiser, D. H. & Selbst, S. M. (1997). *Pediatric emergency & critical care procedures.* St. Louis: Mosby.

Taylor, C., Lillis, C., & LeMone, P. (1997) *Fundamentals of Nursing* (3rd ed.). Philadelphia: Lippincott-Raven.

chapter 51

Somatosensory Testing for Peripheral Nerve Disorders (Foot Care)

CPT Coding:

95925-26 Somatosensory testing: upper limbs ($210–$252)
95926-26 Somatosensory testing: lower limbs ($210–$252)

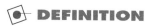 DEFINITION

Testing to screen and monitor peripheral nerve function, usually in the hands or feet

⊙ INDICATIONS

- Monitor for complications in peripheral vascular disease
- Monitor for extent of neuropathy caused by diabetes or alcoholism every 6 months
- Detection of skin ulcers
- Prevention of foot injury due to loss of sensation
- Determine the level of risk for foot injury based on sensation level
- Institute a preventive foot care program based on risk level

⊙ PATIENT EDUCATION

- Discuss the importance of good glucose control with diabetes.
- Discuss the importance of examining the feet every day.
- Stress the importance of regular foot examinations by a health care professional.
- Prevention for development of ulcers includes:
  - Avoiding walking barefoot.
  - Inspecting the feet, including between the toes every day.
  - Bathing the feet daily in warm water. Dry feet carefully, especially between toes. Apply topical moisturizers to help keep skin lubricated.
  - Changing shoes at least twice daily.
  - Avoiding potential trauma: heating pads, hot water, hydrogen peroxide, witch hazel.
  - Contacting the health care provider if any new abnormalities of the feet develop.
  - Stopping smoking.

– Cutting the toenails straight across and not too short.
– Wearing properly fitted clean socks or stockings.

ASSESSMENT

1. Determine whether the patient has had a history of a previous foot ulcer, prior metatarsal surgery, or intermittent claudication.
2. Identify any familial neuropathies.
3. Assess the patient's ability to do foot self-care.
4. Identify any foot problems since last visit.
5. Assess for signs and symptoms of infection.
6. Assess pulses, skin (shiny or thin), temperature (elevated or decreased) presence of hair on the lower leg (absent), nails (thickened), redness of foot when dependent, and pallor when foot is elevated
7. Determine the amount of soft tissue over the metatarsal heads by gently stroking a finger across the plantar surface of the foot.
8. Foot hygiene (cleanliness, fit of shoes).
9. Assess for calluses (plantar callus indicates high pressure), bunions, deformities, and ulcers.
10. Muscle weakness (lift and lower foot against pressure of hand)
11. Determine whether or not the patient's shoes fit properly: Trace foot during weight bearing and compare the shape of the shoes being worn.

DEVELOPMENTAL CONSIDERATIONS

- Distal symmetric polyneuropathy is seen in about 58% of patients with long-standing diabetes mellitus (DM). Neuropathy is present in more than 82% of diabetic patients with foot wounds.
- Patients at high risk for peripheral vascular disease include
  – All diabetic patients (older than 40 years of age)
  – People of any age who have had diabetes for more than 10 years
  – History of alcoholism
  – Patients with human immunodeficiency virus (HIV) and associated neuropathies
- The lack of protective sensation, along with foot deformities, increases the pressure on plantar bony prominences, such as the metatarsal heads. Once the patient has had a foot ulcer, he or she is permanently at high risk for developing another foot ulcer, progressive deformity, and ultimately lower limb amputation.
- In diabetic autonomic neuropathy, several factors are seen:
  – Denervation of dermal structures leads to reduced sweating.
  – Dry skin and fissure formation result, predisposing to the individual to infection.
- A patient with an intact vascular system may have compensatory increased blood flow, leading to the development of Charcot's joint and severe foot deformity.

Elderly: Barriers to carrying out daily foot care noted by elderly subjects include

- Lack of motivation
- Forgetfulness
- Vision problems
- Joint and knee problems
- Family responsibilities

The ability of elderly people to identify foot lesions was investigated in a matched comparison, controlled study. Findings showed that 43% of patients with a history of foot ulcers could not reach and remove simulated lesions on their toes; more than 50% of the older subjects reported difficulty trimming their toe nails; and only 14% had sufficient joint flexibility to allow inspection of the plantar aspect of the foot. Elderly patients who are unable to perform daily self-care of the feet benefit more from regular foot care given by others than from intensive education (Thompson & Masson, 1992).

This procedure describes evaluation of the foot, which is the most common somatosensory testing done. The same procedures can be followed to evaluate other portions of the body.

⊙ EQUIPMENT

- Nylon monofilament device (see figure below)

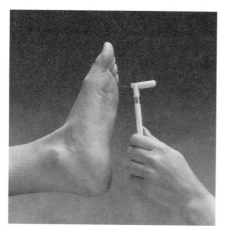

Nylon monofilament device. (Courtesy of North Coast Medical)

- Screening form to identify sensation loss (see next page)

Screening Form for Diabetes Foot Disease

Name: _____

Date: _____

ID #: _____

I. Medical History (Check all that apply.)

☐ Peripheral Neuropathy   ☐ Peripheral Vascular Disease
☐ Nephropathy   ☐ Cardiovascular Disease
☐ Retinopathy

(For sections II & III, fill in the blanks with an "R," "L," or "B" for positive findings on the right, left, or both feet.)

II. Current History

1. Any change in the foot since the last evaluation?
☐ Yes _____ ☐ No

2. Current ulcer or history of a foot ulcer?
☐ Yes _____ ☐ No

3. Is there pain in the calf muscles when walking that is relieved by rest?
☐ Yes _____ ☐ No

III. Foot Exam

1. Are the nails thick, too long, ingrown, infected with fungal disease?
☐ Yes _____ ☐ No

2. Note foot deformities
_____ Toe deformities   _____ Prominent Metatarsal Heads
_____ Bunions (Hallus Valgus)   _____ Amputation (Specify date, side
_____ Charcot foot   and level.) _____
_____ Foot drop   _____

3. Pedal Pulses (Fill in the blanks with a "P" or an "A" to indicate present or absent.)
Posterior tibial: _____ Left _____ Right   Dorsalis pedis: _____ Left _____ Right

4. Skin Condition (Measure, draw in and label the patient's skin condition, using the key and the foot diagram below.)

C = Callus	W = Warmth	F = Fissure
U = Ulcer	M = Maceration	S = Swelling
R = Redness	PU = Pre-ulcerative lesion	D = Dryness

IV. Sensory Foot Exam

Label sensory level with a "+" in the five circled areas of the foot if the patient can feel the 5.07 Semmes-Weinstein (10-gram)nylon filament and "-" if the patient cannot feel the filament. To obtain a monofilament, see the *Resource List* or the *Order Form*.

Screening form to identify sensation loss.

Notes   Notes

Right Foot   Left Foot

V. Risk Categorization (Check appropriate item.)

☐ Low Risk Patient
All of the following:
Intact protective sensation
Pedal pulses present
No severe deformity
No prior Foot ulcer
No amputation

☐ High Risk Patient
One or more of the following:
Loss of protective sensation
Absent pedal pulses
Severe foot deformity
History of foot ulcer
Prior amputation

VI. Footwear Assessment

Does the patient wear appropriate shoes? ☐ Yes ☐ No

Does the patient need inserts? ☐ Yes ☐ No

Should therapeutic footwear be prescribed? ☐ Yes ☐ No

VII. Education

Has the patient had prior foot care education? ☐ Yes ☐ No

Can the patient demonstrate appropriate self-care? ☐ Yes ☐ No

VIII. Management Plan (Check all that apply.)

☐ Provide patient education for preventive foot care. Date: _____

Diagnostic studies: ☐ Vascular laboratory ☐ Other: _____

Footwear recommendations:
☐ None
☐ Athletic shoes
☐ Accommodative inserts

☐ Custom shoes
☐ Depth shoes

Footwear recommendations:
☐ Primary Care Provider
☐ Diabetes Educator
☐ Orthopedic Foot Surgeon
☐ RN Foot Specialist
☐ Orthotist
☐ Podiatrist

☐ Pedorthist
☐ Endocrinologist
☐ Rehab. Specialist
☐ Vascular Surgeon
☐ Other: _____
☐ Schedule follow-up visit.

Date: _____ Provider Signature: _____

Screening form to identify sensation loss (*continued*).

PROCEDURE	SPECIAL CONSIDERATIONS
The patient's foot to be tested should be resting on a padded surface.	The patient should not be able to see his or her foot.
Visually inspect the foot and diagram any calluses, bunions, ulcers, or any other lesions.	When buckling of the monofilament occurs, a known force has been applied to the skin. Inability to feel the stimulus correlates with decreased sensation of the foot.
The patient should be asked to respond when the stimulus is applied.	
Test the stimulus in an area where sensation is known to be normal.	
Begin with the smallest monofilament (5.07 filament = 10 g of force).	If the patient is not able to feel the stimulus, increase the size of the monofilament. Do not apply to ulcer, callus, scar, or necrotic tissue. Do not slide across skin or make repetitive contact at test site.
Apply the monofilament in one smooth motion at a right angle to the extremity surface until the monofilament bends (see Figure 51-1). Touch for approximately 1/2 second, hold for 1/2 second, and lift in 1/2 second.	

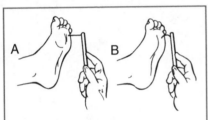

A: Apply monofilament at right angle to surface.
B: Apply until monofilament bends. (From: *Feet Can Last a Lifetime.* National Diabetes Clearinghouse.)

Repeat in each location up to three times to elicit a response.	Most patients lose sensation first in the great toe.
Repeat this process over the plantar surface.	This test has been found to be 97% sensitive and 83% specific for identifying sensation loss if the patient cannot feel the stimulus at 4 of 10 sites (Armstrong & Lavery, 1998, p. 1327).
Document the identified areas of normal and decreased sensation on the screening form.	Using vibration testing (with 128-cycle tuning fork) in addition to monofilament may increase specificity (Armstrong, Lavery, Vela, Quebedeaux, & Fleichli, 1998).

(procedure continued)

PROCEDURE	SPECIAL CONSIDERATIONS

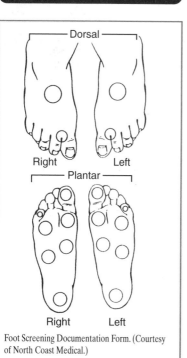

Foot Screening Documentation Form. (Courtesy of North Coast Medical.)

Determine the risk category for ulceration and sensation based on findings.

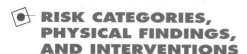 RISK CATEGORIES, PHYSICAL FINDINGS, AND INTERVENTIONS

Risk Category	Physical and Diagnostic Findings	Intervention
Low-Risk Patient Normal, no pathology.	Normal monofilament test. No history of ulcer. No evidence of decreased pulses, intermittent claudication, shiny skin, decreased hair, thickened toenails (arterial vascular occlusion).	Daily foot care. Foot examination by provider a minimum of 2 times a year. Properly fitted shoes with soft inserts and soles.

(table continued)

Risk Category	Physical and Diagnostic Findings	Intervention
High-Risk Patients: Increased risk for ulceration ——— Neuropathy (no previous ulcer, no deformity, callus, no weakness, no pre–ulcer).	Abnormal monofilament test.	As above, plus protective footwear (commercially available athletic shoes and thick, absorbent socks) Check feet at every visit. Identify patient as being high risk. Place "high-risk feet" stickers on chart.
Increased risk for ulceration ——— Neuropathy plus deformity.	Abnormal monofilament. Foot deformity (bunions, calluses, hammer toes, abnormally prominent joints, rigid deformities, or limited range of motion at the subtalar or metatarsophalangeal joints). In shoe, conduct pressure measurements.	As above, plus custom shoe (orthotic referral, (covered now by Medicare Part B when risk factor is identified for ulcer formation and documentation is submitted.) Surgical correction of deformity.
Increased risk for ulceration ——— History of previous ulcer.	No evidence of decreased pulses, intermittent claudication, shiny skin, decreased hair, or thickened toenails (arterial vascular occlusion).	As above, plus check feet more frequently.

Adapted from Armstrong, D., Lavery, L. (1998); Caputo, G., Cavanagh, P., Ulbrecht, J., Gibbons, G., & Karchmer, A, 1994; North Coast Medical; Patient Screening Form, National Diabetes Information Clearinghouse: Feet Can Last a Lifetime.

- If an ulcer is found, the following steps should be taken or the patient should be referred depending on the health care provider's experience in working with ulcers:
- Use adequate débridement to assist in evaluation of the ulcer.
- Remove all necrotic tissue and callus until a healthy bleeding edge is found.
- Probe the ulcer with a sterile blunt instrument for involvement of tendon, joint capsule, or bone.
- Perform a foot x-ray study to look for soft tissue gas, foreign bodies, or bone involvement.
- Check albumin and complete blood count (CBC): Good wound healing requires albumin levels higher than 3.5g/dL and absolute lymphocyte count higher than 1500 mm^3.
- Weight bearing must be stopped. This can be accomplished by the application of a total contact cast. (For more details, see Caputo, Cavanagh, Ulbrecht, Gibbons, & Karchmer, 1994.)

Charcot's Joint
• Custom footwear or corrective surgery
• Periodic x-ray study to monitor joint deterioration
• Referral to a foot specialist

Infected Ulcer
• Débridement, x-ray study, bone scan to rule out osteomyelitis
• Antibiotic therapy
• Hospitalization may be necessary if no improvement is seen.

Peripheral Arterial Disease
• Conduct ankle-brachial index, transcutaneous oxygen measurement, and absolute toe systolic pressure testing.
• Follow the same interventions as appropriate if ulcer or infection is present (Armstrong & Lavery, 1998).

RESOURCES

Information
National Diabetes Clearing House "Feet Can Last a Lifetime Kit" (includes sensory testing monofilament, provider guide, foot screening forms, reference materials and patient education booklet)
1-800-get-level
Web site: http://www.niddk.nih.gov (go to Diabetes, under Health Information and Education)

American Association of Diabetes Educators
1-800-team-up4
http://www.aadenet.org

American Diabetes Association
1-800-diabetes
http://www.diabetes.org

American Podiatric Medical Association,
1-ST800-footcare
http://www.apma.org

Juvenile Diabetes Foundation International
1-800-jdf-cure
http://www.jdfcure.com

Pedorthic Footwear Association
1-800-673-9447

Monofilaments
North Coast Medical "Touch Test Sensory Evaluator"
1-800-821-9319
GWL-HDC, LEAP Program
5445 Point Clair Rd
Carville, LA 70721
fax: 504-642-4738

Center for Specialized Diabetes Foot Care
1-800-543-9055
Smith and Nephew, Inc.
1-800-558-8633

Curative Health Services
1-516-689-7000
Sensory Testing Systems
1-504-923-1297

Evaluation of Foot Pressure
AliMed Company, Foot Imprinter
Dedham, MA
1-800-225-2610

BIBLIOGRAPHY

Ahroni, J. (1993). Teaching foot care creatively and successfully. *The Diabetes Educator, 19*(4), 320–325.

American Diabetes Association. (1997). Standards of medical care for patients with diabetes mellitus [Position Statement]. *Diabetes Care, 20*(Suppl), S11–S12.

American Medical Association. (1998). *Physicians' current procedural terminology: CPT.* Chicago: American Medical Association.

Armstrong, D. & Lavery, L. (1998). Diabetic foot ulcers: prevention, diagnosis and classification. *American Family Physician, 57*(6), 1325–1334.

Armstrong, D., Lavery, L., Vela, S., Quebedeaux, T., & Fleischli, J. (1998). Choosing a practical screening instrument to identify patients at risk for diabetic foot ulceration. *Archives of Internal Medicine, 158,* 289–292.

Birrer, R., Dellacorte, M., & Grisafi, P. (1996). Prevention and care of diabetic foot ulcers. *American Family Physician, 53*(2), 601–612.

Caputo, G., Cavanagh, P., Ulbrecht, J., Gibbons, G., & Karchmer, A. (1994). Assessment and management of foot disease in patients with diabetes. *New England Journal of Medicine, 331,* 854–860.

DCCT Research Group. (1993). The effect of intensive treatment of diabetes on the development and progression of long-term complications in insulin-dependent diabetes mellitus. *New England Journal of Medicine, 329*(14), 977–986.

Dorgan, M., Birke, J., Moretto, J., Patout, C., & Rehm, K. (1995). Performing foot screening for diabetic patients. *American Journal of Nursing, 95*(11), 32–36.

Duffy, J. & Patout, C. (1990). Management of the insensitive foot in diabetes: lessons learned from Hansen's disease. *Military Medicine, 155*(12), 575–579.

Healthcare Consultants of America. (1998). *1998 Physicians' fee and coding guide.* Augusta, GA.

Isakov, E., Susak, Z., Budorgin, N., & Mendelevich, I. (1992). Self-injury resulting in amputation among vascular patients: a restrospective epidemiological study. *Disability and Rehabilitation, 14,* 78–80.

Lavery, L., Ashry, H., van Houtum, W., Pugh, J., Harkless, L., Basu, S. (1996). Variation in the incidence and proportion of diabetes-related amputations in minorities. *Diabetes Care, 19*(1), 48–52.

Ledda, M. A. & Walker, E. A. (1997). Development and formative evaluation of a foot self-care program for African Americans with diabetes. *The Diabetes Educator, 23*(1), 48–51.

Lehto, S., Pyorala, K., Ronnemaa, T., & Laakso, M. (1996). Risk factors predicting lower extremity amputations in patients with NIDDM. *Diabetes Care, 19*(6), 607–612.

Marchand, L. H., Campbell, W., & Rolfsen, R. J. (1996). Lessons from "Feet Can Last a Lifetime": A public health campaign. *Diabetes Spectrum, 9*(4), 214–218.

Mayfield, J. A., Reiber, G. E., Nelson, R. G., & Greene, T. (1996). A foot risk classification system to predict diabetic amputation in Pima Indians. *Diabetes Care, 19*(7), 704–709.

Murray, H. J., Young, M. J., Hollis, S., & Boulton, A. J. (1996). The association between callus formation, high pressures and neuropathy in diabetic foot ulceration. *Diabetic Medicine, 13*(11), 979–982.

Pecoraro, R. E., Reiber, G. E., & Burgess, E. M. (1990). Pathways to diabetic limb amputation. Basis for prevention. *Diabetes Care, 13*(5), 513–521.

Peters, S. (1998). Diabetic foot ulcers. Advance for *Nurse Practitioners, 6*(6), 59–62.

Quebedeaux, T. L., Lavery, D. C., & Lavery, L. A. (1996). The development of foot deformities and ulcers after great toe amputation in diabetes. *Diabetes Care, 19*(2), 165–167.

Reiber, G. E., Boyko, E. J., & Smith, D. G. (1995). Lower extremity foot ulcers and amputations in diabetes. In *Diabetes in America* (2nd ed.). National Institutes of Health, NIDDK, NIH Pub. No. 95-1468.

Rith-Najarian, S. J., Stolusky, T., & Gohdes, D. M. (1992). Identifying diabetic patients at high risk for lower extremity amputation in a primary health care setting. A prospective evaluation of simple screening criteria. *Diabetes Care, 15*(10), 1386–1389.

Sanders, L. J. (1994). Diabetes mellitus—prevention of amputation. *Journal of the American Podiatric Medical Association, 84*(7), 322–328.

Thompson, F. J. & Masson, E. A. (1992). Can elderly diabetic patients cooperate with routine foot care? *Age and Aging, 21,* 333–337.

chapter 52

Glucose Testing

CPT Coding:

82950 Finger stick blood glucose ($12–$15)

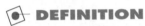
DEFINITION

- Glucose testing is the measurement of blood glucose using the finger stick method. Monitoring of blood glucose can be interpreted with a visual reading or glucose meter.

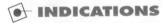
INDICATIONS

- Screening test for hyperglycemia or hypoglycemia
- Monitoring pregnant diabetics or prenatal patients with gestational diabetes
- Method of management and control of diabetes

PATIENT EDUCATION

- Explain the purpose of the test and the procedure.
- Reinforce the importance of home glucose monitoring.

ASSESSMENT

1. Perform history and physical examination.
2. Monitor patient for signs of hypoglycemia: headache, dizziness, weakness, fainting, or irritability.
3. Identify patient's last meal.

 ALERT: Need to follow universal blood and body fluid precautions.

EQUIPMENT

- Gloves
- Reagent test strip
- Lancet or puncture device
- Alcohol swab

PROCEDURE	SPECIAL CONSIDERATIONS
Put on gloves.	Patients with various blood disorders may have inaccurate results.
Examine the hand for a puncture site.	Patients with multiple punctures may have rough skin, making the test more difficult to obtain.
Lower the patient's hand and massage the puncture site.	Gravity and stimulation facilitate blood flow to the area.
Remove cap from lancet or insert needle into the puncture device.	
Grasp the lancet and quickly prick the site or place puncture device against the site and push the release mechanism.	
Remove the first drop of blood with gauze pad.	**This drop has large amount of serum that dilutes the blood.**
Squeeze the finger proximal to the puncture site.	
Place the test strip next to the puncture site to obtain a drop of blood or allow a drop to fall onto strip.	**Do not smear the blood.**

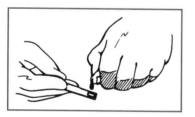

Remove the strip and begin the mechanism for timing. (Follow the manufacturer's directions.)

Place gauze over the puncture site until bleeding stops.

Follow manufacturer's instructions for visual reading.

If using a glucose monitor, need to follow manufacturer's directions.

◉ FOLLOW-UP

- Educate the patient on following the manufacturer's instructions for testing.
- Explain that errors occur if the procedure is not done accurately.
- Patients should keep a record of glucose readings and bring them to each office visit.
- Patients may need assistance performing home monitoring owing to various health problems.

BIBLIOGRAPHY

American Medical Association. (1998). *Physicians' current procedural terminology: CPT*. Chicago: American Medical Association.

Earnest, V. V. (1993). *Clinical skills in nursing practice* (2nd ed.). Philadelphia: J. B. Lippincott.

Healthcare Consultants of America. (1998). *1998 Physicians' fee and coding guide*. Augusta, GA.

chapter
53

Incontinence Evaluation

CPT Coding:

51725-26 Simple cystometrogram (CMG) ($154–$188)
51726-26 Complex CMG (eg, calibrated equipment) ($183–$220)
51736-26 Simple uroflowmetry (UFR) (eg, stopwatch flow rate, mechanical flowmeter) ($67–$79)
51741-26 Complex UFR (calibrated electronic equipment) ($96–$113)
51772-26 Urethral pressure profile studies (UPP) (urethral closure pressure profile, any technique) ($165–$200)
51795-26 Voiding pressure (VP) studies; bladder voiding pressure, any technique ($169–$207)
90911 Biofeedback training, perineal muscles, anorectal or urethral sphincter, including electromyography (EMG) or manometry ($169–$209)

⦿ DEFINITIONS

- Urinary incontinence is involuntary loss of urine.
- Stress incontinence (SUI) is involuntary loss of urine during coughing, sneezing, or other activities due to increased intra-abdominal pressure.
- Urge incontinence is an involuntary loss of urine when the patient feels the urge to urinate but cannot make it to the bathroom in time before leakage begins. The person cannot inhibit the contractions of the detrusor muscle.
- Overflow incontinence is loss of urine from incomplete bladder emptying.
- Nocturnal enuresis is urinary incontinence when the patient is asleep.
- Spontaneous incontinence is leakage of urine without a perceived urge or stressful activity.
- Postvoid dribbling involves small amounts of urine that leak after urination due to urine trapped in the vagina or labia that drips out when the woman stands up.
- Mixed urinary incontinence involves more than one type of incontinence.
- Postvoid residual urine is the amount of urine remaining in the bladder after the patient urinates.
- Cystometry is the test for urge incontinence.
- Provocative stress test identifies loss of urine when the bladder is stressed when full, such as during coughing.

INDICATIONS

- Identification of type of incontinence
- Early diagnosis and treatment before quality of life is affected
- Assessment of pelvic muscle support and strength
- Testing should used to evaluate persistent urinary incontinence
- Determine whether or not urinary incontinence is caused by transient problems, such as urinary tract infections (UTI), stool impaction, atrophic vaginitis, adverse drug effects, urinary retention, and conditions that cause decreased mobility or delirium.

PATIENT EDUCATION

- Discuss the importance of a voiding diary (daily fluid intake, number and amount of voids, and number of incontinence episodes).
- The testing is not invasive and takes approximately 10 to 15 minutes to complete.
- Explain the various components of the testing.
- Although such infections are uncommon, make sure that the patient knows the symptoms of an UTI and to call if these symptoms occur after the testing.

ASSESSMENT

1. Gather data related to history of urinary incontinence:
   - How long has the incontinence been present?
   - When is the loss of urine noted: with activity, coughing, and so on?
   - Do you wear protective clothing for incontinence?
   - Do you have the need to urinate so urgently that you might not make it to the bathroom in time?
   - Is there urinary frequency or urgency?
   - Need to alter activities due to urine leakage?
   - How much urine is lost: a few drops or enough to soak a pad or soil clothing?
   - How many times a day do you urinate?
   - Do you awaken at night to urinate?
   - What is your normal fluid intake: coffee, tea, colas, acidic fruit juices, spicy foods?
   - How much does the urine leakage bother you?
   - Have you undergone any previous treatment for urinary leakage?
   - How many pregnancies and vaginal deliveries have you had?
2. Sexual history:
   - Determine whether or not the patient has any associated symptoms: Hot flashes, irritability, decreased sleeping, sweating (menopause)
3. Past medical and family history:
   - Osteoporosis, history of heart disease (patient or family), history of neurologic disease
4. Have the patient keep a bladder diary for 2 days including the following information:

Your Daily Bladder Diary

This diary will help you and your health care team. Bladder diaries help show the causes of bladder control trouble. The "sample" line (below) will show you how to use the diary.

Your name: _____ Date: _____

Time ☼	Drinks What kind? / How much?	Urine How many times? / How much? (circle one)	ACCIDENTS		
			Accidental leaks How much? (circle one)	Did you feel a strong urge to go? Circle one	What were you doing at the time? Sneezing, exercising, having sex, lifting, etc.
Sample	coffee | 2 cups	✓✓ ⊙sm ○med ●lg	💧💧 ⊙sm ○med ●lg	Yes (No)	Running
6–7 a.m.	|	○ ◒ ●	💧💧 ◒ ●	Yes	No	
7–8 a.m.	|	○ ◒ ●	💧💧 ◒ ●	Yes	No	
8–9 a.m.	|	○ ◒ ●	💧💧 ◒ ●	Yes	No	
9–10 a.m.	|	○ ◒ ●	💧💧 ◒ ●	Yes	No	
10–11 a.m.	|	○ ◒ ●	💧💧 ◒ ●	Yes	No	
11–12 noon	|	○ ◒ ●	💧💧 ◒ ●	Yes	No	
12–1 p.m.	|	○ ◒ ●	💧💧 ◒ ●	Yes	No	
1–2 p.m.	|	○ ◒ ●	💧💧 ◒ ●	Yes	No	
2–3 p.m.	|	○ ◒ ●	💧💧 ◒ ●	Yes	No	
3–4 p.m.	|	○ ◒ ●	💧💧 ◒ ●	Yes	No	
4–5 p.m.	|	○ ◒ ●	💧💧 ◒ ●	Yes	No	
5–6 p.m.	|	○ ◒ ●	💧💧 ◒ ●	Yes	No	
6–7 p.m.	|	○ ◒ ●	💧💧 ◒ ●	Yes	No	
7–8 p.m.	|	○ ◒ ●	💧💧 ◒ ●	Yes	No	
8–9 p.m.	|	○ ◒ ●	💧💧 ◒ ●	Yes	No	
9–10 p.m.	|	○ ◒ ●	💧💧 ◒ ●	Yes	No	
10–11 p.m.	|	○ ◒ ●	💧💧 ◒ ●	Yes	No	
11–12 midnight	|	○ ◒ ●	💧💧 ◒ ●	Yes	No	
12–1 a.m.	|	○ ◒ ●	💧💧 ◒ ●	Yes	No	
1–2 a.m.	|	○ ◒ ●	💧💧 ◒ ●	Yes	No	
2–3 a.m.	|	○ ◒ ●	💧💧 ◒ ●	Yes	No	
3–4 a.m.	|	○ ◒ ●	💧💧 ◒ ●	Yes	No	
4–5 a.m.	|	○ ◒ ●	💧💧 ◒ ●	Yes	No	
5–6 a.m.	|	○ ◒ ●	💧💧 ◒ ●	Yes	No	

I used _____ pads. I used _____ diapers today (write number).

Questions to ask my health care team: _____
_____

Let's Talk about Bladder Control for Women is a public health awareness campaign conducted by the National Kidney and Urologic Diseases Information Clearinghouse (NKUDIC), an information dissemination service of the National Institute of Diabetes and Digestive Kidney Diseases (NIDDK), National Institutes of Health.

- How often voided
- How often leaked urine and why
5. Identify which activities cause leakage of urine
6. The presence of nocturia
7. Measure all urine with each voiding during this same time period
8. Physical examination:
   - Abdominal examination: suprapubic fullness or tenderness, costovertebral angle tenderness (CVAT)
   - Neurologic exam: deep tendon reflexes (DTRs) of lower extremities, motor strength
   - Pudendal nerve (S2–S4) provides innervation to the pelvis. Assess function by assessing sensory and motor functions in the lower extremities.
   - Assess bulbocavernosus and clitoral reflexes: stroke the labia majora or tap the clitoris: a visible contraction of the levator ani muscles and anal sphincter should be seen. (This reflex may be absent in up to 20% of neurologically intact women.)
   - Pelvic examination: perineal skin conditions, lesions, discharge, evidence of hypoestrogenism, uterine or vault prolapse, cystocele or rectocele. Also determine the ability of the patient to contract the pelvic floor muscles. Palpate the levator muscles from the margin of the sacrum and coccyx to the fibromuscular attachment of the lateral pelvic sidewall to the superior margin of the pubic symphysis (as below).

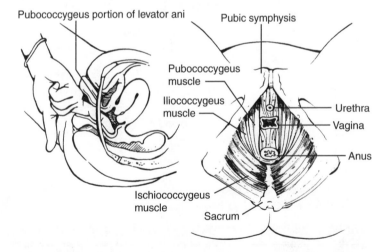

With one finger deep in the vagina, palpate the levator muscles to assess the strength of the pelvic floor muscles. Begin at the margin of the sacrum/coccyx, and follow the muscles along to the fibromuscular attachment of the lateral pelvic sidewall to the superior margin of the pubic symphysis. Ask the woman to tighten the muscles she would use to stop the flow of urine. If she can isolate these muscles from the gluteal, inner thigh, and lower abdominal muscles, she is a good candidate for a self-directed program of pelvic muscle exercises.

- Using the posterior blade of a Pederson's speculum to depress the posterior vaginal wall, the resting position of the urethra, bladder, and uterus can be visualized. Then ask the patient to cough; evaluate the anterior wall for the extent it moves in response to the increased intra-abdominal pressure.

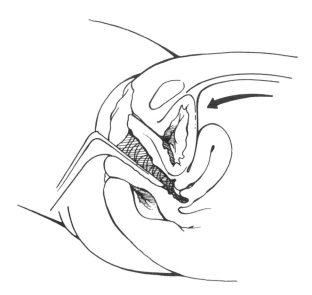

Evaluate the anterior wall for the extent it moves in response to the increased intra-abdominal pressure.

- Rectal: Check rectal tone. Check for rectal impaction if that is indicated.
9. It should be determined that urinalysis and urine culture are normal before other testing is performed.

◉ DEVELOPMENTAL CONSIDERATIONS

Elderly: Incontinence is a classic syndrome in elderly patients. It affects approximately 13 million persons in the United States (Weiss, 1998). In women older than 60 years of age, the most common type of incontinence is a mixed type of stress and urge incontinence (55%).

Women: Approximately 10% to 30% of women 15 to 64 years of age have incontinence. That figure increases to 25% to 35% in women older than 65 years of age.

Diagnostic test options*

Type of UI	Mechanism	Associated Factors	Diagnostic Test Options
Urge	Unstable bladder or detrusor instability (DI)	No neurologic deficit	Simple or multichannel CMG with or without EMG
	Detrusor hyperreflexia (DH), detrusor sphincter dyssynergia (DSD)	With neurologic lesion such as stroke, supraspinal cord lesions, multiple sclerosis	Simple cystometry or multichannel
	Detrusor hyperactivity with impaired contractility (DHIC)	Elderly, usually also associated with obstructive or stress symptoms	Multichannel CMG with or without EMG Videourodynamics
Stress	Hypermobility of bladder neck (female)	Detachment of bladder neck with concomitant hypermobility of the urethra	Provocative stress test (direct visualization) Tests for bladder neck hypermobility Simple or multichannel CMG (to exclude DI) UPP or leak point pressure Videourodynamics
	Intrinsic sphincter deficiency (ISD)	Postoperative (after prostatectomy or anti-incontinence surgery), trauma, aging, radiation, congenital (epispadias)	Same as above
	Neurogenic sphincter deficiency	Neurogenic, sacral, or infrasacral lesion (eg, myelomeningocele)	Same as above EMG
Overflow	Overflow from underactive or acontractile detrusor	Neurogenic (low spinal cord lesion, neuropathy, postradical pelvic surgery), idiopathic detrusor failure	Elevated PVR volume Uroflowmetry Voiding CMG (pressure flow) with EMG Cystourethroscopy
	Overflow from outlet obstruction	Male: prostate gland disease, urethral stricture Female: postoperative	Same as above Videourodynamics

*The urodynamic tests listed here are not recommended for routine use but are options for patients who require further evaluation. For details on various tests, see text.

CMG = cystometrogram, EMG = electromyogram, PVR = postvoid residual, UPP = urethral pressure profilometry

 ## URETHRAL HYPERMOBILITY TEST, OR COTTON SWAB TEST (Q-TIP TEST)

Equipment
- Povidone-iodine (Betadine) solution
- Anesthetic lubricant
- Sterile cotton applicator

PROCEDURE	SPECIAL CONSIDERATIONS
Position woman in supine position. Cleanse urethral meatus with Betadine solution. Insert the sterile lubricated applicator into the bladder and pull back gently until some resistance is met (the applicator will be at the urethrovesical junction).	Urethral hypermobility is the most common cause of stress incontinence. This hypermobility permits downward displacement of the proximal urethra. More intra-abdominal pressure is then transmitted to the bladder than the urethra, causing stress incontinence.

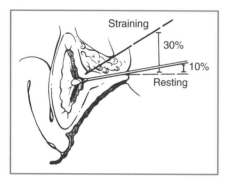

| A goniometer is used to measure the angle between the applicator and the horizontal plane (resting angle). | |
| The patient is then asked to perform a Valsalva maneuver (cough, laugh) This creates the straining angle. The angle is measured during the Valsalva maneuver. | Urethral hypermobility is diagnosed when the angle changes by 30 degrees or more from resting to standing, OR when the straining angle is greater than 30 degrees. The specificity is 53% (many patients who have urethral hypermobility do not have SUI). However, the sensitivity of this test is 90% for patients who complain of SUI. |

STRESS TEST

Equipment
• Absorbent pad

PROCEDURE	SPECIAL CONSIDERATIONS
A stress test can be completed now if the patient has a full bladder, or this portion of the exam may be completed after the cystometry	If urine leaks onto the absorbent pad, a presumptive diagnosis of stress incontinence is made.

(procedure continued)

PROCEDURE	SPECIAL CONSIDERATIONS
test. Have the patient lie supine on the exam table with the full bladder. Place an absorbent pad in front of the urethra. Have her cough forcefully.	
Place your fingers on either side of the woman's urethra and elevate the structure. Ask the patient to cough again.	In patients with stress incontinence, elevation of the urethra prevents further urine leakage.
These maneuvers can be repeated in the standing position if no incontinence is demonstrated.	
Begin the test when patient feels her bladder is full. Have her wear a small absorbent pad. Have the patient cough forcefully several times while standing.	Leakage of urine with coughing is positive for stress incontinence. Prolonged loss of urine is not indicative of stress incontinence.

 ## POSTVOID RESIDUAL URINE VOLUME

Equipment
• Straight catheter kit
• Gloves

PROCEDURE	SPECIAL CONSIDERATIONS
Cleanse the vulvar area using antiseptic pads. Obtain a midstream urine specimen (see text). Have the patient urinate into a measuring device (measuring container in the toilet or other container) and completely empty bladder.	Quantify volume of urine. Submit specimen for urine dipstick or culture, or both, as appropriate. Normal bladder capacity is 400 to 600 mL.
Using the straight catheter kit, catheterize the patient within 5 to 10 minutes of voiding.	Normal residual volume is less than 50 mL. Residual volume less than 200 mL is considered abnormal. Volumes of 50 to 200 mL are considered equivocal, and the test should be repeated. Inability to pass the catheter may indicate bladder obstruction. PVR can detect urinary retention by potentially reversible factors.

ALTERNATIVE PROCEDURE

- Post-void residual (PVR) can be measured with pelvic ultrasound using a portable ultrasound machine. This is helpful in evaluating men with suspected prostate obstruction because it may be difficult to catheterize these patients and may cause a UTI afterward.

Procedure
- Office cystometry

Equipment
- Urinary catheterization kit with:
  - 14 French catheter
  - 50-mL syringe, bayonet tip
  - Sterile water

PROCEDURE	SPECIAL CONSIDERATIONS
The bladder is catheterized using a 14 French catheter. The bladder is emptied. Use the 50 mL syringe with the plunger removed. Insert the tip into the end of the catheter.	First sensation to void is approximately 150 mL. Fullness is noted at approximately 200 to 300 mL. Maximum capacity is 400–700 mL.
Hold the syringe about 15 cm above the urethra. Instill 50 mL of sterile water into the syringe and allow it to flow into the bladder.	Keep track of the total amount of water used. Do not fill the bladder more than 500 mL.

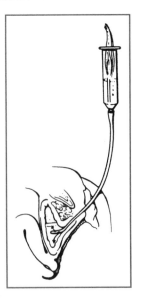

(procedure continued) ──────────────────────────────

PROCEDURE	**SPECIAL CONSIDERATIONS**
Continue to add water in 50-mL increments until the patient experiences the urge to urinate. Continue to add water in 25-mL increments until the patient experiences extreme urgency.	Stop instilling water if bladder contractions occur. Contractions are detected by a rise and fall in the level of fluid remaining in the syringe, indicating a pressure change (contractions).
	Severe urgency at greater than 300 mL is considered presumptive urge incontinence. This test has a 75% to 100% sensitivity, a 69% to 89% specificity, and a 74% to 91% positive predictive value when compared with multichannel cystomegraphy (Weiss, 1998).

 FOLLOW-UP

- Depending on the test results, the following interventions may be appropriate.
- Urge incontinence:
  - 1st line: bladder training and bladder drill
  - 2nd line: medications such as oxybutynin (Ditropan)
  - 3rd line: surgical procedures (rarely used)
- Stress incontinence:
  - 1st line: Kegel's exercise, bladder training
  - 2nd line: medications: alpha adrenergic or estrogen
  - 3rd line: surgical procedures
- Catheterization:
  - 1st line: intermittent catheterization
  - 2nd line: indwelling catheter
  - 3rd line: surgical procedures
- Other interventions for incontinence include
  - Pessaries
  - Electric stimulation devices
  - Biofeedback
  - Vaginal cones
  - Intraurethral inserts
- Patients should be referred to urologic or gynecologic specialists for formal or complex urodynamic testing if any of the following are present:
  - History of lower urinary tract or pelvic surgery, or irradiation
  - Significant pelvic prolapse
  - Marked prostatic enlargement
  - Hematuria
  - Uncertain diagnosis

– Failure to respond to treatment
– Consideration of surgery

BIBLIOGRAPHY

American Medical Association. (1998). *Physicians' current procedural terminology: CPT.* Chicago: American Medical Association.

Cespedes, R., Cross, C., & McGuire, E. (1998). Pelvic prolapse: Diagnosing and treating cystoceles, rectoceles, and enteroceles. *Medscape Women's Health, 3*(4), 4.

Clayton, J., Smith, K., Qureshi, H. & Ferguson, B. (1998). Collecting patients' views and perceptions of continence services: The development of research instruments. *Journal of Advanced Nursing, 28*(2), 353–361.

Cutner, L., & Cardoza, L. (1991). Urinary incontinence–diagnosis. *Practitioner, 235*(1498), 24.

Czarapata, B. (1997). Urinary incontinence: Proactive management. *Contemporary Nurse Practitioner, 2*(4), 16–26.

Fantl, J., Newman, D., Colling, J., et al. (1996). *Urinary incontinence in adults: Acute and chronic management. Clinical Practice Guideline no. 2. 1996 update.* Rockville, MD: US Department of Health and Human Services, Public Health Service, Agency for Health Care Policy and Research, March 1996, AHCPR publication no. 96-0682.

Fonda, D., Brimage, P., & D'Astoli, M. (1993). Simple screening for urinary incontinence in the elderly: Comparison of simple and multichannel cystometry. *Urology, 42*(5), 536.

Maloney, C. (1995). Urinary incontinence: A guide to the diagnosis of chronic and reversible causes in a primary care setting. *Nurse Practitioner, 20*(21), 74–75.

Turzo, E. & Bavendam, T. (1998). Treatment options for urinary incontinence. *Women's Health in Primary Care, 1*(8), 649–658.

Weiss, B. (1998). Diagnostic evaluation of urinary incontinence in geriatric patients. *American Family Physician, 57*(11), 2675–2684.

Winkler, H. & Sand, P. (1998). Stress incontinence: Options for conservative treatment. *Women's Health in Primary Care, 1*(3), 279–294.

chapter 54

Determining Sexual Abuse in Children and Adolescents

CPT Coding:

N/A

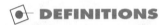 **DEFINITIONS**

Genital examination is a physical examination (inspection) of the external genitalia and anal area of children as part of routine well-child assessment, in the presence of nonspecific findings of concern to parent, or when sexual abuse is suspected.

 ALERT: Because state statutes vary, especially with regard to age, the nurse practitioner should be familiar with definitions in the official code of the state in which practice occurs.

- Child molestation is an immoral or indecent act to, with, or in the presence of any child younger than 16 years of age.
- Aggravated child molestation is that which physically injures the child or involves an act of sodomy.
- Sodomy is the performance of a sexual act that involves sexual organs of one person and the mouth or anus of another.
- Sexual battery is physical contact with the intimate body parts of another without consent.
- Aggravated sexual battery involves penetration with a foreign object or injury.
- Statutory rape is sexual intercourse with a female younger than 16 years of age who is not one's spouse.
- The hymenal orifice is the collar-like or semi–collar-like tissue that surrounds the vaginal opening that varies in structure and appearance depending on the individual's age and extent of estrogenization. Hymenal tissue is thickened and redundant secondary to estrogen's effects in girls up to age 3 from perinatal exposure and again at puberty. Normal configurations of the hymen include:

- Annular: hymenal tissue completely encircles the vaginal orifice
- Crescentic: tissue is crescent shaped with insertion points superior to the 11 and 1 o'clock positions. Most common in girls older than 24 months of age
- Septated: hymen has two distinct openings with bands of tissue between
- Cribriform: hymen has multiple small openings in the tissue
- Fimbriated: hymen has a redundant or fixed nature, seen in girls older than 12 months
- Bumps and vestibular bands: hymen has multiple bumps or vestibular bands; found in up to 21% of girls

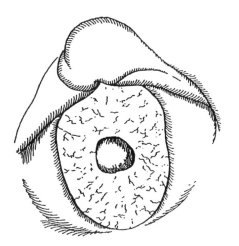

Annular hymen. (Berenson, A. B., Heger, A., Hayes, J. M., Bailey, R. K., & Emans, S. J. [1992]. Appearance of the hymen in prepubertal girls. *Pediatrics, 89*[3]: 387–394.)

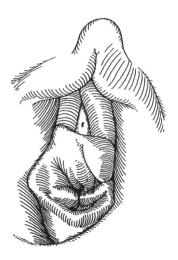

Fimbriated hymen. (Berenson, A. B., Heger, A., Hayes, J. M., Bailey, R. K., & Emans, S. J. [1992]. Appearance of the hymen in prepubertal girls. *Pediatrics, 89*[3]: 387–394.)

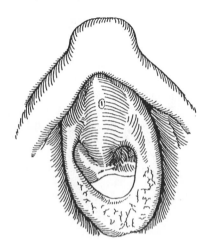

Crescentic hymen. (Berenson, A. B., Heger, A., Hayes, J. M., Bailey, R. K., & Emans, S. J. [1992]. Appearance of the hymen in prepubertal girls. *Pediatrics, 89*[3]: 387–394.)

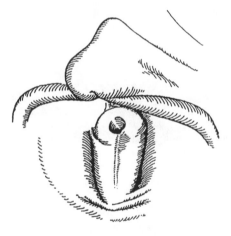

Sleeve-like hymen. (Berenson, A. B., Heger, A., Hayes, J. M., Bailey, R. K., & Emans, S. J. [1992]. Appearance of the hymen in prepubertal girls. *Pediatrics, 89*[3]: 387–394.)

– The primary care provider must appreciate that most lay people and some medical personnel perceive the hymen as an impermeable membrane in which any opening is abnormal before sexual intercourse.
- A sexual assault nurse examiner (SANE) is an RN with special classroom and clinical education for comprehensive care of sexual assault victims. The SANE is competent in the aspect of forensic nursing that involves rape-kit protocol to collect medicolegal evidence; assessment of injuries, pregnancy, and the risk of sexually transmitted disease (STD); provision of immediate treatment and documentation; prophylaxis against pregnancy and STDs; crisis counseling; and testifying in court, as needed. The SANE is certified by the educational program attended.
- Videocolposcopy is an examination using a colposcope equipped with a 35-mm camera with photographic and video capability under 4 to 30×

magnification. There is a scale that allows precise measurement of structures and a red-free filter that enables visualization of vascular patterns and interruption in the integrity of internal mucosa. The colposcope provides a noninvasive and less intrusive examination that reduces the amount of time that the genital area is exposed. Because photographs and videotapes are possible, corroboration of findings and confirmation or dismissal of sexual abuse is more likely.

- In the sexual abuse of children, a continuum of sorts exists along which nontouching, touching, and exploitative behaviors exist; placement on the continuum does not imply seriousness of offense or predict a child's perception of or response to an event. It does serve, in part, to explain why injury is not always associated with sexual abuse in children.

Nontouching Behaviors	Touching Behaviors	Exploitation Behaviors
Exposing genitals to child	Fondling	Using child in pornography
Exposing child to pornography	Directing child to touch adult genitals	Using or soliciting child for prostitution
Deliberately exposing child to sex acts of others	Penetration by penis/other sodomy	
Masturbation in front of child		

- A normal physical exam does NOT rule out sexual assault. Even in the presence of known sexual assault (admitted by offender), 80% of exams are normal for the following reasons:
  - There has been a delay in reporting by child because of fear and threats.
  - The abuse was not recognized by a nonabusing adult.
  - Small injuries heal quickly. New epithelial tissue generates in 4 to 7 days; tissues have remarkable elasticity, especially with lubrication.
  - Perpetrators usually do not use enough force to cause tissue trauma; instead, they try to gain the child's cooperation and silence so participation is ensured over time.
  - The nature of abuse along the continuum does not always leave evidence.

◉ INDICATIONS

- Anogenital exam is appropriate in the following circumstances:
  - As part of routine well-child exam
  - When a child has disclosed sexual abuse or there is compelling history when the attending parent has suspicions about abuse
  - When child presents with complaints of genital injury, rectal or vaginal bleeding, vaginal or penile discharge, dysuria, enuresis, encopresis, pelvic pain, or undue irritation of area
  - When the child exhibits behavioral changes associated with sexual abuse,

such as depression, regressive behavior, sleep problems, appetite changes, anger, aggression and acting out, including abuse, running away, school problems like sudden poor performance, truancy, conduct problems, drug use, and sexualized behavior or knowledge level of sexual matters greater than usual for developmental level

ALERT: *Suspicions of child sexual abuse require mandatory reporting by health providers in all 50 states. If the primary care provider has cause to suspect that abuse has occurred and reports in good faith, immunity from prosecution is ensured. The agency to which reports are made varies from one jurisdiction to another, so the provider should be familiar with regulations for the particular practice site.*

- If there is a history of sexual abuse, the child should be referred to a center that specializes in assessment and treatment. Such centers have specially trained forensic nurse providers who can help substantiate abuse by collection of evidence, following evidentiary procedures, and testifying in court. Such centers enable the child to tell the story only once via videotape and to have an exam facilitated by videocolposcopy, decreasing the number and intrusiveness of examinations.
- **If the most recent alleged sexual abuse occurred less than 72 hours before the clinic visit, refer immediately for assessment and treatment of injury and to ensure that forensic evidence is not lost.**
- If the most recent alleged incident occurred more than 72 hours before, nonemergent referral is appropriate.

PATIENT EDUCATION

- Explain the procedure for the exam in language that is understandable to child.
- Allow play. Explain that, for the young child, most of the exam can be done with him or her seated on the parent's lap.
- If the exam table is necessary, consider drawing the child's outline on paper to make a paper doll.
- Ask the parent what will make the exam easier for the child and incorporate suggestions. Give the child as much control as possible.
- Determine what the child calls particular body parts and use those terms during exam.
- Determine what child knows about "good touch/ bad touch" or "uh-oh" feelings. Reinforce that the body belongs to him or her and why it is okay for you to look at body parts and touch—that there is a grown-up he or she trusts there with the child; that as a nurse, it is important to know that all body parts are healthy; and that no one is asking that this be kept secret. Remind the child that looking at and touching private parts and being told to keep that secret is not all right.

- If child has disclosed sexual abuse or does so at this time, offer praise for telling and remind the child that what happened was not his or her fault—that it happens to many children. Tell the child what actions will be taken to ensure his or her safety.
- Provide anticipatory guidance for the parent about age-appropriate sexuality, realizing that self-touching behaviors are almost universal, albeit more overt at some times than others.

ASSESSMENT

1. The patient's history will determine how the nurse practitioner should proceed with this visit. Spontaneous statements made by the child to non-leading questions have significant legal potential and should be obtained and preserved with the same caution as other forms of forensic evidence. Consequently, if data collection yields suspicions of abuse, refer the child to a specialized center and provide anticipatory guidance to the parent and child. Discuss with the parent the plan to report the alleged abuse to child protective services.
2. Approach the child with simple language.
3. Allow time for play and getting acquainted before any exam takes place. Be sensitive to child's developmental level.
4. Ascertain information about general health and development.
5. Ask about acute and chronic medical problems, allergies, and current medications.
6. Question about presenting complaint, such as the location, duration, timing, effects on usual activity, what improves or exacerbates the problem, and any coexisting symptoms.
7. Determine whether the parent has questions or concerns.

DEVELOPMENTAL CONSIDERATIONS

Child: These questions can help differentiate between sexuality associated with normal development and that associated with sexual abuse (Reece, 1994):
- Does the particular behavior or knowledge level match the child's age and developmental level?
- Is the behavior consensual, or has coercion been involved?
- What motivation is involved ?
- What are the ages of the individuals involved?
- Is there a significant age difference, or are they peers?
- How has the child responded to the events?

Adolescent: The teenage girl with a history of vaginal penetration will need a speculum and bimanual exam, which includes collection of specimens for STDs (VDRL, chlamydia, GC, human immunodeficiency virus (HIV), hepatitis screen). A pregnancy test may also be necessary.

The adolescent male with a history of anal penetration will need anoscopy and evaluation for STDs (as mentioned earlier).

Teens need prophylaxis against STDs and possibly against pregnancy (if within 72 hours of assault).

 ALERT: Referral to a specialized center for sexual abuse assessment and treatment is appropriate for the adolescent as well as younger children to ensure comprehensive care and collection of forensic evidence that can facilitate intervention by child protection services.

If the primary care provider determines that sexual abuse does NOT appear to be involved, the following procedure is appropriate.

⊙ EQUIPMENT

• Usual equipment for a complete physical exam

PROCEDURE	SPECIAL CONSIDERATIONS
Perform complete physical exam, saving genital area to last.	When examiner inspects anogenital region outside context of usual physical exam, it gives an inappropriate focus on that segment of the exam.
Position child to facilitate inspection; sitting on the parent's lap may lend comfort. Older child: lithotomy position. Separation technique: With the child in frog-leg position, separate tissues adjacent to labia at 5 and 7 o'clock positions; exert gentle pressure downward until labia separate.	Varied positions enable effective visualization of different structures, taking advantage of relaxation. **Never use play to direct positioning for this portion of exam.**

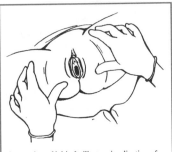

Separation of labia facilitates visualization of vestibule.

(procedure continued)

PROCEDURE	**SPECIAL CONSIDERATIONS**

Labial traction technique: With the child in supine frog-leg position, grasp labia gently between thumb and index finger of each hand, exerting gentle pressure in the posterior and lateral directions.

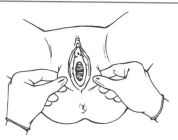

With girl in frog-leg position, gently grasp labia and pull outward and posterior to enhance visualization.

Knee-chest position: Place thumbs on buttocks at 10 and 12 o'clock positions and gently elevate buttocks in lateral and superior direction.

Remember that in this position, clock face descriptions assume a supine position.

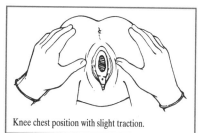

Knee chest position with slight traction.

In male, assess the following:
Tanner's stage.
Normalcy of anatomy: penile shaft, foreskin, glans, scrotum, and testes.
Determine presence of rashes, discharge, lesions.

In female, assess the following:
Tanner's stage.
Normalcy of anatomy: vulva, mons, labia, ure-

Normal variants of hymenal tissue include tags, bumps, mounds, redundancy, perihymenal and periurethral bands, midline avascular lines, erythema, and extreme sensitivity of hymenal tissue to touch.

Do not chart "hymen intact," "virginal hymen," or "nonmarital hymen" because these are meaningless terms. Document descriptions of structures visualized.

(procedure continued)

PROCEDURE	SPECIAL CONSIDERATIONS

thra, posterior fourchette, vaginal/hymenal orifice.
Check for lesions, rashes, discharge, foreign body such as toilet paper.

 ## ALTERNATIVE PROCEDURE

• Magnification can be helpful during this exam. Although an otoscope has been suggested as an appropriate light source with magnification, one should consider the comfort level of the child with the examiner that close to the genitalia for visualization.

 ## FOLLOW-UP

• The child or adolescent who was seen at a specialized center where sexual abuse was diagnosed is often followed in the local community. A 2-week follow-up may include repeat STD or pregnancy testing, or both. At 12 weeks, depending on the patient's history, tests for syphilis, HIV, and hepatitis should be completed.
• At 6 and 12 months, depending on history, follow-up testing for HIV is appropriate.

Indications for STD Follow-up
• Discharge from vagina or rectum
• Evidence of other STDs, including genital warts
• Parental request
• High-risk behavior of perpetrator or known STD in perpetrator
• More than one or a single unknown perpetrator
• Each follow-up visit will include assessment of the child's emotional condition, response to victimization, and any sequelae of the experience. Psychological care is essential.

BIBLIOGRAPHY

Adams, J., Harper, K., Knudson, S. & Revillaa, J.(1994). Examination findings in legally confirmed child sexual abuse: It's normal to be normal. *Pediatrics, 94,* 310–317.
American Medical Association. (1998). *Physicians' current procedural terminology: CPT.* Chicago: American Medical Association.
Berenson, A. B., Heger, A., Hayes, J. M., Bailey, R. K. & Emans, S. J. (1992). Appearance of the hymen in prepubertal girls. *Pediatrics, 89*(3), 387–394.
Girardin, B. W., Faugno, D. K., Seneski, P. C., Slaughter, L. & Whelan, M. (1997). *Color atlas of sexual assault.* St. Louis: C.V. Mosby.

Hatmaker, D.(1997). A SANE approach to sexual assault. *American Journal of Nursing, 97*(8), 80.

Healthcare Consultants of America. (1998). *1998 Physicians' fee and coding guide.* Augusta, GA.

Murram, D. (1989). Child sexual abuse: Relationship between sexual acts and genital findings. *Child Abuse and Neglect, 13,* 211–216.

Reece, R. M. (1994). *Child abuse: Medical diagnosis and management.* Philadelphia: Lea & Febiger.

Sexual Assault Training Program Focus on Pediatrics. Atlanta: Scottish Rite Children's Medical Center, February 17–21, 1997.

chapter 55

X-Ray Interpretation

CPT Coding:

Various codes and costs depending on body part radiographed ($79–$169)

 DEFINITION

- X-rays are radiant energy that can pass through opaque objects with the residual energy landing on x-ray film (exposure). The films can be taken with the patient in a variety of positions:

Position	Definition	Comments/Example
Posterior	X-ray beam penetrates the body from the back (posterior) to the front (anterior).	Normal chest x-ray study.
Anterior	X-ray beam penetrates the body from the anterior to the posterior.	Portable chest x-ray study.
Lateral	The patient is seated or standing with one side of the body against the x-ray film.	Chest x-ray study with left side of chest placed next to film. Used to identify abnormalities behind another organ.
Cross table lateral	Patient is in a supine position, and the x-ray beam is perpendicular to the film.	Cross table lateral spine film used to look for spine fractures.
Lateral decubitus	Patient is in a recumbent position lying on the side. The film is supported upright next to the patient, and the beam is directed perpendicular to the film.	Helps assess fluid and air levels in the pleural or peritoneal cavities.
Oblique	Permits visualization of the body at an angle. Right oblique places the right anterior side of the chest against the film, whereas a left oblique places the left side of the chest against the film.	Used to rule out some bone fractures.
Lordotic	The patient or x-ray machine is positioned at a 45-degree angle.	Helps provide a better view of the right and left middle lung fields.

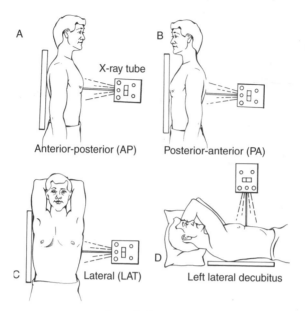

Positions for obtaining x-rays.

- Appearance of densities seen on an x-ray study (see example of densities). Denser tissues absorb more of the x-ray beam than less dense tissues. When a tissue absorbs more radiation, it appears more opaque or white.

Density (most dense to least dense)	Appearance	Examples
Metal	Bright white	Necklace, fillings in teeth
Bone	Slightly less bright white than metal	Bones: calcium
Fluid or Tissue	Medium brightness	Blood vessels, heart
Fat	Less black than air	Breast tissue, fat around rib cage
Air	Appears black, radiolucent	Lungs; increased air as seen in emphysema makes the lungs appear more radiolucent

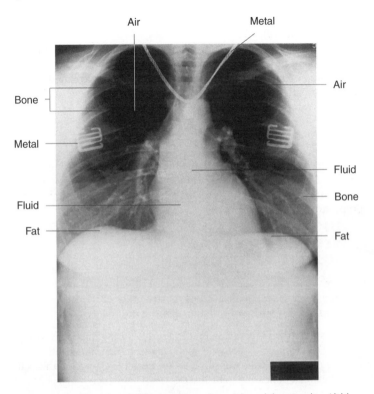

Densities on a radiograph include metal (the brightest white or radiopaque), bone, which contains calcium (slightly less white or radiopaque than metal), blood vessels like the heart, which is fluid or water density (less radiopaque than metal), fat (even less radiopaque than metal or fluid), and air (radiolucent or black). Used with permission from DeHenmeir, Patricia A. (1995). *Radiographic assessment for nurses.* St. Louis: Mosby.

INDICATION

- X-ray studies should be performed whenever the body part in question needs to be evaluated.

PATIENT EDUCATION

- The radiation absorbed from most x-ray studies is minimal and is closely monitored.
- Annual radiation of a healthy individual is about 200 mrad/year.
- Patients most at risk from radiation should be shielded:
  - Gonads of children, men and women of reproductive age are protected by lead aprons.
  - Pregnant women should avoid radiation if possible in the first trimester.
- Safety is dependent on time of exposure, distance of exposure, and shielding.

- Remove ornaments or jewelry before the x-ray study (including dental work as appropriate).
- If the test is a mammogram, the woman should not wear deodorant because it can interfere with the films
- Let the patient know that there will be some instructions related to holding his or her breath. The quality of the x-ray study is dependent on the patient's ability to follow directions.

ASSESSMENT

1. Obtain a complete history related to the problem, including mechanism of injury for potential fractures or soft tissue injuries.
2. Determine past medical history, family history, and social history as appropriate to the problem

DEVELOPMENTAL CONSIDERATIONS

Child: Bones are not completely ossified, so the epiphysis is evident on x-ray studies. Obtain comparison films of extremities of children so that the injured part can be compared with the opposite normal part.

Elderly: Osteoporosis is common in the elderly, causing the bones to appear less dense (less white). Loss of joint spaces may be seen, along with kyphosis or stress fractures. Arthritis will show as degenerative changes with calcific bridging between bones and joint spaces.

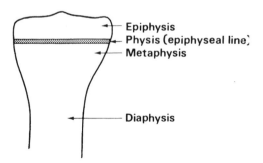

Normal anatomic divisions of the end of a typical growing bone. (Juhl, John H., Crummey, Andrew B., and Kuhlman, Janet E. [1998]. Paul and Juhl's Essentials of Radiographic Imaging. Philadelphia: Lippincott Williams & Wilkins).

EQUIPMENT

- X-ray view box (back lit by fluorescent bulbs)
- Bright light to examine specific areas of the x-ray study (hot light)

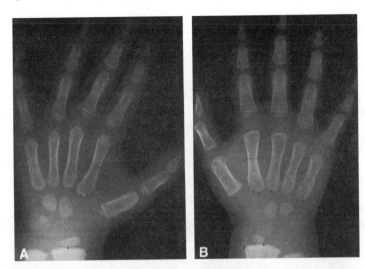

A: Hand of a normal 2-year-old girl. B: Hand of a normal 2-year-old boy. The differences in the appearance of the bones are subtle at this age. Note that the epiphyseal ossification centers of the proximal phalanges and distal radius of the girl in A are larger than those of the corresponding epiphysis of the boy in B. Epiphyseal ossification centers are present in the distal phalanx of the third and fourth fingers of the girl but are not present in the boy. (Juhl, John H., Crummey, Andrew B., and Kuhlman, Janet E. [1998]. *Paul and Juhl's Essentials of Radiographic Imaging*. Philadelphia: Lippincott William's & Wilkins).

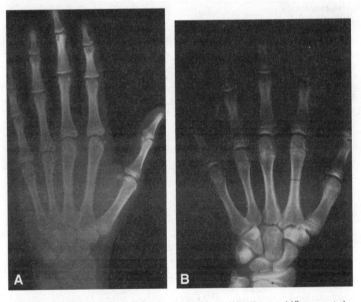

A: Hand of a normal 13 ½-year-old girl. B: Hand of a normal 13 ½-year-old boy. The principal differences are in the width of the epiphyseal plates, the relative size of the carpal ossification centers and the configuration of the epiphyses. Note in A that there is almost complete fusion of the proximal epiphysis of the second and third metacarpals. Compare with the corresponding epiphysis of the boy in B. (Juhl, John H., Crummey, Andrew B., and Kuhlman, Janet E. [1998]. *Paul and Juhl's Essentials of Radiographic Imaging*. Philadelphia: Lippincott Williams & Wilkins).

PROCEDURE	SPECIAL CONSIDERATIONS
It is vital to obtain correctly done views that show the area of interest adequately. In most cases, this means an anteroposterior (AP), a lateral, and in some cases, another view to visualize the area best.	See chart below for specifics related to major body areas. If you are unsure of what to order, order the body part (ie, wrist) and then identify what you are looking for (to rule out fracture). The radiology technician will then take the appropriate views.
Development of a systematic method to analyze x-ray studies: Initial evaluation Make sure patient's name/date and time are correct. Is the x-ray study in the correct position in the viewbox? Right and left marker correct?	Develop pattern to follow routinely. Have an understanding of normal anatomy. Compare views with previously taken films if possible.
Identify the quality of the film: Correct position Proper exposure: Over-exposure/under-exposure Any objects obscuring area?	Repeat inadequate films.
Systematic approach: Look at the entire film. Look at area of interest last. Assess in the following manner: External to internal Side to side Top to bottom Example: Look at the entire area. Assess soft tissue, then look at bony structures. Go completely around the outside edge of the bone for bone continuity. Finally, look at the internal structures.	
Compare clinical findings with radiologic findings.	Examine the patient first before ordering x-ray studies to make sure all needed x-ray studies are obtained.
Obtain postreduction films after a dislocation or fracture is reduced.	Done to make sure bone is in good alignment.

INFORMATION ABOUT SPECIFIC X-RAY STUDIES

Lungs

- Read as though the reader was looking at the patient: patient's right side is to your left.
- Look at soft tissues, bones, and diaphragm first; then lungs from apex to base; and finally, the outline of the heart and aorta.

- Approximately eight to nine ribs should show on film. If there are fewer than eight ribs, it is suggestive of a poor inspiration or poor volume. Look at clavicles for symmetry, usually located at second or third intercostal space. If the clavicular heads are not positioned over the posterior spine, the film is rotated.
- Check the contour of the diaphragm; it should be rounded, with sharp-pointed costophrenic angles. The dome of the diaphragm is located at the level of the sixth rib. The right side should be slightly higher than the left side. If blunting of the costophrenic angles is noted, consider pleural effusion.
- Evaluate the cardiac structures, looking at the cardiac size, configuration, and location. Look at the position and size of the great vessels.
- Lung fields: One can see the fissures between the lobes; the trachea should be midline over vertebrae; check hilar area.

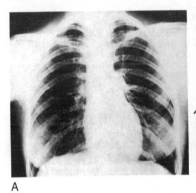 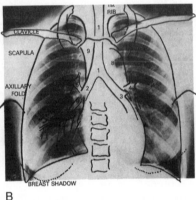

A

B

(A) Normal PA chest radiograph. (B) Outline of structures visible on normal PA chest radiograph. The diagrammatic overlay shows the normal anatomic structures: (1) trachea, (2) right main bronchus, (3) left main bronchus, (4) left pulmonary artery, (5) right upper lobe pulmonary artery, (6) right interlobar artery, (7) right lower and middle lobe vein, (8) aortic knob, (9) superior vena cava. [Adapted from Fraser RG, Pare JAP et al: Diagnosis of Disease of the Chest, pp 288–290. Philadelphia, WB Saunders, 1988]

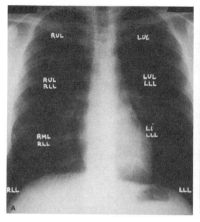 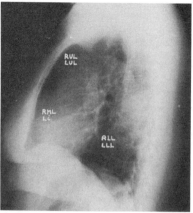

(A) Location of the lung lobes on the frontal chest radiograph. Because some lobes are anterior and some posterior, an abnormality in a certain area on a frontal chest radiograph can be in one of two lobes. Obtaining a lateral film or noticing whether an anterior or posterior structure is obliterated by an abnormal density can help with localization. (*RUL,* right upper lobe; *RLL,* right lower lobe; *LLL,* left lower lobe; *RML,* right middle lobe; *LUL,* left upper lobe; *Li,* lingula) (B) Location of lung lobes in a lateral radiograph. Abnormalities of the right middle lobe and lingula would go undetected with posterior chest auscultation. (Woods, S.L., Sivarajan Froelicher, E.S., Halpenny, C.J., Motzer, S.U. [1995]. *Cardiac Nursing.* Philadelphia: J.B. Lippincott.)

Abdomen

- The most common evaluation of the abdomen is the kidney, ureter, and bladder (KUB), which is taken when the patient is in the anterior to posterior supine position.
- A properly exposed film of the abdomen will show in detail the anatomy of the lumbar vertebrae. Compare the overall density of the central third of the abdomen with the lateral thirds and bones.
- Look for the splenic tip, the liver edge, and renal outlines.
- Identify all bones.
- Identify all the air contained within the bowel. Look for air outside the bowel. Identify the stool and gas pattern.
- Look for any calcifications. Look at the bases of the lungs, if they are included.

Bone

- Cervical spine: Anteroposterior (AP) and lateral views. The lateral film is the most critical view in the case of trauma. Always count the vertebrae.
- Lumbar spine: AP and lateral views. These x-ray studies are rarely ordered because they provide the same amount of gonadal radiation as one chest x-ray study every day for 3 years. In addition, they rarely contribute anything of value to the acute management of back pain or strain.
- Pelvis: AP view. This film must be examined carefully because a fracture may be nondisplaced and very subtle.
- Hip: Standard views (AP and true lateral) are sufficient to find hip fractures. A frog-leg lateral view is useful for evaluation of developmental dys-

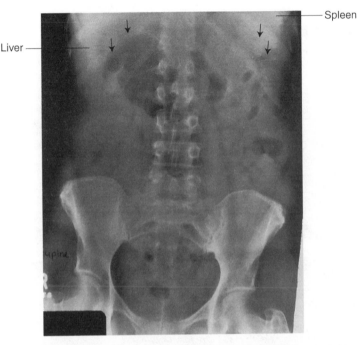

Abdomen AP supine radiograph. Normal-sized liver and spleen. The intestinal gas (*straight arrows*) demarcates the inferior liver and spleen margins. (Erkonen, W.W. [1998]. *Radiology 101*. Philadelphia: Lippincott-Raven Publishers.)

plasia of the hip. Look at the shape of the femoral head, the articulation with the pelvis, the surgical neck, and the femur.

- Long bones: Femur, humerus, tibia and fibula: AP and lateral views are needed. The entire bone (including the joints above and below) must be seen. The ends (include epiphyses, if applicable) should be evaluated. Look at the shaft of the bone for cortex, angulation, and lesions.
- Knee: Standard views include AP and lateral. A sunrise view of the knee is performed when trauma to the patella is involved. A tibial plateau fracture may be seen with an oblique view of the knee. Look at the alignment, tibial plateau, joint space, patella, and proximal fibula.
- Tibia and fibula: AP and lateral views are standard. The entire length of the bones must be visualized.
- Ankle: AP and lateral views, mortise view (this view shows the horizontal space between the tibial joint surface and the talar joint surface). This joint should be consistent 3 to 4 mm over the talar surface. Widening of 2 mm or more is abnormal.
- Hand and foot: Three views are needed: AP, oblique, and lateral views. Identify each individual bone. Look at the alignment, angulation and rotation, and the articulation with adjacent structures (carpals or tarsals).

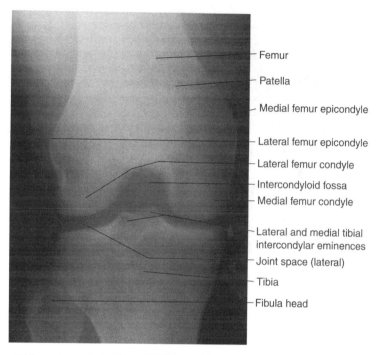

Femur
Patella
Medial femur epicondyle

Lateral femur epicondyle
Lateral femur condyle
Intercondyloid fossa
Medial femur condyle

Lateral and medial tibial intercondylar eminences
Joint space (lateral)
Tibia
Fibula head

Right knee, antero-posterior view. (Erkonen, W.W. [1998]. *Radiology 101*. Philadelphia: Lippincott-Raven Publishers.)

Knee of child aged 12 years: Antero-posterior and lateral views. The outstanding feature in these radiographs is the presence of radiolucent cartilaginous growth plates between the metaphyses and epiphyses of the long bones. (1) Flared femoral metaphysis; (2) Distal femoral epiphysis which has been present since birth; (3) Radiolucent cartilaginous growth plates; (4) Patella, which ossifies from several centers in about the third year; (5) Proximal tinial epiphysis which appears immediately after birth; (6) Tibial shaft; (7) Tibial tuberosity which ossifies in early adolescence. The epiphyses unit with the main mass of bone in the late teens or early twenties and the site of fusion is often marked by a white line on the adult radiograph. (Keogh, Bruce and Ebbs, Stephen. *Normal Surface Anatomy with Practical Applications*. Philadelphia; JB Lippincott).

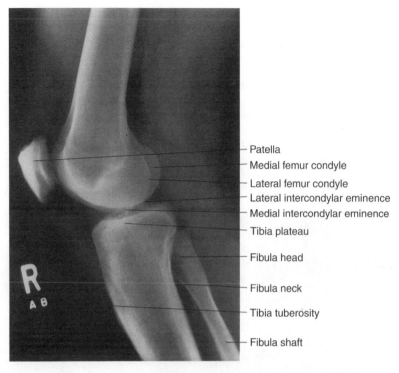

Patella
Medial femur condyle
Lateral femur condyle
Lateral intercondylar eminence
Medial intercondylar eminence
Tibia plateau
Fibula head
Fibula neck
Tibia tuberosity
Fibula shaft

Right knee, lateral view. (Erkonen, W.W. [1998]. *Radiology 101*. Philadelphia: Lippincott-Raven Publishers.)

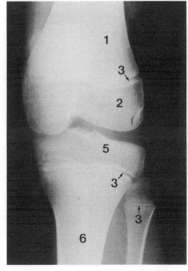

Anteroposterior view

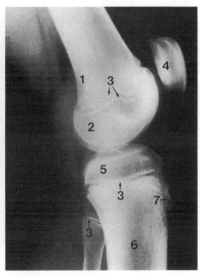

Lateral view

- Elbow: standard views (AP, lateral, and two obliques). Look at alignment, look for fat pad signs, and look at the radial head. The presence of a fat pad sign indicates joint effusion and most likely indicates a fracture, especially in children. The fat pads are more clearly seen by tilting the film to view it obliquely. Nursemaid's elbow films are usually normal.
- Wrist: Standard views (PA, lateral, and two obliques). Look at each individual bone. Examine the cortex of each bone. Evaluate the relationship and alignment of bones. Determine the articulation with adjacent structures (metacarpals, radius and ulna). Navicular views elongate the profile of the scaphoid bone and may assist in identifying a scaphoid fracture. This fracture may not be seen until healing is seen by callus formation (7 to 10 days). These fractures should be presumptively diagnosed and treated based on clinical findings.

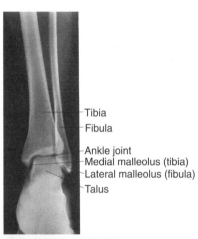

Tibia
Fibula

Ankle joint
Medial malleolus (tibia)
Lateral malleolus (fibula)
Talus

A

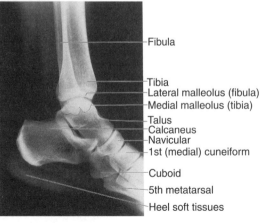

Fibula

Tibia
Lateral malleolus (fibula)
Medial malleolus (tibia)

Talus
Calcaneus
Navicular
1st (medial) cuneiform

Cuboid

5th metatarsal

Heel soft tissues

B

Left ankle. Antero-posterior and lateral views are usually taken. The antero-posterior view is taken with the foot pointing slightly medially in order to rotate the shadow of the lateral malleolous away from the talofibular joint to demonstrate the ankle mortise clearly. (Erkononen, W. W. [1998]. *Radiology 101*. Philadelphia: Lippincott-Raven Publishers.)

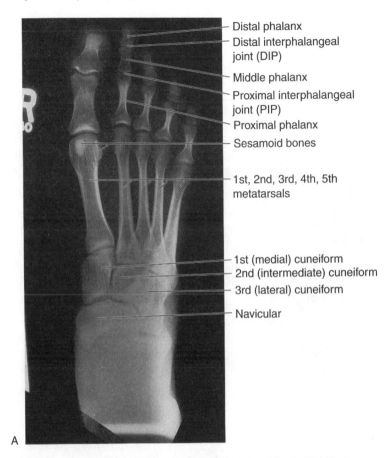

- Distal phalanx
- Distal interphalangeal joint (DIP)
- Middle phalanx
- Proximal interphalangeal joint (PIP)
- Proximal phalanx
- Sesamoid bones
- 1st, 2nd, 3rd, 4th, 5th metatarsals
- 1st (medial) cuneiform
- 2nd (intermediate) cuneiform
- 3rd (lateral) cuneiform
- Navicular

A

Right foot antero-posterior and oblique view (next page). (Erkonen, W. W. [1998]. *Radiology 101*. Philadelphia: Lippincott-Raven Publishers.) (figure continued)

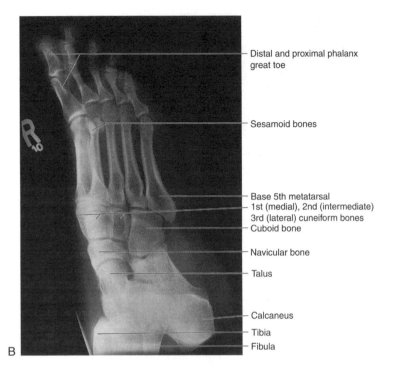

Distal and proximal phalanx
great toe

Sesamoid bones

Base 5th metatarsal
1st (medial), 2nd (intermediate)
3rd (lateral) cuneiform bones
Cuboid bone

Navicular bone

Talus

Calcaneus

Tibia
Fibula

B

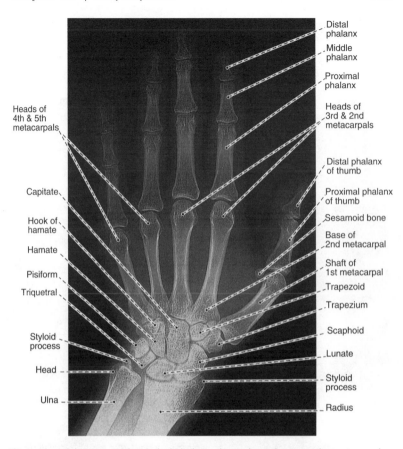

Heads of
4th & 5th
metacarpals

Capitate

Hook of
hamate

Hamate

Pisiform

Triquetral

Styloid
process

Head

Ulna

Distal
phalanx

Middle
phalanx

Proximal
phalanx

Heads of
3rd & 2nd
metacarpals

Distal phalanx
of thumb

Proximal phalanx
of thumb

Sesamoid bone

Base of
2nd metacarpal

Shaft of
1st metacarpal

Trapezoid

Trapezium

Scaphoid

Lunate

Styloid
process

Radius

This view taken with the patient resting his or her hand palm down on the x-ray plage. In those younger than twenty years, who may demonstrate incomplete ossification, and in patients with suspected bone disease, pictures of both hands should always be taken for comparison, preferably on the same film. (Radiograph courtesy of Dr. Thurman Gillespy). (Rosse, C., Gaddum-Rosse, P. [1997]. *Hollinshead's Textbook of Anatomy.* Philadelphia: Lippincott-Raven Publishers).

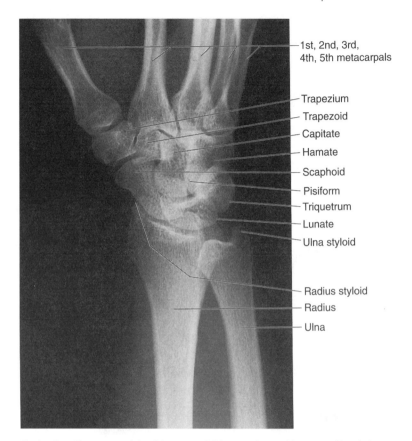

1st, 2nd, 3rd,
4th, 5th metacarpals

Trapezium
Trapezoid
Capitate
Hamate
Scaphoid
Pisiform
Triquetrum
Lunate
Ulna styloid

Radius styloid
Radius
Ulna

Wrist, lateral view. This view is particularly useful in patients with dislocations or fractures of the wrist. It is of limited value in evaluating the phalanges and metacarpals. (Erkonen, W. W. [1998]. *Radiology 101*. Philadelphia: Lippincott Williams & Wilkins.)

⊙ FOLLOW-UP

• Determine what your organization's policy is for re-reading of x-ray studies. It may be prudent to have all x-ray studies reviewed by either your collaborating physician or radiologist.

BIBLIOGRAPHY

American Medical Association. (1998). *Physicians' current procedural terminology: CPT*. Chicago: American Medical Association.

Amorosa, J., Novelline, R., & Squire, L. (1993). *Chest, abdomen, bone and clinical skills* (3rd ed.). Philadelphia: W. B. Saunders.

Bergus, G., Franken, E., Koch, J., Smith, W., Evans, E., & Berbaum, K. (1995). Radiologic interpretation by family physicians in an office practice setting. *The Journal of Family Practice, 41*(4), 352–356.

Dettenmeier, P. (1995). *Radiographic assessment for nurses*. St. Louis: Mosby.

Eisengerg, R. (1992). *Clinical imaging: An atlas of differential diagnosis,* Gaithersburg: Aspen.

Freij, R., Duffy, T., Hackett, D., Cunningham, D., & Fothergill, J. (1996). Radiographic interpretation by nurse practitioners in a minor injuries unit. *Journal of Accident and Emergency Medicine, 13*(1), 41–43.

Hart, R., Rittenberry, T., & Uehara, D. (1999). *Handbook of orthopedic emergencies.* Philadelphia: Lippincott-Raven.

Healthcare Consultants of America. (1998). *1998 Physicians' fee and coding guide.* Augusta, GA.

Huseby, J. (1995). Radiologic examination of the chest. In S. Woods, E. Froelicher, C. Halpenny, & S. Motzer (eds.). *Cardiac nursing* (3rd ed.). Philadelphia: Lippincott.

Meek, S., Kendall, J., Porter, J., & Freiz, R. (1998). Can accident and emergency nurse practitioners interpret radiographs? A multicentre study. *Journal of Accident and Emergency Medicine, 15*(2), 105–107.

Overton-Brown, P., Anthony, D. (1998). Towards a partnership in care: nurses' and doctors' interpretation of extremity trauma radiology. *Journal of Advanced Nursing, 27*(5), 890–896.

Tachakra, S., Freij, R., Mullett, S., & Sivakumar, A. (1996). Teleradiology or teleconsultation for emergency nurse practitioners. *Journal of Telemedicine Telecare, 2*(Suppl 1), 56–58.

chapter 56

Basic Electrocardiogram Interpretation

CPT Coding:

> 93000 Electrocardiogram (EKG), routine with at least 12 leads, with interpretation and report ($57–$68)
> 93005 EKG, tracing only without interpretation and report ($37–$44)

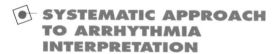 SYSTEMATIC APPROACH TO ARRHYTHMIA INTERPRETATION

- To avoid overlooking an important aspect of arrhythmia interpretation, the following format may be useful when interpreting a rhythm.

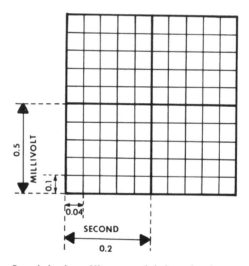

Time and voltage lines on ECG paper, at standard voltage and speed: vertically, 1 mm = 0.1 mV; 5 mm = 0.5 mV; 10 mm = 1 mV; horizontally, 1 mm = 0.04 second; 5 mm = 0.2 second; 25 mm = 1 second; 1500 mm = 60 seconds. (Woods, Froelucher, Halpenny and Underhill Motzer [1995]. *Cardiac Nursing.* Philadelphia: Lippincott-Raven Publishers.)

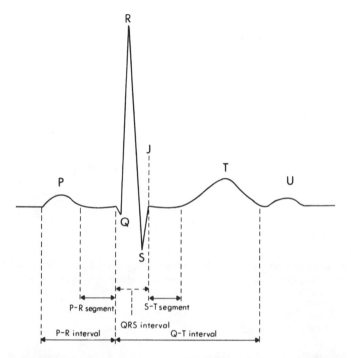

Principal time intervals of PQRSTU. (Wagner, G. S. & Marriott, H. J. [1994]. *Marriott's practical electrocardiography.* Baltimore: Williams & Wilkins.)

EKG CHARACTERISTICS:

P wave
Configuration:
- Do all the P waves look alike?
- Are they upright in lead II?
- Is one P wave seen for each QRS complex?
- Does the P wave precede the QRS complex?

Rate: What is the atrial rate?

Rhythm: Is the P-P interval regular?

P-R Interval
- What is the P-R interval?
- Does it remain the same throughout the strip?

QRS Complex
Configuration:
- Do all the QRS complexes look alike?
- Does a QRS complex follow each P wave?

Rate: What is the ventricular rate?

Rhythm: Is the R-R interval regular?

Duration: What is the QRS interval?

Interpretation:
• Is an arrhythmia present?
• Which kind?

Treatment
• What treatment should be anticipated?
• Which medications are usually needed for this arrhythmia?
• Is cardioversion or defibrillation warranted?
• Should cardiopulmonary resuscitation (CPR) be initiated?

Implications for Practice:
• What actions are required?
• Should the client's activity level be restricted?
• Is the client positioned properly (for instance, a supine position to combat hypotension or a high-Fowler's position to counter dyspnea)?

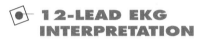 12-LEAD EKG INTERPRETATION

Overview
• The heart is a three-dimensional organ, and its electrical activity must be understood in three dimensions as well. The standard EKG consists of 12 leads, with each lead determined by the placement and orientation of various electrodes on the body. Each lead views the heart at a unique angle, enhancing its sensitivity to a particular region of the heart. The more views, the more information.
• The 12-lead electrocardiogram (EKG) records electrical information from different surfaces of the heart.
– Each lead "sees" the electrical activity in a different way (see table on next page).

Normal Electrocardiogram Waveform Configurations in Each of the 12 Leads

LEAD	P WAVE	Q WAVE	R WAVE	S WAVE	T WAVE	ST SEGMENT
I	Upright	Small	Largest wave of complex	Small (less than R or none)	Upright	May vary from +1 to −0.5 mm
II	Upright	Small or none	Large (vertical heart)	Small (less than R or none)	Upright	May vary from +1 to −0.5 mm
III	Upright, diphasic, or inverted	Usually small or none (for large Q to be diagnostic, a Q must also be present in a VF)	None to large	None to large (horizontal heart)	Upright, diphasic, or inverted	May vary from +1 to −0.5 mm
aVR	Inverted	Small, none, or large	Small or none	Large (may be QS complex)	Inverted	May vary from +1 to −0.5 mm
aVL	Upright, diphasic, or inverted	Small, none, or large (to be diagnostic, Q must also be present in I or precordial leads)	Small, none, or large (horizontal heart)	None to large (vertical heart)	Upright, diphasic, or inverted	May vary from +1 to −0.5 mm
aVF	Upright	Small or none	Small, none, or large (vertical heart)	None to large (horizontal heart)	Upright, diphasic, or inverted	May vary from +1 to −0.5 mm

table continued

(table continued)

Normal Electrocardiogram Waveform Configurations in Each of the 12 Leads

LEAD	P WAVE	Q WAVE	R WAVE	S WAVE	T WAVE	ST SEGMENT
V_1	Upright, diphasic, or inverted	None or QS complex	Less than S wave or none	Large (may be QS)	Upright, diphasic, or inverted	May vary from 0 to +3 mm
V_2	Upright	None (rare QS)	Less than S wave or none (larger than V_1)	Large (may be QS)	Upright	May vary from 0 to +3 mm
V_3	Upright	Small or none	Less, greater, or equal to S wave (larger than V_2)	Large (greater, less, or equal to R wave)	Upright	May vary from 0 to +3 mm
V_4	Upright	Small or none	Greater than S (larger than V_3)	Smaller than R; (smaller than V_3)	Upright	May vary from +1 to −0.5 mm
V_5	Upright	Small	Larger than R in V_4; less than 26 mm	Smaller than S in V_4	Upright	May vary from +1 to −0.5 mm
V_6	Upright	Small	Large; less than 26 mm	Smaller than S in V_5	Upright	May vary from +1 to −0.5 mm

U waves may follow T waves, particularly in leads V_2 to V_4; are upright; and are of lower amplitude than T waves.

Adapted from Goldschlager, N., Goldman, M. J. (1989). Principles of clinical electrocardiography (13th ed.). Norwalk, CT: Appleton & Lange.

– The 12-lead EKG provides 12 different views of the electrical activity of the heart.
– The interpreter must know what is "normal" or expected in any given lead before any abnormal activity can be analyzed.
– The location of each lead's positive pole must be known.

Leads of 12-Lead EKG

Standard or Bipolar Leads—I, II, III:

• Three electrodes equal distance from the heart to form an equilateral triangle (Einthoven's triangle)
• Electrodes placed at right arm (RA), left arm (LA), and left leg (LL)
• Lead I is created by making the left arm positive and the right arm negative
• Lead II is created by making the legs positive and the right arm negative
• Lead III is created by making the legs positive and the left arm negative

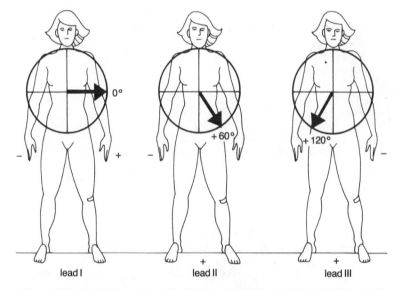

Lead I is created by making the left arm positive and the right arm negative. Its angle of orientation is 0°. Lead II is created by making the leg positive and the right arm negative. Its angle of orientation is 60°. Lead III is created by making the legs positive and the left arm negative. Its angle of orientation is 120°. (Thaler, M. S. [1995]. *The Only EKG Book You'll Ever Need.* Philadelphia: J.B. Lippincott.)

Unipolar or Augmented Limb Leads—aVR, aVL, aVF:

• All unipolar leads referred to as "V" leads
• Augmented leads have no negative electrode
• The heart is the electrical center and is at zero potential
• Called augmented because removal of the negative electrode augments or enhances the tracing size by 50%

- Lead aVL is created by making the left arm positive and all the others negative.
- Lead aVR is created by making the right arm positive and all others negative.
- Lead aVF is created by making the legs positive and all the others negative

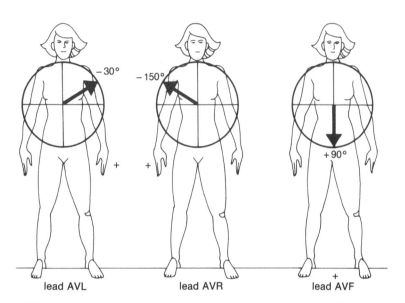

Lead AVL is created by making the left arm positive and the other limbs negative. Its angle of orientation is −30°. Lead AVR is created by making the right arm positive and the other limbs negative. Its angle of orientation is −150°. Lead AVF is created by making the legs positive and the other limbs negative. Its angle of orientation is +90°. (Thaler, M. S. [1995]. *The Only EKG Book You'll Ever Need*. Philadelphia: J.B. Lippincott.)

Precordial Leads or Unipolar Chest Leads—V_1–V_6:

- Allows you to observe the anterior and posterior electrical forces of the heart
- Forces traveling toward one of these electrodes result in a positive deflection, whereas forces traveling away from one of these electrodes result in a negative deflection
- V_1–V_2 lie directly over the right ventricle (V_1: 4th intercostal space [ICS], right sternal border [RSB]; V_2: 4th ICS, left sternal border [LSB])
- V_3–V_4 lie over the interventricular septum (V_3: halfway between V_2 and V_4 sites; V_4: 5th ICS, MCL)
- V_5–V_6 lie over the left ventricle (V_5: Same level as V_4 anterior axillary line [AAL]; V_6: Same level as V_4 midaxillary line [MAL])
- Leads V_1–V_6 are often referred to as the anterior leads, and V_5–V_6 join I and aVL as left lateral leads

Leads	Group
V_1, V_2, V_3, V_4	Anterior
I, aVL, V_5, V_6	Left lateral
II, III, aVF	Inferior
aVR	—

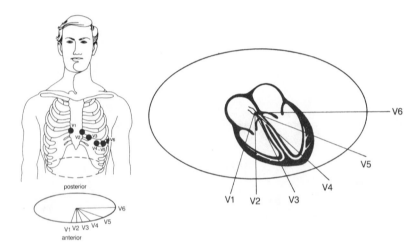

The precordial leads define a horizontal or transverse plane, and view electrical forces moving anteriorly and posteriorly. (Thaler, M. S. [1995]. *The Only EKG Book You'll Ever Need*. Philadelphia: J.B. Lippincott.)

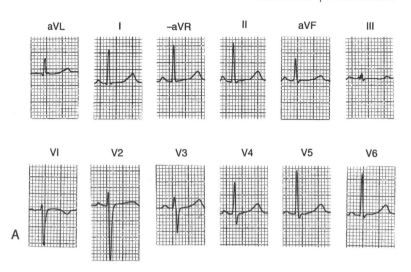

The panoramic display of the 12 standard leads is presented in their orderly sequences in both the frontal (aVL-III) and transverse (V1-V6) planes. Lead aVR is included in its position as -aVR. All 12 leads appear in a single horizontal display. (Wagner, G. S., & Marriott, H. J. [1994]. *Marriott's Practical Electrocardiography*. Baltimore: Williams & Wilkins.)

⬦ DIAGNOSING AN ACUTE MYOCARDIAL INFARCTION (AMI) USING 12-LEAD EKG INTERPRETATION

Location	Leads Affected	Change	Vessel
Anterior MI	V_1–V_4	ST elevation	LAD
Inferior MI	II, III, aVF	ST elevation	RCA
Lateral MI	I, aVL, V_5–V_6	ST elevation	LCX
Posterior MI	V_1–V_2	ST depression	RCA or LCX
		Tall R wave	
		Tall upright T wave	

LAD, left anterior descending; RCA, right coronary artery; LCX, left circumflex

EKG Abnormality	Onset	Disappearance
ST-segment elevation	Immediately	1 to 6 weeks
Q wave more than 0.04 second	Immediately or in several days	Years to never
T wave inversion	6 to 24 hours	Months to years

NURSING IMPLICATIONS

- EKG confirms a clinical impression. Clinical impression includes signs and symptoms (ie, radiating chest pain, nausea, shortness of breath, and so on).
- The ST segment is normally isoelectric but may deviate −0.5 to 1 mm from baseline in standard and unipolar leads.
- Depression of ST or T-wave inversion, or both, indicates ischemia.
- ST elevation indicates injury.
- New wide Q wave indicates an infarct (greater than 0.04-second duration and greater than 4 mm depth), which means necrosis.
- Q waves are normally wide and deep in aVR. Ignore Q waves in this lead because it is a negative lead.
- Localization of an EKG is based on the principle that EKG signs of infarction occur in the leads whose positive terminals face the damaged surface of the heart.
- EKG changes occur in the leads facing the infarct, but at the same time, reciprocal changes (opposite) changes occur in those leads opposite the leads facing the infarct.
- Evolution of an AMI can be mapped through serial EKGs.
- Persistent ST elevation after 6 weeks may indicate a ventricular aneurysm.
- The most commonly seen type of AMI is the anterior MI.
- Most frequently missed AMI is the posterior MI.
- Conduction defects are most commonly seen in an inferior MI.

SUPRAVENTRICULAR TACHYCARDIA

- Supraventricular tachycardia (SVT) is a term used to describe a tachycardia that is being generated somewhere above the ventricles. It should only be used when it is impossible to determine where the tachycardia is coming from. SVT could be sinus or atrial tachycardia with the P wave hidden in the preceding T wave. It could be junctional tachycardia with no visible P wave. Or it could be atrial flutter with 1:1 or 2:1 conduction that obscures the flutter waves.

Causes
- Stimulation of the sympathetic nervous system
- An elevated metabolic rate

• A decrease in the oxygen-carrying capacity of the blood, as seen in clients with anemia, hypoxia, and respiratory disease

Differential Diagnosis Between PSVT and Sinus Tachycardia

• PSVT begins abruptly with a single PAC or PJC, whereas sinus tachycardia moves gradually into a tachycardia in response to physiologic needs.

• PSVT usually has a rate in excess of 160 beats/min, whereas sinus tachycardia usually does not exceed 150 beats/min.

• PSVT may be abruptly terminated by a vagal maneuver, whereas sinus tachycardia is slowed down only momentarily.

• The P wave morphology in PSVT differs from that of the normal sinus P wave.

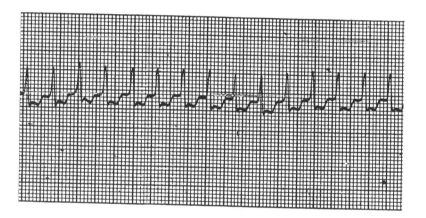

EKG Characteristics

• P wave

Configuration: The atrial activity is probably present, but is not visible.

Rhythm: The rhythm in SVT is monotonously regular.

P-R interval: The P-R interval is not measurable

QRS complex: The QRS complex may be narrow and normal, or wide and bizarre, but each QRS is identical to all of the others.

Rate: The ventricular rate is faster than 150 beats/min.

Rhythm: The rhythm is monotonously regular.

Effects on the Client

• SVT produces all of the hemodynamic alterations that occur with any fast rate dysrhythmia. SVT is a dysrhythmia that occurs frequently in persons with a normal heart, and is caused by stress or anxiety. Usually, it does not cause any real problems in these individuals, although the person may become short of breath and may feel weak or dizzy, depending on how fast the rate is.

Treatment

- The therapy for atrial tachycardia is aimed at controlling the ventricular rate and converting the patient back to normal sinus rhythm (NSR). The course of the therapy depends on the patient's hemodynamic response to the tachycardia. If the patient's blood pressure is dropping or he is showing signs of acute left ventricular failure, immediate intervention is needed, most likely in the form of synchronized cardioversion.
- If the client's clinical picture is not one of deteriorating hemodynamic status, medical therapy will be used first. Traditional drug therapy includes
  - Digitalis
  - Quinidine
  - Procainamide
  - Propranolol
  - Verapamil
- Many times, some form of vagal maneuver may be attempted before drug therapy is instituted. Common procedures such as Valsalva's maneuver or carotid sinus massage may be used to try to increase the vagal tone and stop the tachycardia.

Implications for Practice

- Use caution in performing carotid sinus massage in patients older than 65 years of age. Before the maneuver, listen for carotid bruits, and examine the patient's medical history for any transient ischemic attacks. Try the right carotid artery first, because the rate of success is somewhat better on this side. If this method fails, however, try the left carotid artery. Never compress both arteries simultaneously. Be sure that a rhythm strip is running during the entire procedure so that you can see what is happening. Always have equipment available for resuscitation; in rare cases, carotid massage may induce sinus arrest.

⊡ WOLFF-PARKINSON-WHITE SYNDROME

- In Wolff-Parkinson-White syndrome (WPW), an accessory conduction pathway is present between the atria and the ventricles. The bypass pathway has been named the bundle of Kent. It is a discrete aberrant conducting pathway that connects the atria and ventricles. It can be left sided, connecting the left atrium and left ventricle, or right sided, connecting the right atrium and right ventricle.

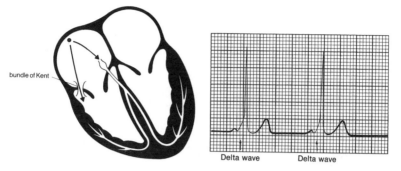

Wolff-Parkinson-White syndrome. Current is held up by the normal delay at the AV node but races unimpeded down the bundle of Kent. The EKG shows the short PR interval and delta wave. (Thaler, M. S. [1995]. *The Only EKG Book You'll Ever Need.* Philadelphia: J.B. Lippincott.)

- This pathway allows impulses to be conducted to the ventricles faster than by way of the atrioventricular (AV) node. WPW is characterized by a shortened P-R interval, as the impulse conducts rapidly to the ventricles via an accessory pathway; a slurring of the initial portion of the QRS (the delta wave), as one ventricle is depolarized rapidly through an abnormal conduction pathway and the other often through the normal pathway; and often a widened QRS complex, when both ventricles are depolarized solely by conduction through the accessory pathway. There are varying degrees of slurring and widening, depending on the contribution of each conduction pathway to ventricular activation. WPW is associated with SVTs that tend to mimic ventricular tachycardia because of the widened QRS complex.

The Following Criteria Are Used for Recognition of WPW

- The P-R interval is short because of conduction through an accessory pathway to the ventricles. The criterion for diagnosis is a P-R interval less than 0.12 second.
- The QRS complex is widened to more than 0.1 second. Unlike bundle branch block, in which the QRS complex is widened because of delayed ventricular activation, in WPW it is widened because of premature activation. The QRS complex in WPW actually represents a fusion beat: Most of the ventricular myocardium is activated via the normal conduction pathways, but a small region of the myocardium is depolarized early via the bundle of Kent. This region gives the QRS complex a characteristic slurred initial upstroke called a delta wave. A true delta wave may be seen in only a few leads, so scan the entire EKG.

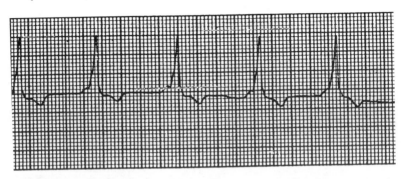

WPW displaying the shortened PR interval and delta wave. The PR is short but constant, ruling out AV dissociation. The shortened PR and the delta wave differentiate this from bundle branch block. (Davis, Dale. [1992]. *How to quickly and accuately master ECG interpretation.* Philadelphia: J.B. Lippincott Company.)

Effects on Client
- If it were not for the potentially fatal arrhythmias associated with the short P-R interval and broad QRS complex, WPW syndrome would be nothing more than an EKG curiosity. Persons with this condition are prone to the following subjective symptoms: palpitations, dyspnea, anginal pain, fatigue, anxiety, dizziness, and polyuria.

Treatment
- Surgery in conjunction with an experienced electrophysiologist has evolved as the treatment of choice for symptomatic patients. The success of surgery has allowed this approach to take precedence over electrophysiologic serial drug testing and a lifetime on medication. Surgical ablation of the accessory pathway is used on an individual basis. Some patients may only require epicardial dissection, others may require an endocardial approach, and a percentage may need cryoablation.

BIBLIOGRAPHY

American Heart Association, (1994). *Textbook of advanced cardiac life support.* Dallas: The Association.

American Medical Association. (1998). *Physicians' current procedural terminology: CPT.* Chicago: American Medical Association.

Davis, D. (1992). *How to quickly and accurately master arrhythmia interpretation.* Philadelphia: J. B. Lippincott.

Dubin, D. (1998). *Rapid interpretation of EKGs* (5th ed.). Tampa: Cover Publishing.

Healthcare Consultants of America. (1998). *1998 Physicians' fee and coding guide.* Augusta, GA.

Huff, J., Doernbach, D. P., & White, R. D. (1997). *ECG workout: Exercises in arrhythmia interpretation.* Philadelphia: J. B. Lippincott.

Seidel, J. C. (Ed.). (1986). *Basic electrocardiography: A modular approach.* St. Louis: C. V. Mosby.

Thaler, M. S. (1995). *The only EKG book you'll ever need.* Philadelphia: J. B. Lippincott.

Wagner, G. S. & Marriott, H. J. (1994). *Marriott's practical electrocardiography.* Baltimore: Williams & Wilkins.

Index